PRAISE FOR *The LDN*

"Since the first volume of *The LDN Book* was released, I have had the privilege of learning from and collaborating with the best clinicians and researchers in the field of integrative medicine. Through these collaborations, we continue to build upon the already vast applications of this low-dose but high-power medication. I am thrilled to see so many trusted colleagues, who have also become friends, contribute to this important body of work. Thank you, again, Linda Elsegood, for bringing together a tribe of like-minded people who continue to find solutions to challenging medical issues with this simple and inexpensive intervention."

—**Dr. Nasha Winters**, ND, FABNO,
author of *The Metabolic Approach to Cancer*

"As a pharmacist, I often wish for a 'miracle' drug that would be safe, effective, and inexpensive and could help the masses take back their health. While no drug is right for everyone, I have seen LDN transform the lives of countless people with autoimmunity. For some, LDN has truly been a miracle drug. I highly recommend both volumes of *The LDN Book* as valuable resources for patients and clinicians alike to explore the best practices for using LDN."

—**Dr. Izabella Wentz**, Pharm.D., FASCP,
New York Times bestselling author of *Hashimoto's Protocol*

"A fantastic resource. All the latest research on low dose naltrexone and its various uses in clinical practice is compiled in this easy-to-use volume—*The LDN Book, Volume 2*. I will definitely be keeping this book in my office for reference."

—**Jill C. Carnahan**, MD, ABIHM, ABoIM, IFMCP

"Even if you think you know about the benefits of LDN for certain conditions through practical experience or otherwise, this book will expand your understanding and amazement. It is a remarkable finding that a drug designed for a specific condition can be applied to so many other systems at lower and lower doses. Interestingly, this has shown us that many other drugs may also have unexpected benefits at lower-than-intended doses. There are many layers of complexity that remain to be uncovered!"

—**Dr. Angus Dalgleish**, professor of oncology, St. George's,
University of London; principal, Institute for
Cancer Vaccines and Immunotherapy (ICVI)

"Over the years, a wealth of clinical trials and studies on LDN have given us better information about how and why LDN actually works. Through this research, we have uncovered many new uses of LDN in medical treatment. Reviewing *The LDN Book, Volume 2* and seeing how other experts prescribe LDN in their clinics has been a great treat for me. My clinic, Clinic 158, has been prescribing LDN for 12 years. We have thousands of very happy patients who have found success with the medication for a myriad of ailments, and we are still learning new information."

—**Dr. Andrew McCall**, director, Clinic 158

"Since inflammation is a major contributor to almost all chronic disorders, LDN therapy bridges nearly every medical specialty. In *The LDN Book, Volume 2*, the authors provide an excellent overview of LDN's mechanism of action, review the vast evidence base supporting clinical applications, and, most importantly, report actual cases in which LDN was instrumental in the successful treatment of patients. This book is a must-have for every clinician, and LDN should be considered in the treatment of the many disorders outlined therein."

—**Sahar Swidan**, Pharm.D., R.Ph., ABAAHP, FAARFM, FACA, president and CEO, Pharmacy Solutions

The
LDN
Book

VOLUME TWO

The Latest Research on How
— Low Dose Naltrexone —
Could Revolutionize Treatment for
PTSD, Pain, IBD, Lyme Disease,
Dermatologic Conditions, and More

EDITED BY
Linda Elsegood
FOREWORD BY Dr. Phil Boyle

Chelsea Green Publishing
White River Junction, Vermont
London, UK

Project Manager: Alexander Bullett
Project Editor: Michael Metivier
Developmental Editor: Natalie Wallace
Copy Editor: Laura Jorstad
Proofreader: Diane Durrett
Indexer: Linda Hallinger
Designer: Melissa Jacobson
Page Layout: Abrah Griggs

Printed in the United Kingdom.
First printing September 2020.
10 9 8 7 6 5 4 3 2 1   20 21 22 23 24

Library of Congress Cataloging-in-Publication Data
Names: Elsegood, Linda, 1956- editor.
Title: The LDN book. Volume 2. The latest research on how low dose naltrexone could revolutionize treatment
    for PTSD, pain, IBD, Lyme disease, dermatologic conditions, and more / edited by Linda Elsegood.
Other titles: Latest research on how low dose naltrexone could revolutionize treatment for PTSD, pain, IBD,
    Lyme disease, dermatologic conditions, and more
Description: White River Junction, Vermont : Chelsea Green Publishing, [2020] | Includes bibliographical
    references and index.
Identifiers: LCCN 2020026302 (print) | LCCN 2020026303 (ebook) | ISBN 9781603589901 (paperback) | ISBN
    9781603589918 (ebook)
Subjects: MESH: Naltrexone—therapeutic use | Naltrexone—pharmacology | Dose-Response Relationship,
    Drug | Narcotic Antagonists—therapeutic use | Opioid Peptides—metabolism
Classification: LCC RM328 (print) | LCC RM328 (ebook) | NLM QV 89 | DDC 615.1/9—dc23
LC record available at https://lccn.loc.gov/2020026302
LC ebook record available at https://lccn.loc.gov/2020026303

Chelsea Green Publishing
85 North Main Street, Suite 120
White River Junction, Vermont USA

Somerset House
London, UK

www.chelseagreen.com

To my late mother, who was the best mum in the world!

CONTENTS

FOREWORD

In the fields of observation chance favours only the prepared mind.
—LOUIS PASTEUR (1822–1895)

How does a fertility doctor (or any doctor) become a low-dose naltrexone prescriber? Quite by chance, at least in my case. In 2002 my sister's husband was diagnosed with progressive multiple sclerosis (MS). He was prescribed LDN by Dr. Bernard Bihari, a neurologist in New York credited with discovering the immune-modifying effects of LDN, and his MS stabilized after just a few weeks. About nine months later I attended a small meeting in Galway, Ireland, presented by Robert, an MS patient who had had a similarly "miraculous" response to LDN treatment. His testimony was striking. He had poor mobility, extreme fatigue, and brain fog with progressive deterioration—until he started LDN. His story made a deep impression on me. I was excited to hear how effective this treatment could be for autoimmunity. I decided I would recommend LDN if I had an infertility patient with an autoimmune condition. But first, I needed to find out more about this interesting medication. At that time, the LDN Research Trust did not exist, and there was very little to find in peer-reviewed publications.

The key points for me were:

- LDN is a licensed medication that is safe and well tolerated at 50 mg with no limitation on the duration of use at this dose.
- The recommended doses of 3 to 4.5 mg are less than one-tenth of the licensed dose, so they are clearly safe.
- It is important to avoid combining with opioid medications, codeine, or alcohol.
- Sleep disturbance and vivid dreams are common side effects, but settle within one to two weeks of use.

Within a month I had an infertility patient with new-onset rheumatoid arthritis. She was seeing a rheumatologist who recommended methotrexate, as she was not responding to non-steroidal anti-inflammatory drugs (NSAIDs). A significant problem with methotrexate is that you cannot conceive while taking it. I suggested we could try LDN, which might improve her symptoms while still allowing her to conceive. I explained this would be off-label use, and that while there were no publications to support the treatment, growing clinical observations in the United States were promising. Pregnancy was her first priority, so she agreed to try LDN, as it was unlikely to be harmful and she could always try conventional treatment if LDN did not help. Her response was amazing. Her fatigue lessened dramatically, her joint pain and swelling significantly improved, and she conceived within two months of starting treatment. Despite her incredible response, her neurologist was hostile to the idea of LDN treatment and refused to accept it or explore it further. That was surprising and disturbing to me.

Since 2004 my practice has evolved and changed so that today I prescribe LDN to over 50 percent of couples who attend for fertility treatment—about 2,000 patients in the past 10 years. LDN contributes significantly to my patients' general health improvement and better fertility outcomes. This has been a gradual evolution over time based on clinical experience and direct feedback from patients receiving treatment. Initially I stopped my patients from taking LDN during pregnancy as I was unsure of its safety, but today I have them continue until 37 weeks and see improved outcomes for both mother and baby.

LDN is not beneficial for everybody with infertility. I target its use to those with clinical endorphin deficiency. When patients have low mood, fatigue, anxiety, sleep disturbance, PMS, painful periods, endometriosis, or an autoimmune condition—symptoms of endorphin deficiency—they are much more likely to respond favorably to LDN. When endorphin levels are normal, LDN can be overstimulating and contribute to unpleasant side effects that persist beyond the typical two-week transitional phase. Enduring side effects indicate LDN is causing excessive endorphin production, hindering rather than improving health and well-being. Such side effects include persistent vivid dreams, sleep disturbance, nausea, headache, and dry mouth. In these cases, we try even lower doses of LDN or stop its use altogether.

Unlike the vast majority of licensed immune-modifying treatments, LDN does not suppress the immune system and its many important functions, thereby mitigating the potential for activating silent tuberculosis (TB) or triggering additional autoimmune conditions or cancer. LDN does not lead to any of these complications. Remarkably, LDN balances the immune system by stimulating endorphin production, which has multiple immune-regulating effects that help control a wide range of autoimmune and inflammatory conditions. In addition, LDN is inexpensive and has very few side effects or interactions with other drugs. As doctors, our guiding principle for treatment is always *"Primum non nocere"*—first, do no harm. LDN is the safest immune-modifying treatment available.

Clinically I have found that about 70 percent of autoimmune conditions respond favorably to LDN, whereas placebo is effective 30 percent of the time. Patients respond better when they avoid wheat and dairy foods and supplement with vitamin D_3 and omega-3. It is important to recognize that not everybody will respond to LDN. I have seen non-responders who absolutely require immunosuppressive treatment with their specialist. It is important to encourage patients to be open to this possibility when LDN treatment doesn't work.

Off-label prescription of LDN represents an approach to medical treatment that is in danger of disappearing in our current climate of evidence-based medicine and medico-legal concerns. Doctors are rightly afraid of harming patients with unproven treatments, and litigation is a very real concern. However, medical thinking is becoming overly tele-scopic, less holistic, and fearful. Many doctors think if it is not published, we shouldn't risk trying it at all—except in the context of a strict clinical trial. This approach will ultimately lead to poorer care of our patients and hinder the development of new medical treatments. Many fertility doctors commonly use the diabetes medication metformin to treat women with polycystic ovaries, and it frequently improves their patients' health and fertility outcomes. The oral contraceptive pill is not licensed as a treatment for painful periods, but this off-label use is widely recommended. Letrozole is licensed to help prevent the spread of breast cancer, but is widely used off-label to stimulate ovulation. Currently more than 100 medications are commonly used for something completely different from what they were licensed to treat. When doctors see unexpected improvements in one condi-tion while using a medication licensed for something else, these chance findings favor the prepared mind. If doctors must wait for published studies before prescribing reasonable off-label medications, advances in medical treatment will be very slow indeed. The most important thing is for doctors to let patients know if a treatment is new or off-label, and allow the patient to decide whether they'd like to try it. Most of my patients are excited to try a safe, new, and "experimental" treatment when they are fully informed.

Many doctors like to go by the book, developing confidence only when a sizable group of other practitioners recommends a novel treatment. However, the Bolam principle provides legal protection for doctors when a responsible body of medical opinion supports their treatment strategy, even if other doctors adopt a different practice. This is reassuring for doctors who are wary of being the first to try something new. Thankfully, many doctors now use LDN as an immune-modifying treatment.

This second book from the LDN Research Trust covers a wide range of conditions treated by practicing doctors with many years of successful clinical experience. Their positive experiences will hopefully inspire more doctors to consider LDN for suitable patients. This book should be a valuable guide for doctors interested in learning how to treat patients correctly with the safest immune-modifying treatment available.

DR. PHIL BOYLE

PREFACE

In December 2003 Dr. Bob Lawrence, a general practitioner in Wales, prescribed me low dose naltrexone. I have multiple sclerosis, and I was going downhill rapidly at the time. I started taking LDN on December 3, and the results were amazing. After only three weeks the awful fog I'd been living in for so long finally lifted. I could think clearly again and speak coherently. My 15-year-old daughter had been feeding, clothing, and bathing me; now, the caretaking roles were reverting back to their natural positions. By Christmas 2004 my liver tests were back to normal, and I was fully functioning again. LDN had given me my life back.

Following my success with LDN, I founded the LDN Research Trust as a U.K. nonprofit registered charity in 2004. The LDN Research Trust is run purely by volunteers; we receive no funding and rely on donations. We liaise closely with prescribers, pharmacists, and patients, offering support and education. Our website, www.ldnresearchtrust.org, features lists of clinical trials and studies involving LDN, conditions for which LDN is used, global LDN prescribers and pharmacists, prescriber/patient guides, and more. We have our own *LDN Radio Show*, which listeners can access on Mixcloud, Apple Podcast, iTunes, and Spotify. The shows are now being transcribed and set alongside video, which can be found on our Vimeo and YouTube channels. We have made five documentaries, which have been huge successes. Additionally, we arrange LDN conferences both large and small, and host seminars in conjunction with pharmacies. In short the LDN Research Trust strives to spread the word about LDN, and to encourage and support ongoing research about the drug.

The LDN Book, Volume 1 covered the latest research, trials, and studies on LDN. Its chapters discussed the following conditions, for which LDN has been shown to have positive benefit:

- Multiple sclerosis and lupus
- Inflammatory bowel disease

- Chronic fatigue syndrome and fibromyalgia
- Thyroid disorders
- Restless legs syndrome
- Depression
- Autism spectrum disorder
- Cancer

Awareness of LDN has expanded exponentially since *The LDN Book, Volume 1* was published in 2016. There have been numerous new trials, studies, and papers on its uses in treating the above conditions as well as a host of others. This volume therefore serves as a follow-up to *Volume 1*, showcasing new information and providing further resources for both medical professionals and patients suffering from conditions such as traumatic brain injury, Lyme disease, endometriosis, chronic pain, and more.

Readers of *The LDN Book, Volume 1* will notice that chapter 1, "The History and Pharmacology of LDN," has been updated and adapted from the first volume. We have chosen to reinclude this chapter, authored by J. Stephen Dickson, due to its comprehensive and accessible discussion of LDN's background and mechanisms.

The LDN Research Trust continues to grow in strength. We have astounding advisers who are a great asset and amazing volunteers who give their time freely to help others. Without all this help, we wouldn't be able to carry out the work we do. A big thank-you to all of the authors in this book, and to everyone who has supported us.

I wouldn't be here today without LDN. I am endlessly grateful to Dr. Lawrence for all his support in helping me get my life back: the most valuable gift you can give anyone!

LINDA ELSEGOOD
FOUNDER, LDN RESEARCH TRUST

ONE

The History and Pharmacology of LDN

J. STEPHEN DICKSON, BSC (HONS), MRPHARMS

Naltrexone belongs to a class of drugs called opioid antagonists, a relatively new class of medicines that were first formally theorized in the 1940s. Antagonists, including opioid antagonists, block the physiological activity of other drugs, as well as naturally occurring hormones, catecholamines, peptides, and neurotransmitters.

Among the first classes of antagonists to be developed were the beta-blockers, discovered by Sir James W. Black in 1964. Beta-blockers, such as propranolol, are adrenergic blocking drugs, used to control the fight or flight response in human beings. The discovery of propranolol is widely heralded as the most important contribution to pharmacology in the 20th century.[1]

Being able to modify endogenous biological mechanisms in a clinically relevant way was so important to medicine that in 1988 the decision was made to award Sir Black with the Nobel Prize in Medicine, not only for his development of antagonists but also for his follow-up work, which showed how blocking receptor sites (in this case adrenergic receptors) could be used for the management of debilitating conditions, including high blood pressure, angina pectoris, and heart failure. To this day beta-blockers are the mainstay of treatment for patients with cardiac problems, preventing millions of deaths worldwide since their development, making them one of the most successful classes of drugs ever produced.[2] The scientific excitement generated by the potential of receptors to treat disease led researchers to look closely at how opioid painkillers actually worked in relation to opioid receptors in the body.

Painkillers based on the opium poppy (*Papaver somniferum*) have existed for millennia, as evidenced in literature by Homer's *Odyssey*, written nearly 3,000 years ago: "Presently she cast a drug into the wine of which they drank to lull all pain and anger and bring forgetfulness of every sorrow."[3] Although Theophrastus in 300 BC, and Dioskourides in AD 60, both argued that the wine in question was actually an extract of the henbane plant, which contains several active tropane alkaloids (notably scopolamine, hyoscine, and atropine, the latter of which will be discussed later in this chapter), this has been refuted in modern times, with pharmacologists Schmiedeberg (1918) and Lewin (1931) making a convincing case that Helena's drink in the *Odyssey* was made from the extract of the opium poppy.[4]

Archaeologists have also uncovered many references to painkillers made from the opium poppy. Six-thousand-year-old Sumerian texts and 2,000-year-old Egyptian hieroglyphs contain similar symbols referring to *gil*, which, when translated into modern language, stands for "joy" and is derived from *hul gil*, whose pictograph is unmistakably an opium poppy.[5]

Many references throughout history support the common use of opioids for a variety of ailments. The Ebers Papyrus, dated approximately 1500 BC, recommends a particular remedy to "prevent excessive crying of children" and includes instructions for how to make it: "Spenn, the grains of the spenn [poppy]-plant, with excretions of flies found on the wall, strained to a pulp, passed through a sieve and administered on four successive days. The crying will stop at once."[6]

The Greco-Roman fascination with opium is clear in many historical records. In ancient Greece, Hippocrates (460 BC) made many medicinal treatments from herbs, including the opium poppy seed.[7] Opium abuse is also widespread in every time period from which records exist. Notably, Roman emperor Marcus Aurelius displayed many of the symptoms and side effects of opium addiction.[8] The decline of the Roman Empire, which began in about AD 500, took with it many trade routes, and widespread knowledge of the opium poppy appears to have retreated to the Arab world for the next few hundred years.

The opium poppy has been cultivated in the Arab world continuously since ancient times. Records of cultivation most often point to the country now known as Iraq, previously Sumeria, with good evidence of post–Roman

Empire trade networks for opium poppies and their extracts beginning to India and China in AD 800 and farther into what is now Europe by AD 1500.[9] The spread of opium as a recreational drug, which was most often smoked, is frequently attributed to this exponential growth and advance of Arabian influence from AD 500 to AD 1000. With the foundation and rise of Islam, Arab peoples commonly used both opium and hashish recreationally due to the prohibition of alcohol in the Koran.[10] Manuscripts referring to widespread common usage of opium, both medicinal and recreational, start to appear more regularly in the historical record from AD 1500 onward.[11] Paracelsus, a Swiss doctor often heralded as the father of modern medicine, first standardized an alcoholic extract of the opium poppy, known as laudanum, in 1527.[12] This standardized laudanum has been in use right up to the modern era, with the first branded laudanum making an appearance in England in as early as 1680.[13]

It is notable, and very important to the development of naltrexone, that the use of opium extracts was commonly known to result in addiction as well as death by overdose. Surgeons routinely used opioid extracts to dull pain or perform surgery, but due to the unpredictable strength of the opioids in medicines, death from overdose during surgery occurred frequently. The use of *spongia somnifera* (a sponge soaked in opium used locally during surgery, considered to be a safer alternative to large oral doses of opium) was commonplace until modern times, but was often ineffective due to lack of absorption, or too effective, causing complications.[14]

It was not until the Georgian era (1714–1830) that the modern science of chemistry was sufficiently advanced to allow fractional distillation, as well as extraction and identification, of active components. German pharmacist Friedrich Sertürner first isolated opium's active component in an extract called papaverine in 1806 and named it morphine, after the Greek god Morpheus, the god of dreams.[15] Morphine belongs to a class of substances known as alkaloids. The term *alkaloid* was first used in 1819 by Swiss botanist Carl Meissner when he referred to a plant known as *al-qali*.[16] Sodium carbonate, first extracted from this plant, was known as *al-kali* in Arabic. The term has come to refer to a chemical's pH and, unsurprisingly, alkaloids are slightly alkaline.

The discovery of a natural, active component that could be extracted and purified generated much scientific excitement. But at this stage of history, the science of receptors was nonexistent, and an understanding of how the drug worked was less important to the scientists of the day than producing stronger, more powerful versions with fewer side effects.

Morphine continued to be extracted and widely used throughout the first part of the 19th century. Additionally, the use of morphine as an adjunct to chloroform for anesthesia started to become widespread in the 1850s after being popularized by French physiologist Claude Bernard.[17] Bernard's experiments on animals demonstrated empirically that less chloroform was needed to keep an animal anesthetized when it was premedicated with morphine.[18]

However, over the next 50 years it became increasingly apparent to doctors that morphine had several drawbacks, including breathing suppression, constipation, addiction, and even death by overdose. As morphine's problems became more widely known and understood, an intense search began to find safer alternatives.

English scientist Charles Romley Alder Wright first synthesized diacetylmorphine in 1874 by chemically adding two acetyl groups to the morphine molecule, now commonly known as diamorphine or, when abused, heroin.[19] Over the next few decades, many such chemical analogs of the original morphine were made, each one heralded as the "new morphine" without the side effects or drawbacks. None of these new compounds were found to be free of side effects, and it is now known that the beneficial effects of morphine analogs are directly tied to the side effects through the same receptors.

Research continued, but during World War I (1914–1918) many developed countries found it difficult to access morphine due to disrupted trade. The lessened availability of morphine intensified the scientific search for a way to synthesize the drug. Throughout World War II difficulties obtaining morphine during the previous war were acutely remembered, but by this time another chemical took the spotlight: atropine.

Atropine is extracted from the belladonna plant (*Atropa belladonna*), a perennial plant native to parts of Europe and western Asia. Historically, it was used in medieval times to increase the size of women's pupils, which led to its name (*bella*: beautiful, *donna*: woman), but it would later prove to have much more important uses. At the time of the war effort, atropine was the only anti-cholinergic agent available to medics to counteract an attack with nerve gas. Since an inability to source sufficient atropine would significantly disadvantage any army, huge resources were applied to find an alternative to plant-derived atropine on both sides of the war.

It was through this intense scientific effort that a German scientist, Dr. Otto Eisleb, first synthesized a molecule that he called meperidine, in 1939. Meperidine failed to successfully replace atropine, but was soon recognized by Dr. Otto Schumann (who was working for a German chemical company, IG Farben) as a powerful analgesic, similar in action to morphine.[20] Meperidine, also known as pethidine, is still used today during childbirth. Pethidine represented the first opioid drug with a chemical structure completely divergent from that of morphine (see figure 1.1).

The door to chemical synthesis of new drug compounds was now well and truly open, with scientific laboratories working around the clock to do so. The next most widely known nonmorphine opioid to be discovered was 1,1-diphenyl-1 (dimethylaminoisopropyl) butanone-2, now commonly known as methadone, synthesized just a few short years later between 1940 and 1946.[21]

Working in the research laboratories of Merck & Co., two scientists, Weijlard and Erickson, synthesized a compound that puzzled everyone.[22] In certain circumstances this compound seemed to exert the opposite effect of morphine, reversing the latter's negative effects. They called this compound nalorphine (chemical name N-allylnormorphine). Weijlard and Erickson discovered that this compound actually had mixed effects: It had a slight analgesic action in animals, a bit like morphine, but when given

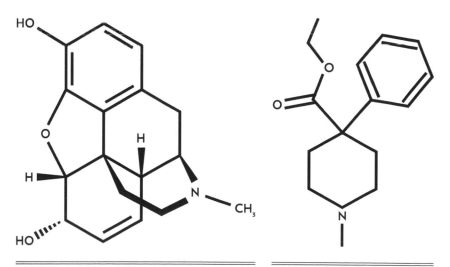

FIGURE 1.1. Structure of morphine.   FIGURE 1.2. Structure of pethidine.

to an animal pretreated with an overdose of morphine, the effects of the morphine (such as breathing suppression) were reversed. This discovery presented a bit of a conundrum, as medical science did not yet understand the concept of receptors.

However, unhindered by the confusing effects of this compound, and recognizing that a drug that completely blocks the negative effects of morphine would be very useful, many laboratories and companies continued to synthesize different molecules. The first patent for a pure morphine-blocking drug was recorded in Great Britain in 1963, and in the United States in 1966.[23] The discovered compound was naloxone.

Naloxone was a panacea for opioid overdose. Upon intravenous injection, it appeared to immediately block all effects of morphine. More than 50 years later, naloxone is still on the World Health Organization's international list of essential medicines.[24]

More important to the background of low dose naltrexone (LDN), naloxone's discovery led to other researchers discovering, in 1967, an analog that could be taken orally named Endo 1639A.[25] Endo 1639A is now commonly known as naltrexone.

Historical Use of Naltrexone

Addiction to opioid drugs has long been a societal problem. People become addicted to opioid medications for a number of reasons: They numb physical and psychological pain; with long-term use, they cause biological changes that result in side effects upon withdrawal; and they create pharmacological tolerance, requiring ever-larger doses to produce a similar effect.

It is important to understand some of the underlying biological mechanisms that are involved in the action of opioids in order to understand the importance of the naltrexone molecule. Opioid medications, as well as opioid-acting medications that have the same effect but a different structure (such as pethidine, described above), mimic natural neuropeptides. These natural neuropeptides are called endorphins and, specifically in the case of opioid analgesic actions, beta-endorphins. They are synthesized in the brain in the anterior pituitary gland and are released in reaction to a variety of stimuli.

The precursor protein to most endorphins is pro-opiomelanocortin (POMC). In normal physiological function the hypothalamus secretes corticotropin-releasing hormone (CRH) in response to stress on the physiological system. This in turn stimulates the pituitary to make POMC, which, as a large complex molecule, can be enzymatically broken up into neuropeptides such as the endorphins. A negative feedback loop then occurs, which suppresses the release of CRH when the by-products of POMC breakdown reach a certain level. Almost every physiological system in the body contains the necessary enzymes to break down POMC to the component neuropeptides.

When discussing how endorphins work, it is perhaps simplest to focus on their painkilling (analgesic) properties. These are generally well understood and have a sound scientific literature. They may have a much more complex biological role, which is less understood, but this will be discussed later.

There are two main areas of action for analgesia where natural endogenous neuropeptides, such as beta-endorphins, exert a painkilling effect: first, the peripheral nervous system (PNS), and second, the central nervous system (CNS).

The PNS can be thought of metaphorically as the wires connecting every part of the human body between sensors and the brain. These wires are connected together via junctions. However, unlike in an electrical system—where the wires touch one another—nerve junctions speak to one another via the release of chemicals. These chemicals are called neurotransmitters. A nerve can be described as starting with a postsynaptic terminal, which receives messages from the previous nerve, and ending with a presynaptic terminal, to communicate with the next nerve. The nerves that transmit the sensation of pain do so by releasing a neurotransmitter called substance P. In the PNS, opioids bind mainly to the presynaptic terminal and prevent the release of substance P by a cascade reaction. If substance P cannot be released into the nerve junction, the pain signal cannot be transmitted.

Diagrammatically, this is difficult to represent in a simple manner. However, returning to simplified university lecture notes, the reaction can be represented as shown in figure 1.3.

In figure 1.3 we see how communication of the pain signal is interrupted by the naturally occurring endorphins, which act on opioid receptors to suppress pain in a similar way to opioid drugs. In this way a pain signal coming from the peripheral sensing systems can be prevented from being as strong when it makes it back to the brain, or even from making it to the brain at all.

This system is far more complex than is represented here; there are a range of neurotransmitters called tachykinins that act in similar ways to substance

P, along with several different types of opioid receptor, each of which has a slightly different action and all of which are involved in the chemical cascade that fully transmits pain throughout the different nerve fibers in the PNS. However, a subclass of opioid receptors called mu receptors is ubiquitous through the PNS and is the main target for opioid analgesics.

In the CNS, specifically the brain, opioid receptors are very well distributed and are involved in a multitude of different neurochemical actions. Unlike the PNS, opioid receptors centrally act to inhibit pain by modifying the release of the potent neurotransmitter dopamine.

Dopamine is commonly known as the body's natural "happy chemical" and is primarily controlled by the release of another neurotransmitter called gamma-aminobutyric acid (GABA). When opioids bind to the mu-opioid receptor, they cause a reduction in the release of GABA, which in turn reduces the inhibitory effect that GABA activation has on the presynaptic nerve release of dopamine.

In layman's terms, activating a mu-opioid receptor centrally disrupts the normal controls on baseline release of dopamine, meaning that far

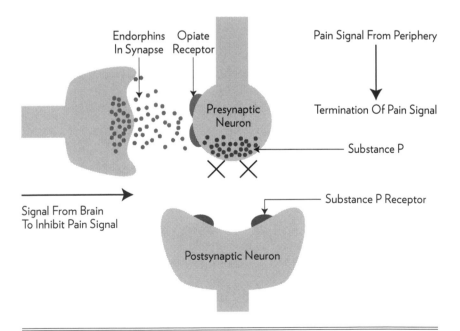

FIGURE 1.3. Communication of pain signal interrupted by endorphins.

more dopamine is released than normal. This has an analgesic effect by suppressing the conduction of pain messages and the response to pain caused by the euphoric effect of excess dopamine. The excess dopamine is largely responsible for the "high" desired by people who abuse opioids, but belongs entirely to a natural system that exists to maintain homeostasis and is activated by naturally occurring endorphins as discussed earlier.

A diagram showing this process at work will help to make this process clearer.

In figure 1.4 normal homeostasis is depicted on the left. On the right, heroin (diamorphine) breaks down to morphine and then attaches to a mu-opioid receptor, inhibiting GABA release, and increasing dopamine release. The mu-opioid receptors on these nerves are activated by biological endorphins.

Receptors are one of the most important discoveries in modern medicine. Although theorized widely in the 1960s, the first opioid receptor was discovered in the early 1970s when the technology of radioisotope labeling became available.[26] Interestingly, the scientists who are widely referred to as

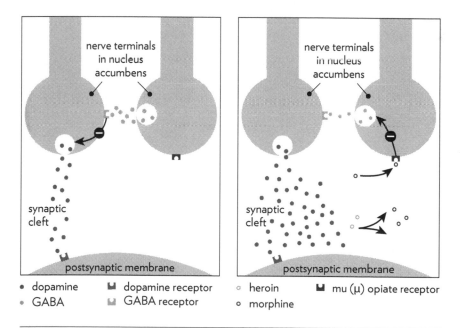

| • dopamine | ᴍ dopamine receptor | ∘ heroin | ᴍ mu (μ) opiate receptor |
| • GABA | ᴍ GABA receptor | ∘ morphine | |

FIGURE 1.4. *Left*, normal function of GABA and mu-opioid receptors. *Right*, effect of heroin on GABA and mu-opioid receptors.

the first to describe and identify an opioid receptor did so using naloxone, which, as discussed earlier, led directly to the development of naltrexone.

It has since been discovered that many receptors are similar in nature, and in fact, opioid receptors belong to a family called G-protein-coupled receptors, which are all generally inhibitory when activated. Structurally, opioid receptors are similar to somatostatin receptors and another class of receptor (discussed later) called toll-like receptors (TLR), which are involved in inflammatory processes.[27]

Returning to the opioid receptors, scientists quickly discovered that many different chemicals could bind to them. Although some chemicals could bind to the receptors and be observed attaching to these receptors via radiological study, they did not all have the same effect. In fact, a huge range of activity was seen, from extreme activation of the receptor, to slight activation, right up to blocking anything else from attaching to the receptor. In pharmacology chemicals that produce these effects are referred to, respectively, as agonists, partial agonists, and antagonists.

Classically, receptors are thought of as locks. Imagine a standard door lock where different keys can fit into the same keyhole. Agonists are keys that fit the lock and open the door fully (extreme activation of the receptor); partial agonists fit the lock but only partially open the door (slight activation); and antagonists fit the lock, but cannot open the door, actively preventing any other keys from trying to open the door (blocking).

Figure 1.5 shows that although the lock (receptor) and key (ligand) analogy is easy to understand, the actual structure of a receptor site is in three dimensions, and different parts of the receptor can be activated or blocked depending on the physical structure of the ligand interacting with it. Endogenous endorphins, such as the beta-endorphins discussed earlier, are agonists; these are mimicked by opioid drugs such as morphine and diamorphine. Naltrexone and naloxone are antagonists: keys that fit the same door, but stop the receptor from being activated by an agonist. It has since been discovered that these receptors are fluid and can become more or less sensitive to agonists and can increase and decrease in active number depending on circumstances.

Based on this knowledge, naltrexone was first licensed as a treatment for addiction to opioids in 1984.[28] Scientists understood that blocking opioid receptors would prevent an addicted patient from being able to obtain the euphoria achieved by taking drugs such as heroin. As such,

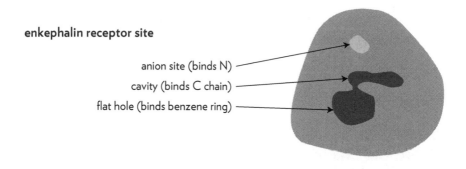

enkephalin receptor site

anion site (binds N)

cavity (binds C chain)

flat hole (binds benzene ring)

FIGURE 1.5. Enkephalin receptor site. Adapted from Fred Senese, "Anandamide," General Chemistry Online!, last revised Feb. 23, 2018, http://antoine.frostburg.edu/chem/senese/101/features/anandamide.shtml.

naltrexone was highly effective; when a patient addicted to high doses of opioids was given naltrexone, all the effects of the opioids were immediately blocked for a number of hours. However, this efficacy proved to be highly dangerous, resulting in large numbers of deaths of patients who were tolerant to opioids and thus were unwittingly pushed into immediate opioid withdrawal.

The problem with attempting to treat addiction to opioids with an antagonist is that as someone becomes a regular user of opioids, the reactivity of the receptors to opioids (natural endorphins included) is greatly reduced, and the physical number of receptors also decreases. This is a natural biological phenomenon caused by physiology always attempting to return to a baseline state (homeostasis). In pharmacology this effect is referred to in terms such as *desensitization* and *downregulation*.

This is a reversible reaction, and naltrexone was used widely in the 1980s and 1990s for assistance with abstinence from opioids, but only once a patient had been gradually titrated down from their regular dose and a level homeostasis had returned. Naltrexone was given in tablet form, orally, in daily doses ranging from 50 milligrams (mg) to 300 mg. The opioid receptor blockade was strong and predictable; should the patient take any opioids while on naltrexone, there was no euphoric effect.

Still, there were several problems that led to naltrexone not becoming the mainstay for opioid addiction management. First, although the drug effectively created an opioid blockade, the patient's underlying psychological addiction to the euphoric feeling of opioids was not reduced. In fact, the cravings were often reported to be higher during naltrexone therapy.

Second, the opioid blockade in patients taking naltrexone also muted the effects of naturally occurring endorphins required to maintain a basic homeostasis. When the brain responds to pleasurable stimuli, the response is mediated by endorphins, so when full opioid blockade is achieved, it theoretically interferes with the ability of the patient to feel or experience happiness and pleasure. Opioid-addicted patients taking naltrexone often describe a "flatness," technically described as dysphoria, which is reported to lead to significant depression. The link between naltrexone and dysphoria has been researched, but results are contradictory, though dysphoria is still listed on the summary of product characteristics as a side effect. Research has suggested that initial symptoms of depression may improve and clinically reported side effects are related to the withdrawal from opioids, or concomitant disease.[29]

Finally, compliance with treatment was often poor due to chaotic lifestyles, or the side effects mentioned, whether real or psychosomatic; patients were often not taking the tablets every day and would therefore be able to regress into addiction. Many drug companies have tried to avoid this problem by developing a slow-release injectable pellet, a few of which are still on the market today, but the uptake has been poor due to the complexity of administration, the price of the injectable, and the overall evidence-based, international move to replacement and slow-reduction therapy with agents such as methadone.

During the period when naltrexone was being used for opioid addiction, it gained favor for treatment in another area: alcoholism. Clinicians postulated that if a patient was to take naltrexone while drinking to excess, as in the case of alcoholism, their brain could be retrained to attain no pleasure from the alcohol, by the same process as described above, blocking the effects of endorphins.

When doctors tried this in patients, they found significant success, and naltrexone has consistently gained momentum over the last 25 years as a treatment to reduce heavy drinking in alcohol-dependent patients. A review study in 2006 showed that 70 percent of clinical trials conducted in this area demonstrated clinically important benefit.

The basic scientific groundwork and standardization for widespread use of naltrexone for alcoholism was set out by John David Sinclair when working at the Finnish National Institute for Health and Welfare in the late 1990s. He demonstrated that a process described as pharmacological extinction showed that concomitant alcohol drinking when being prescribed naltrexone worked by gradually reducing the craving. Statistically, this followed an extinction curve, which was repeatable and predictable. This was named the Sinclair Method and is widely used throughout the world today. Sinclair's groundwork has led to a recent formal license for an analog of naltrexone, nalmefene, to be formally approved for use in patients with alcohol dependence.

Immunological Effects

Naltrexone has a long history of safe use in patients for its opioid receptor and endorphin-modifying properties. Over the last two decades, it has been recognized that naltrexone also has immunological effects that have been reported to be beneficial in autoimmune diseases. Furthermore, clinicians have reported that naltrexone has been useful in treating various types of cancer. This has led many to wonder what is going on. How can a medication with a well-defined and understood pharmacological effect have such a wide range of other possible indications?

Drug companies go to great lengths to modify their products before they reach licensure, to make sure the active molecule is as selective as possible for the intended target. However, despite the best efforts of these companies, most licensed drugs on the market today are not 100 percent selective for their intended target.

Many biologically active chemical substances will interact with more than one area in the human body. The pharmacological term for this is *dirty drug*, which means that although the drug does exactly what it says it does, it also does other things. These are interpreted as "side effects," as often the secondary action is unwanted.

Over the last 55 years, the understanding of receptor structure has greatly improved as the understanding of biological chirality has increased dramatically. Chirality means that receptors, and other target cellular areas, are generally three-dimensional structures that can be "left-handed" or "right-handed." Despite having the same cellular building blocks, they can be put together in different ways, just as our hands have the same number of bones and tendons, but are the opposite of each other.

This concept extends down to the molecular level in physiological systems, and has been discovered to be important in the production of drugs, as these, too, can have a left-handed or right-handed design. Chemically, this "handedness" is described as an L or R isomer.

Unsurprisingly, pharmacologists now understand that each different isomer can actually have a different effect, and the amount of drug of each isomer that is bioavailable can be dose-dependent. However, most drugs, when synthesized, are present in a consistent ratio of L and R isomers in the eventual product.

Figure 1.6 serves to demonstrate that how drug molecules actually affect the human body has yet to be fully understood, and that many molecules that were previously thought to be well explained have been observed to have different effects when examined carefully for their inherent structure, or dosing regimen. As discussed earlier, drugs that alter homeostasis also have the potential for altering those inherent biological systems in different ways depending on how effective they are at modifying the natural control mechanisms.

In the case of naltrexone, the dose that seems to have an effect in autoimmune diseases is significantly lower (10 to 40 times lower) than the dose used for opioid addiction or alcoholism. This is referred to as low dose naltrexone (LDN). Most commonly, LDN is taken daily in doses of between 0.5 mg and 4.5 mg.

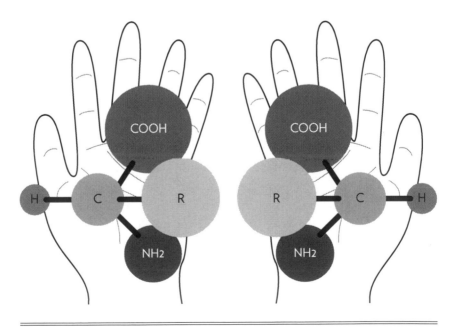

FIGURE 1.6. Demonstration of chirality. Image courtesy of NASA.

LDN should not be confused with homeopathy, where an active substance is mysteriously diluted so many times that few, if any, of the original chemical molecules remain in the eventual product. Even at low doses of 0.5 mg to 4.5 mg, naltrexone still has significant bioavailability and can precipitate immediate short-term opioid withdrawal. That is to say, although the dose is a lot lower than the drug was historically licensed for, clinicians can still demonstrate some of the well-known effects of the drug at this dose. It is still biologically active at these dose ranges.

One of the first hints as to how LDN could potentially affect the immune system came from research into the effects of endorphins conducted in the early 1980s. One influential paper, published in 1985, concluded that "endorphins can be considered as immunomodulators . . . and may become a tool in the field of immunotherapy."[30] It was already known at the time that naltrexone was capable of binding to endorphin receptors, as endorphins are endogenous opioids. What was also known was that interrupting homeostasis, by blocking these receptors, could result in tricking the body to produce more endorphins to compensate.[31]

The first clinician to record immunological effects of LDN was Dr. Bernard Bihari, working in New York City in 1985. He was embroiled in the middle of the HIV/AIDS epidemic at a time when none of the modern treatments had yet been developed. Human immunodeficiency virus (HIV) is an infection that leads to destruction and weakening of the immune system; when patients become immunocompromised, they are then said to have AIDS, the final stage of the infection, and they generally die from complications of the immune system damage. Bihari's practice tried anything and everything in this patient group to improve survival. Previously conducted research had shown that endorphins were significantly involved in the regulation of the immune system, so it was an ingenious step to try treatment with LDN.[32]

First, Dr. Bihari tested a small group of very unwell AIDS patients, whose endorphin levels were about a third of what is considered normal. This endorphin deficiency was something that his clinic felt could be treated with a small dose of naltrexone, so they began a 12-week trial. In the placebo group, 5 out of 16 patients developed opportunistic infections, but none of the 22 in the LDN group did. These results, although on a small scale, were extremely encouraging. Bihari's clinic then proceeded to look at treating larger numbers of patients with LDN.[33]

Dr. Bihari was able to demonstrate, in a reasonably sized HIV/AIDS patient group, that taking LDN regularly largely prevented the gradual destruction of the immune system. He did this by measuring the presence in the blood of a type of immune cell called CD4. CD4 was, and remains, the standard marker for seeing how fast HIV is progressing. What was most interesting and striking in his practice was that the number of deaths in the patient group who took LDN, compared with the patient group who did not regularly take it, was vastly lower. Its success also appeared to be synergistic with the new classes of antiretroviral drugs that became available during the years of treatment, meaning that LDN improved the outcomes in his patients regardless of whether they took the new antiretroviral drugs.[34]

Over the next few years, a plethora of research was conducted on the importance of endorphins and opioids / opioid antagonists to the regulation of the immune system. One of the most important discoveries was published in 1986 by Drs. Zagon and McLaughlin, demonstrating that opioid receptors were present inside multiple types of immune cells, and laterally that messenger RNA (mRNA) inside these cells held coding for endorphin receptors.[35]

Over the next 29 years, Dr. Ian Zagon championed the basic research into endorphins and LDN, publishing nearly 300 papers on the subject. The extent of the research is too overwhelming to present here; however, it has confirmed beyond doubt that the endorphin/opioid receptor system is involved in almost every biological system that regulates immune response.

The mechanism of action of LDN, as proposed by these studies, can be summarized as follows:

1. Many outward diseases are expressions of a malfunctioning immune system.
2. The immune system is regulated by endorphins, which have a primary action on opioid receptors.
3. Blocking opioid receptors briefly using naltrexone causes an upregulation in the production of endorphins, which can act in an immunomodulatory way to correct immune system malfunction.
4. Furthermore, cell growth (proliferation) is also mediated by a subtype of endorphins; cell proliferation can be suppressed by endorphins, and this is applicable to some forms of cancer.[36]

This is a gross simplification of 30 years of detailed work, of course, and to fully understand the concepts within the published papers would take a degree in immunology and a lot of time. However, the experimental models for multiple sclerosis; wound healing; pancreatic, colon, brain, head/neck, liver, breast, and ovarian cancers; ocular surface disease; Crohn's disease; and many other pathways have been shown to be responsive to endorphins in vitro. The wide range of diseases that appear to be responsive to modification of the endorphin system is staggering, none more so than terminal cancers and debilitating autoimmune diseases like multiple sclerosis.

Over the last 30 years, clinical use of LDN has been increasing. However, many researchers currently think that endorphins are not the whole picture. Scientists have long known that naltrexone binds to more than just the opioid receptors; there is also a significant attachment to a group of receptors called toll-like receptors.

Toll-like receptors were first demonstrated in 1985 by Christiane Nüsslein-Volhard.[37] They are an essential part of the innate immune system, providing a first line of defense against microbial invasion, and are present on cells such as white blood cells (macrophages), dendritic cells, neutrophils, B lymphocytes, mast cells, and monocytes, as well as directly on cells of various human organs, such as the kidney and intestines.

When a foreign body invades, such as bacteria or viruses, different subclasses of TLR receptors (TLR-1 to TLR-10 in humans) respond to different parts of the invading organism, including surface proteins, by-products from the cellular metabolism of the bacteria/viruses, physical structures on the surface or inside of the bacterial cell, DNA, RNA, and even the specific sugars that are unique to certain bacteria. This is not an exhaustive list, as research continues to this day. For example, a class of TLR receptor (TLR-10) is known to exist, but the substrate is not presently known.

The role of these receptors appears to be to recognize an intruder—they have a structure complementary to doing so—and then to start an intercellular signaling pathway that triggers an appropriate immune response.

In general, activation of a TLR leads to the production of pro-inflammatory cytokines (a loose class of small proteins), which then mobilize the innate immune system to, for example, send white blood cells to the affected area to engulf the intruder—or in the case of a virus, instruct the infected cell to die. Interestingly, the activation of many types of TLRs has been demonstrated to also produce a highly potent molecule called nuclear factor kappa B (NF-kB) (pronounced *enn-eff-kappa-bee*) as part of the signaling mechanism.[38] NF-kB is currently undergoing intense research and has been shown to be a potent target for the treatment of autoimmune diseases and cancers.[39] NF-kB has even been linked to the expression of cancer oncogenes, which turn off the natural cell-death mechanism, leading to the uncontrolled growth of the cancer.[40]

As with all biological systems, TLRs appear to have more than one way of being activated. As mentioned previously, naltrexone is a potent antagonist of the TLR pathway.[41] This pathway has been shown to be clinically relevant in vivo, by studies showing that naltrexone can inhibit TLR-4 and reverse symptoms of neuropathic pain and in vitro where inhibition of TLR-7, 8, and 9 improved models of auto-inflammatory disease.[42]

A recent paper specifically discussing neuropathic pain was one of the first to demonstrate that the effect of naltrexone is chiral. Returning to an earlier discussion, where left- and right-handed molecules can have different binding sites, a study by Hutchinson and colleagues in 2008 effectively demonstrated that opioid-binding receptors are antagonized by *levo*-naltrexone, whereas the TLR-4 receptor is antagonized by *dextro*-naltrexone.[43] Furthermore, in 2017 Cant, Dalgleish, and Allen found antagonism at TLR-7, 8, and 9 from a racemic mixture of naltrexone.[44]

It is entirely possible, and in fact likely, that the reason naltrexone seems to have such a wide range of activity in different physiological systems is because it behaves as two different drugs, depending on structure of the isomer.

Clinicians and scientists postulate that in some autoimmune diseases, such as lupus, rheumatoid arthritis, and multiple sclerosis, natural mammalian cell by-products may inappropriately activate TLR receptors, directly leading to the inappropriate inflammation.[45] In addition, imiquimod, a drug that has recently reached clinical use for treating skin cancer, has been shown to activate, rather than antagonize, TLR-7, causing so much inflammation in the area that it is very effective at killing basal cell cancer of the skin.[46]

To summarize the data so far:

- Naltrexone, when produced for human consumption, consists of a 50:50 mixture of levo- and dextro-isomers.
- Levo-naltrexone is an antagonist for the opioid/endorphin receptors, and is credited with:

- Upregulation of endorphin release
- Immunomodulation
- Reductions in cell proliferation via endorphins
- Dextro-naltrexone is an antagonist for at least one TLR, if not more, and is reported to:
  - Antagonize TLR, suppressing the cytokine-modulated immune system
  - Antagonize TLR-mediated production of NF-kB, reducing inflammation, and potentially downregulating oncogenes

In this way, it is easy to see how the large number of actions attributed to LDN could be feasible. What is currently lacking is sufficient in vivo, double-blind clinical studies showing that the effects proven in a petri dish and test tube scale up reliably to actions on humans.

Conclusion

Naltrexone has a long history of amelioration and treatment of human disease. Widespread research continues internationally into the relatively new use of LDN for immune, autoimmune, and neoplastic diseases, with sporadic use for a variety of seemingly unrelated conditions. There is significant rationale for a clinician to consider the use of LDN as an adjunct to standard therapy, where standard therapies are unsuccessful. Several clinical trials are either under design or under way as of 2020, and it is highly likely that a licensed form of LDN will be available within five years. Until then, patients and clinicians should make an informed decision on what is most appropriate for them by looking at the currently available evidence, both published and anecdotal, before considering treatment.

Notes

Naltrexone in both standard and low dose forms is often created illegally, manufactured to substandard quality, and sold on the Internet. No reputable pharmacy will sell naltrexone without a prescription. Any patient trying to source a prescriber or supplier for LDN should refer to reputable sources. The only charity in the United Kingdom that promotes research into LDN, and has extensive links to international resources, prescribers, and suppliers, is the LDN Research Trust.

TWO

Chronic Pain

SARAH J. ZIELSDORF, MD, MS,
AND NEEL D. MEHTA, MD

Multiple epidemiologic studies, including the Global Burden of Disease Study (2016), have confirmed that chronic pain and pain-related conditions are the leading cause of disability and disease burden worldwide.[1] The most common of these chronic conditions, affecting 1.9 billion people, is a recurrent tension-type headache. The prevalence of suffering is only increasing, as 1 in 10 people worldwide develop chronic pain each year. When quantifying years lived with disability (the metric most often used is the DALY, or disability-adjusted life year), researchers find that lumbosacral and cervical neck pain are primary causes internationally.[2] Moreover, other chronic pain conditions are represented in the top 10 causes of disability.

Estimates of prevalence for chronic pain conditions vary between 10 and 50 percent of the world's population. Such variance is accounted for by differences in prevalence both between countries and within specific regions of the same country. The global burden of the chronic pain is unequally distributed—low- to middle-income countries are more profoundly affected than high-income countries, as are the lowest socioeconomic and oldest subsets of the population. These populations bear the highest burdens of persistent pain and have fewer management options.[3] Of note, the International Pain Society and Global Health Community concluded in 2004 that "failure to treat pain is viewed worldwide as poor medicine, unethical practice, and an abrogation of a fundamental human right."[4]

Furthermore, chronic pain is deemed a health crisis due to its pervasiveness across diverse populations and its impact on quality of life, both physical and emotional. Epidemiologic studies of chronic pain amplify its complexity through discordant classifications of duration and disease state. This multidimensional condition is defined by the International Association for the Study of Pain (IASP) as pain persisting for more than six months. There is controversy as to whether the definition of chronic pain with respect to symptomology (for instance, anxiety, depression, irritability) or degree is appropriate. An alternative classification for chronic pain is that it is a disease state or injury pertaining to persistent central or peripheral nervous system changes, which results in sensitization. The sensitized nerves lead to both increased amplitude (intensity) and frequency (duration) of the pain response.[5]

In a Brazilian population-based study, nearly 50 percent of participants were dissatisfied with their chronic pain management. Furthermore, in Brazil, as in many therapeutic paradigms worldwide, treatment is not specific to gender. Yet significant gender-associated differences were found in the perception of pain intensity and interference of pain with daily life activities. Women cited pain crises greater in both frequency and duration than those experienced by men, as well as greater interference of pain in the categories of self-care, work, sexual life, and sleep interruption.[6]

Low dose naltrexone (LDN) represents a treatment strategy completely different from the standard of care for chronic pain. There are prejudicial and preconceived attitudes throughout the allopathic, naturopathic, and allied health professions. The knee-jerk response to naltrexone is, "That's used for addicts." Clearly, much work is to be done in the way of educating clinicians to have greater sensitivity toward patients with alcohol or opioid dependence (or overdose), and to understand the therapeutic benefits of naltrexone and naloxone. Almost universally there is little awareness that if we use a low dose of naltrexone, we can achieve pain relief through a brief opioid receptor blockade. Here we will review the current evidence supporting the use of LDN in the management of neuropathic conditions, complex regional pain syndrome, osteoarthritis, autoimmune and rheumatologic diseases, multiple sclerosis, myofascial pain, fibromyalgia, and abdominal pain.

General Considerations for the Management of Chronic Pain

Clinical experience has shown that the use of LDN, in the absence of opioids, works synergistically with other anti-inflammatory agents, including non-steroidal anti-inflammatory drugs (NSAIDs; these should be used judiciously), topical pain relief compounds, therapeutic omega-3 fatty acid supplements, magnesium (especially glycinate or malate oral forms, and topical magnesium chloride preparations), curcumin, resveratrol, glutathione, arnica, and many other herbal compounds (see the appendix for ULDN considerations for the use of LDN with opioid medications). Much as a bucket brigade works to quench a fire, these compounds act as many hands to reduce systemic inflammation. In the past several years, many LDN clinicians and researchers have taken an interest in cannabidiol (CBD), another compound that works synergistically with LDN via the modulation of the endocannabinoid and endorphin pathways.

Of note for all inflammatory conditions: The cornerstone of any treatment plan should be an oligoantigenic (elimination) and an anti-inflammatory diet that emphasizes unprocessed foods, green and nonstarchy vegetables, low-glycemic fruits, wild-caught fish, and olive oil, while most commonly eliminating grains, dairy, sugar, and sometimes nightshade seeds and spices. A variety of anti-inflammatory diet protocols exist, but it is paramount that patients work with a clinician to personalize their own optimal diet that emphasizes nutrient density rather than embark on a restrictive diet plan without guidance, for reasons elaborated below.

Since the popularity of restrictive diets for healing chronic conditions has increased, new research is concerning. Many clinicians, including Dr. Zielsdorf, are seeing a loss of oral tolerance in patients that have utilized restrictive diets for lengthy periods of time (often years). Our gastrointestinal tract is constantly bombarded by potential threats, and in general the term *oral tolerance* represents the ability of the body to recognize previously ingested antigens.

There are several possible reasons for loss of oral tolerance. Restrictive diets can lead to a decrease in microbial diversity. If there is a concomitant imbalance via opportunistic or pathogenic bacteria, yeast, protozoans, or even parasitic infections, then the individual will likely be less able to tolerate food proteins.[7]

Another reason for a loss of oral tolerance and subsequent food sensitivities seems to be overactive dendritic cells. These cells, known as antigen-presenting cells (APCs), sample the proteins that are being broken down in the lumen (inside) of the small intestine. APCs are required for the induction of oral tolerance and help generate regulatory T cells (Tregs), which act as police officers of the immune system. Their aim is to keep the peace—a balance in recognizing benign or potentially dangerous antigens. However, when overstimulated, dendritic cells are more likely to inappropriately activate our immune system, which may respond to self-proteins as foreign invaders and increase the risk of autoimmunity. We can help these hyperactive dendritic cells' response by improving the digestion of proteins (sometimes addressing low stomach acid and other digestive enzymes), and also improving first responders of the gut, antibodies known as secretory IgA (sIgA).[8]

As mentioned above, when undertaken with the guidance of a clinician, an anti-inflammatory diet can have profound benefits for chronic pain management. Because chronic pain is so energy depleting, both at the cellular level and symptomatically, a high-yield strategy is to prioritize an anti-inflammatory diet with a variety of colorful fruits and vegetables. "Eating the rainbow" is the best way to ensure consumption of a variety of phytonutrients (including polyphenols and flavonoids) that maximize mitochondrial energy output, antioxidant support, and detoxification. In addition to eating colorful foods, maintaining an optimal vitamin D level is important in reducing inflammation. Dr. Zielsdorf recommends 60–80 ng/mL 25-hydroxyvitamin D for patients with autoimmune or immune system dysfunction. She is sensitive to the homeostatic physiologic responses with regard to calcium, vitamin D, magnesium, and potential contraindications to higher dose vitamin D supplementation that may be required to achieve these optimal levels.

This is a subject that is fraught with controversy. When supplementing with vitamin D_3, ionized calcium, red blood cell (RBC) magnesium, and 1,25-dihydroxyvitamin D levels should be monitored, with further testing of parathyroid hormone if needed. Much of the concern regarding higher therapeutic doses of vitamin D is over the displacement of calcium and thus potential vascular calcification and loss of bone density. However, many clinicians are using vitamin K_2 (MK4 and MK7) to help mitigate this possible effect. Vitamin K promotes osteoblast (bone-building) maturation and is involved in the upregulation of specific genes in osteoblasts. Increased vitamin K also activates bone-associated vitamin K–dependent proteins, which play critical roles in extracellular bone matrix mineralization.[9] Vitamin D and its metabolites are hormones, which activate hundreds of genes via the expression of the vitamin D receptor (VDR).[10] The influence of vitamin D on the immune system and cellular metabolism, in general, cannot be understated.

There are no known interactions between LDN and any minerals, supplements, vitamins, or hormones. Rarely can an adjunctive pain therapy be so widely considered. For example, a multitude of patients are unable to take traditional NSAIDs or acetaminophen. The NSAID class is notorious for disrupting the GI tract and can cause life-threatening GI bleeding, as well as immune system disruption via the alteration of gut microbiota.[11] Acetaminophen depletes glutathione, which is the body's master antioxidant.[12] These classes of drugs, while sometimes necessary for short-term use, should not be used without understanding the greater implications of possible toxicity. Low dose naltrexone is an important alternative with a much safer profile for chronic pain management.

A multidisciplinary, multi-modality approach to chronic pain must be undertaken for the best result. Such an approach might include medications, acupuncture, local electrical stimulation (e-stim), surgery for structural deficits if necessary, and therapies such as psychotherapy / behavior modification, relaxation techniques, neurofeedback, and biofeedback. Yoga and bodywork—including massage, myofascial release, and condition-specific physical therapy—are useful to address pain resulting from the aging of the musculoskeletal system and chronic inflammation, which accelerates cellular degeneration and mitochondrial insufficiency. Finally, many chronic pain patients have underlying life trauma experience. Newer therapies to address these deep-seated injuries include eye movement desensitization and reprocessing (EMDR) and limbic system modulation therapy.

Neuropathies

One case report has described the off-label use of LDN for the treatment of diabetic neuropathy. The patient had a seven-year history of intractable pain due to bilateral lower extremity diabetic neuropathy that was refractory to multiple pain medications and interventional management. LDN at a daily dose of 4 mg reduced the patient's pain from 90 to 5 on the 0–100 point visual analog scale (VAS).[13] Although this case study was the first to demonstrate the potential for LDN to relieve the pain from diabetic neuropathy, further studies are needed to determine safety, mechanism, and efficacy.[14] In many LDN clinicians' practices, other cases of peripheral neuropathic pain from a variety of etiologies have shown improvement in patient pain scores and quality of life.[15]

Complex Regional Pain Syndrome

Complex regional pain syndrome (CRPS) is a neuropathic condition characterized by pain that is usually disproportionate in severity and duration to the initial insult. Type I CRPS has no known nerve injury etiology, while Type II CRPS develops after an injury resulting in a nerve lesion. Its symptoms include sensory disorders (allodynia and/or hyperesthesia), vasomotor challenges (temperature or skin color changes or asymmetry), edema or sweating, motor dysfunction (weakness, dystonia, tremor), and trophic changes (hair, skin, nails).[16] CRPS is associated with an inflammatory state. Patients with CRPS demonstrate elevated levels of pro-inflammatory cytokines in their cerebrospinal spinal fluid, plasma, and affected tissue.[17] Additionally, postmortem analysis of a CRPS patient demonstrated that microglia and astrocyte activation is implicated in the condition.[18] Thus LDN can theoretically benefit CRPS patients by countering the inflammatory response and microglial activation.

Limited evidence suggests that LDN may be effective in the treatment of CRPS. One case report exists in the literature, describing two patients with CRPS who were successfully treated with LDN after failed conventional medical management. The first patient was a 48-year-old man with a 6-year history of CRPS symptoms in his right lower extremity. Following initiation of LDN at a dose of 4.5 mg nightly, the patient experienced a resolution of dystonic spasms as well as remission of pain. The second patient was a 12-year-old girl with Ehlers-Danlos syndrome who developed right lower extremity CRPS symptoms following a right ankle subluxation. The patient had a remission of all CRPS symptoms (including dystonia of her lower right leg) after receiving LDN at a daily dose of 4.5 mg. CRPS patients using LDN have shown decreases in both acute and chronic inflammation biomarkers—erythrocyte sedimentation rate (ESR) and C-reactive protein (CRP), respectively.[19]

Osteoarthritis

The use of naltrexone for the treatment of pain due to osteoarthritis has been investigated in the context of combination therapy. Oxytrex is an investigational drug that combines a therapeutic dose of oxycodone with microgram doses of naltrexone.[20] One phase II randomized clinical trial that involved 360 patients with moderate to severe osteoarthritic pain of the hip or knee found that Oxytrex was associated with significant pain relief as compared with oxycodone alone.[21] However, valid results could not be obtained in subsequent phases due to a high dropout rate.[22]

Autoimmune/Rheumatologic Conditions

LDN has been studied in conjunction with a small number of autoimmune diseases, including inflammatory bowel disease (IBD) and rheumatoid arthritis. Naltrexone is theorized to play a beneficial role in the treatment of some chronic inflammatory states related to opioid growth factor–opioid growth factor receptor (OGF–OGFr) axis dysfunction, given that it has been shown to modulate this pathway.[23]

Emerging evidence may support the use of LDN in the treatment of IBD, a chronic inflammatory condition that includes Crohn's disease and ulcerative colitis. While initial studies were promising, a 2014 meta-analysis that analyzed two small, randomized control trials concluded that there is insufficient evidence to support the use of LDN in Crohn's disease.[24] However, more recent studies have had positive results. A quasi-experimental pharmaco-epidemiological study found that the initiation of LDN therapy was associated with a reduced dispensation of medication used to treat IBD.[25] A prospective cohort study of 47 patients with IBD found that LDN led to clinical improvement in a majority of patients, as evidenced by endoscopic proof of remission and mucosal healing.[26] Despite these results, a 2018 Cochrane systematic review concluded that there is currently insufficient high-quality evidence regarding the efficacy and safety of LDN in treating Crohn's disease.[27] As approximately 30 percent of patients with inflammatory bowel disease either are refractory to current IBD drugs or relapse, and current treatments have a significant side effect profile, LDN offers a low-risk alternative where other options are not available. As a more radical suggestion, if the disease is mild or in its early stages, it is valid to ask why an LDN regimen coupled with an anti-inflammatory diet should not be tried before other treatment options, given the mounting evidence and case studies attesting to its benefits.

Studies exploring the role of LDN in the treatment of rheumatoid arthritis (RA) and other rheumatologic conditions have been limited to date. One recent, quasi-experimental study exists in the literature. It found that LDN therapy was associated with a reduction in the use of other medications, including analgesics, for the treatment of rheumatoid and seropositive arthritis.[28] Further research is necessary to evaluate the efficacy of LDN in inflammatory arthritis. Clinical experience with RA patients has demonstrated that the combination of an anti-inflammatory diet and LDN has enabled a subset of patients to reduce or eliminate use of disease-modifying anti-rheumatic drugs (DMARDs) such as methotrexate.

A 2018 journal article published in *Thyroid* demonstrated—via an online survey with over 12,000 respondents—that the majority of patients with hypothyroidism are not satisfied with their current therapy or their physicians.[29] Dr. Zielsdorf's practice has a thyroid focus and a reputation for improving quality of life through the use of low dose naltrexone and a personalized approach to thyroid hormone prescription and management. Thyroid disease is most often autoimmune-mediated, and may result in clinical hyperthyroidism due to Graves' disease or hypo/hyperthyroidism secondary to Hashimoto's thyroiditis. The symptoms and resulting disease state depend on the autoantibodies produced toward specific antigens, with subsequent cellular inflammation and destruction of the targeted organs and tissues (in the case of Hashimoto's, the eventual atrophy and loss of function of the thyroid gland). An online survey was sent to clinic patients via email and social media, and to both thyroid and LDN advocacy groups on social media sites. One thousand one hundred and eight respondents completed the 24-question survey (1,610 unique visits and a 68.8 percent completion rate) between February 19 and March 7, 2019.

Participants were asked about expanded treatment options including synthetic T4, synthetic T3, NDT, compounded T4, compounded T3, synthetic T4/T4 combination, glandular thyroid supplements, and iodine, as well as whether they ever used LDN as an adjunct thyroid treatment. Overall, 479 respondents (43.4 percent) used LDN, with 53.6 percent of those using 3.6 to 4.5 mg daily and 53.2 percent taking LDN for a duration over 12 months. In addition, 20.4 percent ranked their symptoms at 10, or "strongly improved," on a scale of 1 through 10. Of the thyroid patients taking LDN, 56.9 percent had reduced pain, 55 percent had improved energy and reduced fatigue, and 41.7 percent had improved mood.[30] The results of this survey highlight the pain relief thyroid patients often experience with the addition of LDN to their medication regimen. LDN is a vital adjunct for lowering inflammation and improving thyroid function, and potentially reversing the autoimmune process in Hashimoto's/Graves' pathology. Clinicians should take a personalized approach to thyroid treatment; no one medication or protocol fits all.

Multiple Sclerosis

Multiple sclerosis (MS) is a chronic inflammatory disease involving demyelination of the central nervous system.[31] Nearly 1 million individuals were afflicted with MS in the United States in 2017.[32]

Preclinical studies have demonstrated OGF–OGFr axis dysregulation as a feature in the pathophysiology of MS, suggesting a role for LDN as a potential therapeutic agent. Mice induced with experimental autoimmune encephalomyelitis (EAE), the accepted animal model of MS, showed a reduction in OGF prior to the onset of clinical signs of the disease.[33] In the same animal model, treatment with LDN or OGF inhibited the progression of EAE.[34] The introduction of LDN therapy resulted in restored levels of OGF in mice with EAE as well as in humans with MS.[35] Furthermore, mice with EAE that were treated with LDN or OGF had decreased levels of interferon-gamma and tumor necrosis factor alpha.[36]

In the clinical setting, the use of LDN in MS treatment has shown some promising, though inconclusive, results. A pilot trial demonstrated that LDN was safe and tolerable for patients with primary progressive MS, and resulted in a significant reduction in spasticity.[37] Subsequent studies also provide evidence that LDN is well tolerated and significantly improves quality of life for patients with MS.[38] However, some studies did not identify much benefit. A randomized control trial found that LDN was safe in MS but had unknown efficacy, and a quasi-experimental before-and-after study reported that LDN therapy was not followed by a reduction in medication used to treat MS.[39] However, the latter study also showed that opioid dispensation was significantly reduced in persistent LDN users. This included a cumulative dose reduction of 42 percent, and a 9 percent reduction in the number of users. In addition, there was an 8 percent decrease in the number of NSAID users.[40] Overall, studies have demonstrated some positive impact from LDN on quality of life for MS patients, particularly in the areas of pain and fatigue management.

Myofascial Pain

There is sparse data on the use of LDN in myofascial pain. A single case report exists in the literature describing the use of LDN for the treatment of chronic back pain. The patient had a two-year history of paraspinal low back pain that was resistant to nonsteroidal anti-inflammatory drugs, anticonvulsants, tricyclic antidepressants, physical therapy, and interventional management. After receiving LDN therapy at a dose of 4 mg daily, the patient's pain decreased from 90–100 to 35 on the 0–100 point visual analog scale.[41] More studies are needed to follow up on the one available case report.

There is also one phase III clinical trial in the literature that investigated the use of Oxytrex in patients with chronic low back pain.[42] Its findings were that adding ultra low dose naltrexone (ULDN) to oxycodone provides superior analgesia and reduces opioid side effects. However, this study has been criticized for its high dropout rate and other limiting factors, which may compromise its clinical significance.[43]

Fibromyalgia

Fibromyalgia is a poorly understood disorder characterized by chronic, diffuse musculoskeletal pain associated with a number of tender points.[44] The prevalence is approximately 2 to 8 percent of the population.[45] Features of fibromyalgia include dysfunction in sleep, pain, and stress response. Patients also report chronic fatigue, cognitive disturbances, headaches, and gastrointestinal symptoms.[46] Unfortunately, this condition, which disproportionately afflicts women, is often treated as a psychosomatic illness.

LDN's anti-inflammatory properties may help with management of fibromyalgia. The pathophysiology of fibromyalgia involves glial activation and the production of pro-inflammatory molecules. These pro-inflammatory molecules cause irritation of nerves and, thus, a hypersensitive pain response.[47] A pilot study examining the effects of LDN on fibromyalgia found that an individual's baseline erythrocyte sedimentation rate was predictive of their response to LDN therapy.[48] Additionally, LDN administration has been associated with reduced biomarkers of inflammation, with concomitant improvement in pain and other symptoms.[49] Dr. Ginevra Liptan, an internist with fibromyalgia herself, founded The Frida Center for Fibromyalgia in Portland, Oregon. She states that "for fibromyalgia, I have found the combination of CBD and LDN to be more effective for pain reduction than either treatment alone. CBD also eases the anxiety that can occur as a side effect of LDN."

Preliminary clinical studies have supported the role of LDN therapy in the treatment of fibromyalgia. Two small clinical trials found that LDN was well tolerated and effectively reduced fibromyalgia symptoms.[50] A recent small, prospective study corroborated these findings.[51] Larger controlled trials are necessary to fully evaluate the efficacy of LDN in treating fibromyalgia.

Abdominal Pain / Pelvic Pain

"Functional" abdominal pain is arguably one of the most overmedicated and one-dimensionally treated conditions. Furthermore, the term *irritable bowel syndrome* is, in one sense, a wastebasket diagnosis, encompassing the "idiopathic" classification. It is rare for a clinician to appropriately seek out the root cause of IBS pain. To give clinicians the benefit of the doubt, conventional biomarker tests such as a complete metabolic panel or complete blood count are rarely abnormal, and it is difficult for patients to describe the location or quality of their pain. It takes a multifaceted approach to find the root causes of pain, constipation, diarrhea, and other symptoms of IBS. It is possible for pain receptors to be activated in either superficial or deep tissues. These may include somatic receptors (encompassing the musculo-skeletal system), or visceral receptors within organs in the chest, abdomen, or pelvis. Any of these receptors, individually or in combination, sound the alarm of damage to the body. In addition, the cure is often more difficult to bear than the symptoms. If medications such as combinations of antispasmodics, antidepressants, benzodiazepines, or opioids are abruptly stopped, the individual may face severe withdrawal symptoms known collectively as discontinuation syndrome. LDN users do not face this dilemma.

LDN was first studied for its effects on IBS in a 2006 pilot study. An Israeli research group enrolled 42 IBS patients in an open-label study using a daily dose of 0.5 mg LDN daily for four weeks. There were no significant adverse effects. Seventy-six percent of patients responded using a global assessment, which measured pain-free days and symptom relief. Patients recorded their degree of abdominal pain and stool urgency, consistency, and frequency. The study was statistically significant, and concluded that a large, randomized, double-blind, placebo-controlled study was justified. More than a decade later, no such study has yet been undertaken.[52]

Other examples of chronic abdominal and overlapping pelvic pain conditions include endometriosis, interstitial cystitis, and vulvodynia. Patients may have one or more of these issues concomitantly. Each of these aforementioned conditions is poorly understood with respect to its pathophysiology. There are theories regarding the way in which immune system activation and microbiome dysbiosis shift the body toward a pro-inflammatory state, and thus, one of chronic pain.

In endometriosis (not yet classified as an autoimmune condition but often expressed in women with other autoimmune conditions), the endometrial tissue thickens and breaks down according to the menstrual cycle, but since this tissue is on the outside of the uterus, it is trapped in the pelvic cavity, causing retrograde menstruation.

Endometrial tissue is fascinating—it can form in utero (congenital endometriosis), or iatrogenically. For example, in the case of cesarean section, when the surgeon irrigates the pelvic cavity, those endometrial migratory cells may be strewn throughout the intra-abdominal cavity. This further accelerates the process of tissue growth, inflammation, and severity of symptoms. Moreover, in females, a small opening in the peritoneum near the ovaries is an opportunity for cell migration to any gastrointestinal organ regardless of surgical intervention. One case study involved a post-hysterectomy patient who required excision of her vaginal vault due to iatrogenic endometriosis. She presented with sudden lower pelvic discomfort and vaginal bleeding 13 months after hysterectomy.[53] If involving the ovaries, cysts known as endometriomas can form, and as a consequence severe pain and infertility may result from chronic irritation and development of scarring and adhesions. This scarring can also lead to painful intercourse (dyspareunia), urinary tract symptoms, and other symptoms.

Dr. Jennifer Mercier, women's health specialist and creator of the gynovisceral manipulation therapy known as Mercier Therapy, discusses the aggressive nature of endometrial tissue and why endometriosis is so devastating: "These migratory cells adhere to structures in the abdominal and pelvic cavity, and as menstruation is occurring, those migratory endometrial cells are weeping fluid into the peritoneal and pelvic cavities causing pain and scar tissue to form, which glues anything down in its wake. Anything that is glued down has inadequate blood flow. In essence, organs need to be freely moving against each other for proper function."[54] Dr. Mercier stumbled upon her novel therapy after many years of suffering with autoimmune thyroid disease and stage IV endometriosis. Lying in bed after enduring three laparoscopic surgeries, she developed her unique methodology by self-manipulating her viscera and observing changes in her own symptoms over time. Eventually, she noticed that her period would start spontaneously without the telltale severe pelvic and vaginal pain that would usually precipitate her cycle, radiating to her legs or a low backache. Patients who use Dr. Mercier's therapy protocol for six hours (one hour per week for six weeks) have shown an 83 percent increase in natural conception. For women with endometriosis, maintenance treatments are encouraged.

Despite the clear benefits of Mercier Therapy, there are no formally accepted alternatives for treating long-term pain without using opioids/analgesics, hormonal birth control, or surgery. The gold standard of therapy for deep pelvic endometriosis, defined as a subperitoneal invasion exceeding 5 millimeters in depth, is laparoscopic surgery. The severe pain from these deep endometriotic lesions is poorly localized due to the lesions' pervasive nature throughout the intra-abdominal cavity and frequent extraperitoneal spread.[55] Referral to gastroenterology is often fruitless, as endoscopy only looks internally, and laparoscopic assessment only allows the doctor to visualize the pelvic organs, but does not physically run through all the loops of the bowel. Cadaveric studies show that endometriosis can be in nasal and brain matter in living women. Endometrial adhesions have been the cause of cyclic headaches and nosebleeds, all previously thought to be unrelated and of unknown etiology in women. Most impressively, in one case, a woman had a nasal nodule that had caused cyclical bleeding since puberty—surgical excision and pathologic analysis confirmed endometriosis.[56]

Clinical trials are under way to assess the therapeutic potential of LDN in chronic abdominal pain from endometriosis. As endometriosis is inflammatory in nature and possibly autoimmune-mediated, it follows that LDN can be used as an adjunctive therapy for pain management.[57]

Insights from Clinical Practice

In clinical practice, patients report a range of experiences with LDN as a treatment for chronic pain. While some patients report no difference in their pain levels, others experience improvement in their quality of life, and sometimes even the complete resolution of their pain. Aside from improved pain management, benefits derived from the use of LDN have included decreased fatigue, improved mood, reduced sleep disturbances, and enhanced cognitive function. We have found that patients may experience a placebo effect upon initiation of the medication. Thus, the individual may need to take LDN consistently for several weeks, or even months, before the true effect of the medication can be elucidated. In general, a trial of six months to one year is recommended for chronic pain conditions before concluding whether the medication has had an effect.

Above all, it must be impressed that LDN is rarely a panacea with regard to chronic pain relief.

In our experience LDN has a low incidence of adverse effects. Infrequent side effects reported by patients taking LDN include transient insomnia, vivid dreams, headaches, nausea, and anxiety. We have not observed any serious adverse events in our patient population.

A wider dosing range of LDN is utilized in clinical practice than is reported in the literature. While the standard dosage in existing research is approximately 4.5 mg, some patients are initially started on a dose as low as 0.5 mg, which is uptitrated to effect in subsequent clinic visits. Patients experiencing side effects at higher doses are often reduced to a dose of 3 mg or less.

While clinical data on the subject is currently sparse, LDN may also be helpful for patients with Ehlers-Danlos syndrome. EDS includes a heterogeneous group of inherited disorders affecting the connective tissue, characterized by joint hypermobility, tissue fragility, and skin hyperextensibility.[58] Patients with EDS may initially present with nociceptive joint pain that may later lead to the development of neuropathies.[59] Patients with EDS-associated chronic pain who started on LDN therapy have reported improved mobility, reduced frequency of flare-ups, enhanced gastrointestinal motility, and improved pain tolerance.

Conclusion

The off-label use of LDN has demonstrated some positive, albeit preliminary, results in the treatment of chronic pain in the clinical literature. Despite limited information on the topic, LDN therapy has grown in popularity both in the United States and abroad. More than 250 pharmacies in the United States compound LDN.[60] In Norway a TV documentary on LDN led to a significant increase in its prescription; 0.3 percent of the country's population has reportedly utilized the drug.[61]

There remains a significant need for proper, large-scale studies to investigate the use of LDN for chronic pain conditions. Additionally, optimal dosing regimens have yet to be elucidated. Despite the demand for high-quality trials, there are obstacles to conducting this research. Naltrexone is off-patent and inexpensive; thus, there is little financial incentive to carry out these trials.[62] Clinicians are not being educated on this treatment option, and patients admitted to hospitals have been met with ill-informed and even discriminatory reactions to their use of LDN. In the meantime little is being done to provide low-risk therapies (rather than only symptom mitigation) for chronic pain conditions that disproportionately affect aging populations, which are rapidly increasing. LDN is a vital adjunctive therapy that fills a gap in a comprehensive therapeutic toolbox of traditional allopathic and complementary treatments.

— THREE —

Gut Health

Leonard B. Weinstock, MD, FACG, and Kristen Blasingame, MA

There are several gastrointestinal (GI) diseases and disorders for which low dose naltrexone has been applied as a therapeutic agent. The pathological factors that allow for the use of LDN in gut disorders and diseases include uncontrolled inflammation, abnormal immunity, increased intestinal permeability, increased visceral hypersensitivity, abnormal motility, and unregulated cellular growth. In this chapter we review publications in the medical literature that illustrate the effect of LDN in GI diseases and the pathway to gut health. These disorders include inflammatory bowel disease, constipation, gastroparesis, irritable bowel syndrome (IBS), mast cell activation syndrome (MCAS), sarcoidosis, and mesenteric panniculitis. A brief discussion of the use of LDN in GI cancers will conclude the chapter. For most of these disorders, we will review our experience and/or present data from our unpublished case series.

The mechanism of action whereby LDN reduces inflammation is well described in the first chapter of this book and applies to some of the GI disorders in this chapter. The potential use of LDN or endorphins to treat motility disorders is not well known by clinicians. If LDN does lead to improved motility, then it could be used to treat constipation, abnormal small intestinal motility, small intestinal bacterial overgrowth, and gastroparesis. Reducing the overactive immune system by reducing T cells can help MCAS, sarcoidosis, and mesenteric panniculitis. Direct toll-like receptor blockade by naltrexone could help reduce neuroinflammatory processes such as visceral hypersensitivity in IBS.

Normal and Abnormal Gut Structure

A number of the aforementioned disorders disturb the balanced structure of the healthy gut. In the healthy gut, there are healthy bacteria adherent to mucus produced by the goblet cells. The mucosa has crypts (involutions) to maximize the absorptive surface area. Enterochromaffin cells are interspersed along the epithelium cells and regulate intestinal motility and secretion. They also modulate neuronal signaling in the enteric nervous system via the secretion of serotonin and other peptides. Zonulin and occludin are proteins that create bridges that maintain the tight junctions between epithelial cells. In the submucosal plexus there are nerves, blood vessels, and dendritic cells. The nerves join in with other nerves and course through the muscle layers, and ultimately connect to the central nervous system.

When there is small intestinal bacterial overgrowth (SIBO) or dysbiosis (imbalanced bacteria colonies), the adherent bacteria create inflammation. Goblet cells consequently produce less protective mucus, allowing for attachment of bacteria to the epithelium. With increased intestinal permeability, the gram-negative bacteria—known as lipopolysaccharides—enter through the mucosal barrier. This can upset the hypothalamic-adrenal-pituitary axis. The tight junctions created by zonulin and occludin are damaged by cytokines produced by inflammatory cells. The dendritic cells respond to this inflammation by recruiting mast cells and T- and B-cell lymphocytes. Mast cells secrete many chemicals that can either contribute to further damage or help mediate the inflammatory process depending on their genetic status. The T-cell lymphocytes secrete cytokines, including interleukins and tumor necrosis factor alpha, which are potent inflammatory chemicals. They can further damage intestinal permeability, which creates a vicious cycle. This inflammatory storm can activate nerves and contribute to abnormal pain sensation and motility. The B cell lymphocytes manufacture antibodies, and it is possible that some of these are the source of autoimmune diseases.

Inflammatory Bowel Disease

In the first volume of *The LDN Book*, chapter 3 describes the effect of LDN therapy in inflammatory bowel disease (IBD).[1] The two main chronic inflammatory bowel diseases are Crohn's disease and ulcerative colitis. They each involve abnormal immunity and inflammation, and often respond to the same medications. They also differ from each other in several ways.

Read that chapter for a detailed discussion of how LDN reduces abnormal immunity and inflammation, and subsequently reduces disease activity of inflammatory bowel disease. Crohn's disease is an inflammatory disease of the intestine that can start in the mouth and extend all way down to the anus, potentially causing perianal disease. It is an ulcerating disease that starts in the mucosa and is caused by abnormal action of lymphocytes, excess cytokines, and altered vascular permeability.[2] An abnormal genome and altered microbiome in the context of an environmental triggering event may be the conditions out of which inflammatory bowel disease develops. Increased depth of inflammation and ulceration can result in fistulas that lead to abscess formation. Inflammation of the intestinal wall will lead to fibrosis, scar tissue, and strictures. Damage to the endoplasmic reticulum, which defines the structure of cells, may play an important role in stricture formation. Crohn's disease is extremely difficult to treat. No one has demonstrated a perfect therapy despite the use of expensive medications. Furthermore, once patients have seen improvements using biologic therapies, these medicines lose their efficacy by 13 to 24 percent. It is thought that 30 to 60 percent of all inflammatory bowel disease patients will have treatment refractoriness, requiring them to turn to surgery or steroid use.[3]

Since the publication of *The LDN Book* in February 2016, there have been several articles published on use of LDN in inflammatory bowel disease. A 2018 review examined articles and abstracts for high-quality research in Crohn's disease, two of which were discussed in the chapter on inflammatory bowel disease in *The LDN Book*.[4] The authors of the review stated that the studies examined have a small sample size, but suggest that LDN leads to a benefit in clinical and endoscopic response in adults. They cautioned that further randomized studies are required to assess how well LDN works in Crohn's disease.[5]

One of the more recent studies referred to in the 2018 review was an animal model study. With respect to inflammatory bowel disease, these kinds of studies are important for multiple reasons. They allow for a controlled situation and precise measurements, and there is generally no placebo effect to worry about. A framework for determining cause and effect can be established in a much more efficient manner. In the aforementioned study, rats were given injections of a nonsteroidal anti-inflammatory medication—indomethacin—to induce inflammation of the small intestine.[6] Indomethacin administered by subcutaneous shots or by mouth has been shown to cause small intestinal ulcers in rats. There is some logic in using this as an experimental model, since nonsteroidal medications will often worsen Crohn's disease in humans. Nonetheless, the NSAID injury in animals is not Crohn's disease, per se.

After indomethacin was administered, the rats received therapy with a placebo (sulfasalazine), naltrexone, or both medications. Two inflammatory markers (C reactive protein and tumor necrosis factor) were measured to determine disease activity. After treatment with indomethacin, the levels of tumor necrosis factor in the rats treated with naltrexone alone were 73 pg/ml, compared with 599 pg/ml in the animals treated with indomethacin alone. There was also a significant improvement in the histopathology of the naltrexone-treated animals.[7]

Studies with human subjects have also demonstrated the efficacy of LDN in treating IBD. A study of 40 inflammatory bowel disease patients examined the effects of administering 0.5 mg of naltrexone daily. They examined the blood and biopsies from seven patients before and after LDN treatment. There was a clinical response in 23 patients, 13 of whom had Crohn's disease and 10 of whom had ulcerative colitis. An in vitro study of the biopsy tissue from these patients examined the effect of stress on the endoplasmic reticulum of the cells. This is a network of cellular membranes that are important in the synthesis and transport of proteins and membrane lipids. The researchers demonstrated that patients treated with LDN had improved cell migration into wounds compared with controls. Endoplasmic reticulum stress, which plays a role in scar tissue formation in inflammatory bowel disease, was improved by naltrexone. Improvement in tumor necrosis factor or interleukin 8 in the blood of patients was not seen in this small study.[8]

In 2013 there was a significant increase in LDN use in Norway thought to have resulted from widespread viewing of a TV documentary on the drug.[9] Subsequently, a study out of Norway examined whether LDN could change the medication profiles of inflammatory bowel disease patients. The authors looked at the medication profiles of a group of 582 patients two years before and one year following the initiation of LDN therapy. Of these patients, 256 became regular users of the medication. In the patients who continued on LDN, there was a significant reduction in the prescription use of intestinal steroids, including a 50 percent reduction for patients with Crohn's disease and ulcerative colitis. This is an important research study given that steroids cause so many serious side effects, and even increase the risk of mortality in patients with inflammatory bowel disease.[10]

The most recent study of naltrexone's use in the treatment of inflammatory bowel disease was carried out in the Netherlands.[11] This study evaluated LDN's potential for inducing remission of inflammatory bowel disease. LDN was used as an add-on or complementary treatment in patients not responding to conventional therapy. Of the 47 patients recruited for this 12-week study, 75 percent showed clinical improvement, and 26 percent went into remission. This study also demonstrated that LDN improved epithelial barrier function by improving wound healing and reducing endoplasmic reticulum stress. The authors stated that their remission rates were less than previously reported by Smith et al. in a 2011 study, though they thought the comparison was difficult to make because their own patients were more ill, and because the other study had a smaller sample size.[12]

Since 2005 I have seen the remarkable effects of LDN on inflammatory bowel disease in my own practice. Some of these outcomes are outlined in my 2014 publication on LDN in ulcerative colitis and Crohn's disease.[13]

Over the last two decades, I have routinely offered LDN to IBD patients and seen a significant benefit in more than 50 percent of them. I have prescribed LDN in concert with biologicals and/or in place of azathioprine, which carries a risk of lymphoma. I have even had several patients for whom LDN monotherapy was beneficial.

Gut Health and Motility

One of the most important basic roles of the GI tract is to transport food down the esophagus into the stomach, where muscle activity and gastric acid start the digestive process. The peristaltic movement then carries food into the small intestine, where pancreatic enzymes further the digestive process and assist with absorption of nutrients, electrolytes, and water. The remaining liquid and debris then migrates into the colon, where water is absorbed and fecal matter forms. The microbiome plays an important role in stool formation, as 50 percent of the fecal weight comprises bacteria. Peristaltic activity moves the stool down for elimination. The fasting state triggers the cyclic migrating motor complexes, which are important to keep the small intestine clean and free of debris and bacteria.[14]

The above process is a well-orchestrated one, involving nerves, muscles, neurotransmitters, hormones, and endorphins.[15] The peristaltic reflex is regulated by cholinergic motor neurons in coordination with tachykinins, such as substance P, and other motor neurons and chemicals, including vasoactive intestinal peptides and endogenous opioids. The release of opioids appears to exert a restraining influence on peristalsis. Endogenous opioids have direct tonic influence over circular smooth muscle and thus reduce peristalsis. Thus, since enteric opioids regulate peristalsis, treatment with an opioid antagonist such as naltrexone could alter that regulation and reduce suppression of peristalsis. The involvement of endogenous endorphins in the physiology of motility suggests that there may be a role for LDN when dysmotility is present.

Endorphin receptors are present in the muscles and the gut lining. When narcotics are administered, these receptors cause constipation due to the reduced secretion and loss of peristalsis that accompanies sustained, nonpropulsive muscular contractions. One would think that increasing natural endorphins by LDN would do the same. Normal bowel functioning is primarily the result of coordinated neuromuscular function and well-balanced secretion and absorption of fluid and electrolyte. Intestinal hormones control chloride and subsequent sodium and water secretions, thus keeping the stool hydrated. The two main drivers for normal motility are (1) normal serotonin levels and (2) a balanced parasympathetic and sympathetic nervous system. Serotonin (5-hydroxytryptamine [5-HT]) is the primary neurotransmitter of the enteric nervous system (ENS).[16] Serotonin is a molecule in the brain-gut axis, with 95 percent present in the enteroendocrine cells of the GI lining and also in GI interneurons. 5-HT's action upon serotonin receptors in the GI tract triggers submucosal intrinsic primary afferent neurons to exhibit peristaltic and secretory reflexes. Vagal nerves release acetylcholine, which results in peristaltic movements that are further enhanced by 5-HT4. The ENS signals to the brain are mediated by 5-HT3.

There have been a few studies of the impacts of methionine enkephalin (an endogenous opioid peptide) and naltrexone on peristalsis and the migrating motor complex. Thirty years ago physiologists examined the role of opioid nerves in the regulation of intestinal peristalsis. In their study it was demonstrated that opioid antagonists increase the frequency and amplitude of peristaltic contractions. Opioid antagonists also increased descending relaxation and decreased ascending contraction.[17]

Another study demonstrated a complex interaction of somatostatin, opioid, GABA, and vasoactive protein neurons in normal motility.

Increased somatostatin due to bowel stretching resulted in the inhibition of opioid neuron activity, leading to a decrease in met-enkephalin. By reducing opioid nerve activity, vasoactive intestinal peptide (VIP) and nitrous oxide production helped activate peristalsis.[18]

One study examined the effects of intravenous met-enkephalin on esophageal motility and the migrating motor complex in 17 human volunteers. This endorphin analog decreased complete relaxation of the lower esophageal sphincter and also decreased gastric fundic accommodation due to distension. The most important finding of this study was that met-enkephalin increased the migrating motor complex, which is one of the problems seen in patients with SIBO. It was suspected that a met-enkephalin analog induced these effects by inhibiting the inhibitory nervous system.[19]

In another study experimental inflammation in mice led to increased mu-opioid receptors in a manner similar to the process observed in humans following abdominal surgery.[20] It was proposed that endogenous opioid peptides participate in the neural control of peristalsis by dampening peristaltic performance via activation of mu and kappa receptors. Furthermore, it is thought that opioid receptor antagonists normalize pathologic inhibition of gut function arising from opioid upregulation and/or overactivity. A more recent study by Holzer's group suggests that blockade of the toll-like receptor 4 (TLR-4) in the colon plays a role in opioid-induced constipation.[21] A synthetic TLR-4 antagonist did not alter the morphine-induced inhibition of peristalsis in the isolated guinea pig small intestine, but morphine-induced inhibition of colonic peristalsis was alleviated by TLR-4 antagonism.

A separate study involved chickens that were given met-enkephalin intravenously.[22] Phase III of the migrating motor complex was triggered, and it started in the distal duodenum and propagated to the ileum. This phenomenon will be important for a disorder discussed later in the chapter —small intestinal bacterial overgrowth.

Constipation

Constipation is defined as having bowel movements less than three times per week, straining to pass bowel movements, and having a hard stool. At least 20 percent of the American population is affected by this disorder. The involved pathophysiology can be attributed to poor peristalsis, reduced secretion of fluids and electrolytes, and/or abnormal pelvic floor function.

A small study was published showing LDN to be a helpful agent in patients with idiopathic constipation.[23] In this report 12 patients with chronic constipation were treated with 2.5 mg of LDN twice a day. Seven patients were markedly improved, one was moderately improved, three were mildly improved, and one was unchanged. Dr. Weinstock was involved in this study, which was not placebo-controlled. The patients were refractory to other treatments, although in 2010 the more sophisticated, FDA-approved chloride channel activating drugs were not yet available.

Subsequently Dr. Weinstock has seen in his practice several patients who have taken 2.5 mg of LDN either daily or twice a day experience reduction of constipation. Of his LDN patients who are refractory to other medical treatments for idiopathic constipation, approximately 25 percent experience significant benefit.

Gastroparesis

There is one online case presentation regarding successful LDN treatments in idiopathic gastroparesis.[24] The physician wrote that the patient had a positive response to LDN, though it is difficult to isolate the effect of the LDN because it was prescribed in conjunction with acupuncture, visceral massage, and medical marijuana. A randomized, placebo-controlled study is being initiated to examine the effect of high dose naloxegol, a peripherally active mu-opioid receptor antagonist, in opioid-related gastroparesis.[25] Reports on the effects of LDN on idiopathic gastroparesis by prescribing clinicians is encouraged.

Irritable Bowel Syndrome

IBS is a disorder of the GI tract characterized by abdominal pain and alterations in bowel function, and is often accompanied by bloating and bowel urgency.[26] The abnormal bowel habits associated with IBS may be constipation-predominant (IBS-C), diarrhea-predominant (IBS-D), or they might involve alternating or mixed periods of both (IBS-M).[27] The prevalence of IBS in North America is estimated to be 10 to 15 percent of the population.[28] The disorder is more prevalent in females than males, but this bias may be less pronounced than practitioners generally perceive since women feel more comfortable, on average, seeing their physicians. In a telephone survey of households, the ratio of IBS prevalence between women and men was 6:4.[29] Although IBS is the most common diagnosis made by gastroenterologists, the disorder often goes unrecognized or untreated, with as few as 25 percent of people with IBS seeking clinical care.[30]

IBS is a complex disorder. It is a "syndrome," meaning there are multiple disorders and factors that cause the same set of symptoms. Accordingly, no one specific treatment will ever be 100 percent effective in a clinical study. It is important, whenever possible, to identify underlying mechanisms that can be treated specifically. The diagnosis of IBS is primarily based on the exclusion of other possible diagnoses (such as inflammatory bowel disease, celiac disease, colorectal cancer, lactose intolerance, pancreatic insufficiency, mast cell activation syndrome, and sucrase-isomaltase enzyme deficiency).[31] There has been a historical tendency to simply view IBS as an idiopathic hypersensitivity syndrome, or as a nonspecific "functional" stress disorder.[32]

Two biologic markers have emerged to identify subsets of IBS. One biomarker is the anti-vinculin antibody. Motility testing in IBS patients with evidence of SIBO determined that the migrating motor complex was damaged.[33] An animal study showed that the rats that developed post-infectious irritable bowel syndrome after inoculation with campylobacter had a loss of nerve cells (interstitial cells of Cajal) that are required for a healthy migrating motor complex.[34] Upon further investigation, it was discovered that anti-vinculin is the autoantibody responsible for this neurologic damage.[35] The nightly cleansing waves that start in the stomach and course through the small intestine are lost upon damage to the migrating motor complex and thus contribute to small intestinal bacterial overgrowth. The subsequent results of SIBO include (1) fermentation of carbohydrates that lead to gas and bloating and (2) inflammation and increased intestinal permeability ("leaky gut").

The other biomarker is hydrogen and methane gas, as measured via breath testing.[36] A 2000 study evaluated lactulose breath testing as a diagnostic method for SIBO, and as a way to measure patients' subsequent response to antibiotic therapy. This study demonstrated that 157 (78 percent) of 202 patients who met the Rome diagnostic criteria for IBS also had SIBO.[37] After receiving oral antibiotic therapy (for example, neomycin, ciprofloxacin, metronidazole, doxycycline) for 10 days, 47 patients were given follow-up breath tests. There was significant improvement in diarrhea and abdominal pain in the 25 patients whose SIBO had been eradicated, compared with those patients for whom SIBO persisted ($P < 0.05$). Twelve of these patients (48 percent) no longer met the Rome criteria for IBS ($P < 0.001$). A subsequent double-blind, placebo-controlled study demonstrated that 93 (84 percent) of 111 patients with IBS had abnormal lactulose breath test results at baseline.[38] After 10 days of treatment with either neomycin or placebo, the patients with abnormal breath test results at baseline who were receiving neomycin achieved a 35 percent improvement in constipation, diarrhea, and abdominal pain symptoms, compared with a 4 percent improvement achieved by those who received placebo ($P < 0.01$).

Furthermore, normalization of the lactulose breath test in response to neomycin correlated with patient-reported normalization of bowel function. Among patients in whom breath testing indicated eradication of SIBO by neomycin, bowel normalization was improved by 75 percent, compared with a 37 percent improvement for patients in whom SIBO had not been eradicated by neomycin and 11 percent for patients who received placebo ($P < 0.001$).[39] Therefore, the results of these studies not only support the administration of lactulose breath tests in IBS diagnosis, but also highlight the connection between antibiotic eradication of SIBO and the relief of IBS symptoms.

Subsequently, several large studies have documented the efficacy of antibiotic therapy with rifaximin (a non-absorbed gut-directed antibiotic) in treating IBS-D. These publications ultimately led to the 2015 FDA approval of antibiotic treatment for IBS-D.[40] A follow-up study showed that an abnormal breath test was predictive of a good response to rifaximin.[41] Finally, in IBS cases associated with SIBO, the underlying cause of SIBO needs to be addressed since repeat antibiotic therapy generally will be needed.[42] A variety of prokinetic medicines have been shown to reduce the recurrence of SIBO.[43]

The first published study that evaluated the use of LDN in patients with IBS was conducted by investigators in Israel.[44] Their theory was that visceral hypersensitivity, or a heightened perception of pain in one's inner organs, can occur when intrinsic endorphins prolong action potential duration, increase calcium influx, and prompt neurotransmitter release. They hypothesized that visceral hypersensitivity would be mitigated by LDN. They enrolled 42 patients in an open-label study. Patients were given 0.5 mg naltrexone daily for one month and were evaluated at baseline, during treatment, and at a follow-up after four weeks. Symptoms evaluated included abdominal pain, urgency, and consistency and frequency of bowel movements. The study determined that overall symptom relief occurred in 76 percent of these patients. The number of pain-free days increased from 0.5 to 1.25, and this was statistically significant.

The study is problematic, however, in that it had a small sample size, it was too brief in duration, and it had an open-label design. There is also known to be a significantly higher rate of placebo effects in IBS patients (circa 30 to 35 percent). In the 42 patients treated, there were 18 adverse events, including stomatitis, various infections, headaches, allergic dermatitis, and migraines. As per the investigators, these side effects were not severe, and the drug was well tolerated overall. The number of pain-free days in response to LDN ranged from 70 to 86 percent. The patients with IBS-C had the best response. This study design was unique in that the IBS subjects could have a diarrhea-predominant type, constipation-predominant type, or mixed type. Generally, drug studies will look at only one subtype at a time with a particular drug therapy.

Dr. Weinstock's experience in treating IBS with LDN concerns two groups: (1) SIBO-positive patients who may or may not have fatigue or extra-intestinal disorders and (2) SIBO-negative patients who have failed FDA-approved medications. His first report on the subject examined IBS patients with SIBO who used naltrexone as a second agent.[45]

Subsequently, Dr. Weinstock performed another chart review of LDN therapy for IBS in other patients, some with and some without SIBO. The patients were asked to rate their clinical response to LDN by saying whether they were markedly improved, moderately improved, mildly improved, unchanged, or worse. Of the 68 SIBO-positive patients who took antibiotics followed by LDN, 15 patients (17.6 percent) were markedly improved, 32 (37.6 percent) were moderately improved, and 11 (12.9 percent) were mildly improved. Of the 13 SIBO-negative patients, 2 (15.3 percent) were markedly improved, 5 (38.5 percent) were moderately improved, 2 (15.3 percent) were unchanged, and 3 (23.1 percent) were markedly worse.

A more recent, unpublished review of Dr. Weinstock's IBS patients who received LDN contains the following observations. Of the 33 IBS-constipation patients who received antibiotics, 19 were markedly improved, 7 mildly improved, and 7 unchanged. LDN was then used by these patients for an average of 10 months. Follow-up data was available for 30 patients. Eighteen patients (47 percent) had a combined marked and moderately improved response, 6 (15.7 percent) were mildly improved, and 11 (28.9 percent) had no response. Five patients had adverse reactions that led to early termination of LDN therapy.

Of 22 IBS-diarrhea patients, 20 received antibiotics. Thirteen (65 percent) of these patients had combined marked and moderate improvement, one (5 percent) had mild improvement, and six (30 percent) saw no benefit. After administering LDN to all 22 patients, there was combined marked and moderate improvement in 12 patients (55 percent), mild benefit in 1 (5 percent), and no benefit in 6 patients (27 percent). Three (13 percent) patients dropped out owing to side effects.

There are no FDA-approved therapies for IBS with mixed stools (IBS-M). Of 24 IBS-M patients treated with antibiotics, 16 (66 percent) had a marked response to antibiotics, 4 (17 percent) had a mild response, and 4 (17 percent) had no response. Eighteen patients received LDN after antibiotic therapy. The clinical responses were as follows: 7 (39 percent) experienced combined marked and moderate improvement, 4 (22.2 percent) had mild improvement, and 5 saw no benefit. Two patients had to discontinue LDN due to side effects.

LDN offers a new approach to therapy for IBS. This is important since the FDA-approved IBS medications generally have less than 40 to 50 percent efficacy, whereas the placebo rate is 30 to 35 percent. Finally, the roles of inflammation and increased intestinal permeability in IBS are gaining more acceptance among physicians, and this suggests a role for LDN in IBS therapy.

Mast Cell Activation Syndrome

Mast cell activation syndrome is a common disorder involving uncontrolled mast cell (MC) activation with multisystemic inflammatory and allergic symptoms.[46] A study of a German control group estimated the prevalence of MCAS in this population to be 17 percent.[47] Of the patients in the study, 74 percent reported similar symptoms in one or more first-degree relatives. The indirect prevalence estimate for MCAS in Americans is 1 percent.[48] Although MCAS is technically an immune disorder with a mutation in the MC control gene, the GI tract is a common site of MC deposition, and activation of these cells produces symptoms both in the gut and systemically. The most common symptoms reported by 50 percent or more of the 413 patients were fatigue, myalgia, conjunctivitis, rhinitis, tinnitus, hives, itching, nausea, heartburn, dyspnea, near syncope, headache, chills, and edema.[49] Virtually all organ systems can be involved in MCAS.[50]

GI symptoms are commonly reported by MCAS patients and often mistaken by physicians for symptoms of functional syndromes, especially in the cases where the term *IBS* is assigned to the patient.[51] In IBS patients, local and systemic effects of mediators released by MCs can account for constipation, diarrhea, and pain.[52] In a study of IBS patients' colon tissue, histamine and tryptase levels were shown to correlate with pain, as was proximity of the MCs to the submucosal nerves.[53] Interestingly, constipation has been linked to the local release of MC mediators near glial cells and filaments.[54] Thus, MC-induced neuropathy may explain reduced peristalsis of the large intestine. GI symptoms can include tingling or burning, aphthous ulcers, globus, heartburn, dysphagia, chest pain, nausea, altered bowels, bloating, and abdominal pain.[55] Dyspepsia may be due to mediator-induced nociception.[56] Gastritis, in the absence of *Helicobacter pylori* and/ or non-steroidal anti-inflammatory medications, could be explained by MC-mediator-induced inflammation.[57] Chronic and acute peritoneal pain has been reported in the setting of epiploic appendagitis, where local increased MC deposition was identified.[58] Studies that demonstrate success with MC-directed therapy in some patients who were labeled with an IBS diagnosis are suggestive of a pathophysiological role of the aberrant MC.[59] SIBO was recently shown to be common in MCAS.[60] Bacterial overgrowth, as determined by an abnormal breath test, was present in 30.9 percent of 139 MCAS subjects versus 10.0 percent of 30 controls.

MCAS is often associated with hypermobile Ehlers-Danlos syndrome (hEDS) and postural orthostatic tachycardia syndrome (POTS), both of which also have extensive GI system involvement.[61] MCAS, both alone and in association with these other disorders, results in significant GI morbidity.[62] MCAS patients pose considerable management challenges due to their pathophysiologic heterogeneity, numerous systemic symptoms and triggers, comorbid conditions, and varied response to therapy. Triggers for MC activation include stress, food, alcohol, excipients in medications, infections, altered microbiome, environmental stimuli (including heat, chemicals, atmospheric changes, electrical changes, and odors), and mold exposure.[63]

The first publication to demonstrate the efficacy of LDN in MCAS looked at a patient who also had POTS and SIBO. In addition to receiving antibiotic therapy for SIBO, the patient received LDN and immunotherapy with intravenous immunoglobulin (IVIg). A dramatic and sustained response in more than 40 severe symptoms of POTS, MCAS, and SIBO was documented. The utility of IVIg in autoimmune neuromuscular diseases has been established, but clinical experience with POTS is relatively unreported, and data on IVIg in POTS and MCAS had not been previously reported. In this case study the patient found significant benefit from IVIg and rifaximin, but it was not until she escalated the dose of LDN from 2 mg to 4.5 mg that she attained complete improvement. Other early experience in our clinic was also discussed in this publication. We looked at 27 patients with POTS, 11 of whom were administered LDN. Seven of the 11 experienced improvement in GI symptoms, and 5 experienced improvements in MCAS and POTS. Out of 15 patients who were administered antibiotics for SIBO, this therapy helped GI symptoms in 10 and POTS symptoms in 4. We did not use an improvement scale.[64] This has been observed in additional POTS patients in our clinic as well.

Owing to the numerous MC mediators and receptors, no single medication currently available will control all symptoms of MCAS. It is a common approach to offer first-line therapy with efforts to identify and avoid triggers and then to prescribe antihistamines, vitamin C, vitamin D, and montelukast. A number of MCAS physicians have seen that LDN helped some of their patients. In a review of a cohort of my own MCAS patients, I found clinical evidence of LDN's efficacy in treating the condition. Out

SYMPTOMS RELIEVED IN MCAS PATIENTS TAKING LDN

- Depression
- Brain fog
- Anxiety
- Nausea
- Insomnia
- Hives
- Rash
- Itch
- Allergies
- Dyspnea
- Edema
- Erythromelalgia
- Fatigue
- Headache
- Dizziness
- Abdominal pain
- Diarrhea
- Constipation
- Bloating
- Pain (joint, nerve, and muscle)

of the 116 MCAS patients who were given daily 4.5 mg LDN, 60 percent reported improvements, 28 percent saw no benefit, and 22 percent had to stop LDN owing to side effects.

Although worthy, it would be difficult to have this data accepted for publication given that the patients involved simultaneously altered their diets and used several medications. Patients in this series could tell that the LDN treatment was effective due to the clinical response they noted as they increased their doses to 4.5 mg. Others noticed the therapeutic impact when they ran out of LDN, or after they had stopped and then restarted the medication.

Sarcoidosis

Sarcoidosis is an idiopathic granulomatous disease that most often involves the lungs and is characterized by the accumulation of T lymphocytes and macrophages.[65] This ultimately results in poor pulmonary function and a need for systemic therapy.[66] The disease is rarely localized to the luminal gut, such as the stomach, but the liver and spleen are frequently involved in cases of systemic sarcoidosis.[67] Prednisone is often administered for many months, carrying a risk for multiple side effects. Infliximab increases the risk of infection, while immunomodulators such as steroid-sparing agents not only carry risks for infections and malignancies but also have a delayed onset of action. In light of these issues, alternative therapeutic options are desirable.

A patient presented to our clinic with severe fatigue, sarcoid rash, and marked radiographic evidence of splenic and liver involvement. We drew comparisons between sarcoidosis and Crohn's disease in that each disease is characterized by unregulated lymphocytic activity—a common pathological feature of non-caseating granulomas—and each is commonly treated with steroids and immunomodulators. Accordingly, we administered LDN to this patient, who subsequently experienced the complete resolution of her symptoms and radiographic abnormalities.[68] Thus far we have used LDN in three other patients, whose pulmonary diseases subsequently improved.

Mesenteric Panniculitis

The mesentery is the tissue within the peritoneal cavity that supports and attaches the small and large intestines to the posterior walls of the abdomen, spleen, and liver. Blood vessels and lymphatic vessels can also course through the mesentery. Mesenteric panniculitis (MP) is a nonspecific inflammatory process affecting the fatty tissue at the root of the mesentery.[69] A more advanced form of this disorder is known as sclerosing mesenteritis, which is a thickening of the mesentery in the abdominal cavity with degeneration, inflammation, and scarring of both the adipose tissue and the surrounding mesenteric vasculature.[70] *Retractile mesenteritis* is a term reserved for advanced sclerosing mesenteritis when there is fibrosis and CT imaging displaying a "pulling in" or tethering phenomenon. Nonspecific panniculitis is commonly seen by radiologists in CT scans being taken for chronic pain, and may or may not have clinical significance. Patients with panniculitis can present with abdominal pain, nausea, and weight loss. When sclerosing mesenteritis progresses to include mesenteric calcification and fibrosis, the risk for tethering the small bowel and causing small bowel obstruction is significant. Significant radiographic sclerosing mesenteritis is much less frequently encountered than nonspecific panniculitis. This is a diagnosis of exclusion; thus, the clinician must first rule out carcinoids, metastases, desmoid tumors, lymphoma, chronic infection, and autoimmune disease.[71]

The largest study to date regarding mesenteric diseases reviewed CT scans and follow-up clinical data on those with mesenteric panniculitis.[72] The investigators reviewed nearly 150,000 CT scans as part of a malignancy staging evaluation, which may have biased the findings since they did not include patients with idiopathic abdominal pain. Mesenteric panniculitis was seen in 359 patients: 22.6 percent had a known history of cancer, and 5.3 percent had a new diagnosis of cancer. Lymphomas were the most common cancers associated with mesenteric panniculitis on CT—this association occurred 36 percent of the time. Other cancers associated with the condition included prostate and renal cancer. CT follow-up was available for 56 of the 359 patients. The mesentery was unchanged in 80 percent of the patients, worse in 11 percent, and improved in 9 percent. A new diagnosis of cancer is uncommon in patients with CT findings suggestive of panniculitis, yet the radiographic changes often remain stable in patients with associated malignancies.

In contrast, another study of 3,820 patients with abdominal pain found 94 patients (2.5 percent) with mesenteric panniculitis. In 48.9 percent of those 94 patients, mesenteric panniculitis coexisted with malignancy (most often prostatic carcinoma).[73] For each subject with MP, two control subjects were selected from the total study population database who did not have MP on their first CT scan. These control patients were matched for age and sex. Coexistent cancer was slightly higher in the patients with MP than in the control patients (n = 188, 46.3 percent). Of the 94 patients with MP, the MP was presumed to be idiopathic. Of these patients, 14.6 percent developed malignancies in the next five years, as compared with 6.9 percent of the controls. The frequency of idiopathic panniculitis or mesenteritis in the presence of chronic abdominal pain is unknown.

The usual treatments for idiopathic panniculitis and mesenteritis include prednisone, colchicine, and immunosuppressants.[74] One case report of retractile mesenteritis was treated successfully with progesterone.[75] Surgery is accompanied by high risks. The largest study to date on sclerosing mesenteritis was by Sharma et al., and reviewed 192 cases.[76] In this study complications included bowel obstruction / ileus / ischemia (n = 10, 23.8 percent) and obstructive uropathy / renal failure (n = 10, 23.8 percent). Twelve (6.3 percent) of the patients died secondary to sclerosing mesenteritis–related complications.

In an open-label study Roginsky et al. reported that two of three mesenteric panniculitis patients treated with 4.5 mg naltrexone per day for 12 weeks had a long-term symptomatic response.[77] These patients had an inflammatory mass, and biopsies showed inflammation, fibrosis, fat necrosis, and calcifications. All three patients had clinical improvement at four weeks, but only two continued to show benefits at eight weeks. The improvement was tracked using a clinical scoring method called the mesenteric panniculitis subjective score. During the study, the mean score decreased from 53 to 21 at week 8.

In a personal communication with Dr. Weinstock in 2020, Dr. David Kaufman noted that one of his MCAS patients with sclerosing mesenteritis experienced symptomatic relief with a combination of mast cell directed therapy and LDN. Dr. Weinstock currently has an abdominal pain patient with pan-systemic symptoms who was found to have mesenteric panniculitis. His workup included high tryptase levels. Treatment with LDN and antihistamines has reduced many of his symptoms, including abdominal pain.

Further studies using LDN and testing for MCAS are indicated. LDN could theoretically reduce MC mediator release (in the mesentery or from a distant site) that cause inflammation and fibrosis.

Gastrointestinal Malignancies

In the first volume of *The LDN Book*, Drs. Angus G. Dalgleish and Wai M. Liu discuss the limited published information that was available at the time for the use of LDN in cancer.[78] On the website www.lowdosenaltrexone.org, there is a review of Dr. Bernard Bihari's experience treating 450 cancer patients with LDN. Unfortunately, his experiences were not placebo-controlled trials using LDN as a sole therapy or as part of a combination therapy, and therefore weren't published in peer-reviewed medical journals. Dr. Bihari's formal publications regarding naltrexone involved alcoholism and AIDS.

However, Dr. Dalgleish and Dr. Liu describe well the information that has been published about the basic science that supports the use of LDN in cancer.[79] The basic mechanism of action involves temporary blockade of the opioid receptors, resulting in rebound production of OGF (also known as met-enkephalin, methionine enkephalin, MENK), which regulates cell growth.[80] Naltrexone-induced OGF production has been demonstrated to reduce the activity of in vitro colon cancer cells.[81] Methionine enkephalin also boosts immunity in immunocompromised patients by inhibiting regulatory T cells.[82] This is another way in which LDN can potentially benefit cancer patients. In other in vitro GI cancer studies, primary hepatocellular cancer cells were evaluated in response to exogenous OGF.[83] This was observed to have a dose-dependent receptor-mediated inhibitory action on cell proliferation. The mechanism of the OGF and OGF receptor interaction on the cell number was related to inhibition of DNA synthesis and not to apoptotic or necrotic pathways. A recent study examined MENK-treated gastric cancer cells and the anti-tumor effect of this endorphin on gastric cancer in animals.[84] MENK inhibited the growth of human gastric cancer cells by arresting the cell cycle and inducing cell death. The ability of LDN to increase MENK represents a potentially important mechanism of action in suppressing cancer.

Concerning GI malignancies in humans, clinical studies that support the efficacy of LDN include one of pancreatic cancer patients who responded to LDN in combination with intravenous alpha-lipoic acid (ALA).[85] One of the patients survived more than four years after being told that he had terminal cancer. In a follow-up to this case report, the authors described three more case studies where patients were treated in the same manner. The original patient was alive two and a half years later, and three others were doing well, including one who presented with metastatic disease to the liver and was alive three years after initial diagnosis.[86] The roles of ALA include reduction of oxidative stress, stabilization of NF-kB, and stimulation of cell death activity.

The direct administration of met-enkephalin lends further evidence to support the benefit of LDN in pancreatic cancer. Investigators at Pennsylvania State University conducted a prospective, open-label trial in 24 patients who failed standard chemotherapy for advanced pancreatic cancer.[87] Patients were treated weekly with 250 µg/kg OGF by intravenous infusion. There was a control group of 166 patients of similar age who failed chemotherapy and were discharged to hospice care. The OGF-treated patients had a threefold increase in median survival time compared with the control group. Tumor size was stabilized or reduced in 62 percent of the patients who received OGF.

In a prospective study by Schwartz et al., LDN was used in combination with ALA and hydroxycitrate in 10 terminal cancer patients, 4 of whom had gastrointestinal cancers (colon, esophageal, and cholangiocarcinoma).[88] Of the 10 patients, 2 died within two months as predicted, 2 needed conventional chemotherapy, and 6 experienced stabilization or slower progression of their cancer. One patient who presented with liver metastases failed to respond to chemotherapy. After the addition of LDN, the patient's liver lesions stabilized for nine months. After that the lesions progressed. A colon cancer patient had liver metastases that progressed with chemotherapy and subsequently failed two months of LDN Rx. A patient with metastatic esophageal cancer relapsed after chemotherapy. Use of LDN Rx as a monotherapy initially failed, but the addition of a new chemotherapy led to tumor shrinkage. Finally, a cholangiocarcinoma patient had advancement of the cancer despite aggressive chemotherapy. LDN Rx was added and a CT scan showed no further progression over the next three months.

In an Israeli study two children with hepatoblastoma had incomplete surgical resection and were treated with OGF/LDN instead of chemotherapy, which was contraindicated or not tolerated.[89] Each child was free of disease and had no symptoms 10 and 5 years later, respectively, at the time of the case report.

As a gastroenterologist, Dr. Weinstock's own experience with cancer and LDN is limited in scope as he does not play a primary role once his patients are referred to an oncologist. He has personally prescribed LDN to four cancer patients. One colon cancer patient required resection of a liver metastasis followed by chemotherapy, while another had postoperative chemotherapy because of a positive lymph node. Thus far (two years out from surgery), both are in remission. A patient with long-standing Crohn's disease, whose lymphoma was thought to be due to prior exposure to azathioprine, has achieved complete control over her Crohn's disease owing to LDN as a monotherapy; she has been in deep remission for the last 10 years (she had chemotherapy for 1 year). Finally, a woman with Waldenstrom's lymphoma is taking LDN preventatively after routine chemotherapy and has been in complete remission doing well for the last four years. This malignancy has a high relapse rate—it returns in 90 percent of patients. Further research is required in this area, though it is encouraging that scientists and clinicians are increasingly evaluating LDN's applications for cancer treatment.[90]

Conclusion

LDN has the potential to restore gut health in several GI disorders and diseases. High-quality research using randomized, double-blind, placebo-controlled studies is the ideal. However, until funding is available for such trials, continued clinical use and reports of case series will benefit many patients.

– FOUR –

Dermatologic Conditions

APPLE BODEMER, MD

All chronic skin conditions are associated with inflammation and/or immune system dysfunction at some level. The specific patterns of inflammation and immune dysregulation differ among disorders related to skin, hair, and nails, but many share similar pathways. Low dose naltrexone (LDN) has been shown to influence both inflammation and immune dysregulation at multiple levels. This, along with the very low side effect profile, makes it an ideal option for patients with a variety of skin diseases. It has been suggested that LDN could be helpful for a number of dermatologic conditions, including alopecia areata and variants, atopic dermatitis, autoimmune-related skin disorders (sclerosis/morphea, lupus, dermatomyositis, et cetera), pemphigus, pemphigoid, psoriasis, lichen planus, lichen sclerosis, pruritus, prurigo nodules, Hailey-Hailey, autoimmune scarring hair loss, vitiligo and pyoderma gangrenosum, among others. At this point there are very few reports in the literature demonstrating the effectiveness of LDN for dermatology patients. Those that do exist consist of case studies, case series, and reviews. This chapter will cover the conditions for which there is evidence regarding the benefits of LDN, including itch, Hailey-Hailey, lichen planopilaris, and psoriasis. It will review what is known about opioid receptors related to the skin and how the known mechanisms by which LDN works could improve skin disorders.

While we generally think of opioid receptors being primarily in the central and peripheral nervous system, they also have important roles within the immune system, the skin, and various other organs. The three predominant types of opioid receptors—mu, delta, and kappa—are transmembrane receptors that are linked to a variety of regulatory enzymes, including adenylyl cyclase—a ubiquitous cellular regulatory enzyme—and to calcium channels, which are essential for maintaining a calcium gradient within all cells that controls a wide variety of cellular processes.[1] Mu, delta, and kappa opioid receptors can be found in varying concentrations on epidermal keratinocytes, epidermal melanocytes, fibroblasts, and peripheral nerve fibers.[2] Within the skin opioid receptors are more concentrated in the basal layer and just above the basal layer, but can be found throughout the epidermis.[3] Interestingly, there are several skin conditions in which we find altered expression of epidermal mu receptors. These include psoriasis, basal cell cancer, and chronic wounds.[4] This supports data suggesting that opioid receptors and opioids play an important role in epidermal cell proliferation and differentiation.[5]

Opioid receptors are present on the surface of keratinocytes and help regulate intercellular adhesion and keratinocyte migration.[6] They have also been shown to be involved in maintaining proteins—including involucrin, loricrin, and filaggrin—that are crucial to the integrity of the stratum corneum.[7]

Other important roles that opioids and opioid receptors play in the skin include regulation of pain and itch—especially in chronic dermatoses—melanin production, and sebum production. The mu receptor, in particular, also appears to be involved in melanocyte proliferation.[8] Additionally, opioids and their receptors regulate functions of a variety of types of cells involved in the immune response, including dendritic cells, macrophages, mast cells, lymphocytes, and polymorphonuclear leukocytes (neutrophils, eosinophils, and basophils).[9]

One of the particularly interesting things about naltrexone is that it can interact with other receptors as well. The toll-like receptor (TLR) family is a group of proteins found in both plants and animals that plays an important role in immunity. These receptors help the body identify pathogenic microbes, initiate an appropriate immune response, and distinguish the "bad" from the "good" when it comes to bacteria, yeast, fungi, and viruses.[10] The immune system is tightly involved in inflammation, so it follows that by interacting with these important immune system receptors, receptor ligands can impact inflammatory pathways. Naltrexone has been shown to decrease tumor necrosis factor alpha (TNF-a), as well as other inflammatory compounds, including interleukin (IL) 6, nitric oxide, and nuclear factor kappa B (NF-kB) via interacting with TLR-4.[11] It is likely that naltrexone interacts with other TLRs as well. Given what we know about the mechanisms of action of naltrexone and LDN, it is clear that there are several points at which it can impact inflammation and immune system function, making it potentially incredibly useful in the treatment and management of skin diseases.

Itch

The sensation of the itch is common in many chronic inflammatory skin conditions. Additionally, there are a number of systemic causes for itch, including thyroid abnormalities, liver disease, kidney disease, cancer, hematologic abnormalities, and disorders of the nervous system. Basic lifestyle adjustments can go a long way toward alleviating itch, and should be assessed and addressed early. Maintaining good skin hydration through appropriate bathing and moisturizing, minimization of exposure to irritants, and appropriate stress management is crucial to alleviating the sensation of itch regardless of the cause. When the itch is localized, topical treatments are often adequate. Once appropriate skin hydration has been addressed, topical steroids are the main first-line treatment when skin inflammation is present. With prolonged use, topical steroids can cause skin atrophy—a superficial fine wrinkling of the skin. If this is noted early and the steroid is stopped, the epidermis typically will regenerate itself and recover. Continued use, however, can lead to permanent skin thinning and fragility.[12] The topical calcineurin inhibitors—tacrolimus and pimecrolimus —topical antihistamines, and topical anesthetics can also be helpful in the management of itch without the potential side effect of atrophy.

Topical capsaicin is an extract from chili peppers that has also been shown to be effective for relieving the itch. When used regularly, it depletes nerve endings of substance P—a neuropeptide known to convey the itch sensation. Because capsaicin initially promotes the release of neuronal substance P, patients may experience increased intensity of itch and burning that can last up to 30 minutes after applying it. This is typically self-limited and will resolve after a few weeks of regular use.[13]

Phototherapy is commonly used for inflammatory skin conditions such as atopic dermatitis and psoriasis, but it can be effective for alleviating itch even in the absence of inflammation.[14] The mechanisms by which photo-therapy alleviates itch are not completely clear, but it is thought to influence the endogenous opioid system, alter epidermal cytokines, and regulate the activity of cutaneous mast cells and nerves.[15]

Widespread, severe itching may require systemic medications. Oral anti-histamines are often used, but except in the setting of urticaria and mast cell disorders, their benefit is unclear. Sedating antihistamines, however, can be very helpful when the itch is most prominent at night and/or inter-feres with sleep.[16] Antidepressants such as mirtazapine, doxepin, and the selective serotonin reuptake inhibitors (SSRIs: paroxetine, fluvoxamine, and sertraline) can be useful for managing itch as well. This effect is likely due to alteration of serotonin and histamine levels.[17] The anticonvulsants gabapentin and pregabalin are often used for generalized itch and are especially helpful for itch related to neuropathic conditions.[18] Thalidomide has immunomodulatory and neuromodulatory properties as well as anti-inflammatory effects, making it an option for people with chronic refrac-tory itching. This is a medication with significant potential side effects and should only be used when other options have been exhausted.[19]

Naltrexone and Itch

Mu-opioid receptors have been found to be decreased in people with chronic skin conditions associated with itch, including atopic dermatitis, prurigo nodularis, and lichen simplex chronicus, suggesting a potential benefit for naltrexone in treating these conditions.[20] Oral naltrexone at doses of 50 mg a day or more has traditionally been used to treat a variety of different types of itch.[21] One literature review found evidence for the varied effectiveness of naltrexone at this higher dose in the management of itch associated with atopic dermatitis, psoriasis, lichen simplex chron-icus, prurigo nodularis, mycosis fungoides, cutaneous B-cell lymphoma, uremic pruritus, cholestatic pruritus, aquagenic pruritus, and pruritus of unknown origin.[22] The benefit of this higher dose protocol is that insur-ance typically will cover these doses, but doesn't cover the compounding of low dose capsules. When cost is an issue, it is reasonable to try naltrex-one at 50 mg to 100 mg a day. At these doses, liver function tests should be monitored.

Topical Naltrexone and Itch

Topical 1 percent naltrexone has been shown to be effective in patients with atopic dermatitis and severe itch. A placebo-controlled crossover study that included 40 patients found that 70 percent of those treated with topical naltrexone experienced significant reduction in itch, while 40 percent of the placebo group had a reduction in itch. The high rate of response in the placebo group demonstrates the significant impact skin hydration has on itch. This study involved skin biopsies of 11 of the 40 patients before and after the application of topical naltrexone. Increased staining of mu-opioid receptors was seen in the skin after the application of topical naltrexone. There were not enough samples to make any specific conclusions, but it appeared that the intensity of mu-opioid receptor staining correlated with decreased sensation of itch.[23]

Low Dose Naltrexone and Itch

LDN can be very useful for the management of itch. Additionally, when thyroid abnormalities are responsible for the itch, LDN can be used to treat the underlying thyroid disorder (see chapter 5 in the first volume of *The LDN Book*).[24] There are two published case series that look at the effectiveness of LDN for itch related to specific skin conditions. One case series includes three patients with systemic sclerosis and disease-related itch. All three were started at 2 mg naltrexone before bed for one month. The dose was then increased by 1 mg each week, up to a maximum of 4.5 mg (the dose escalation for the last week was 0.5 mg). One of the three patients maintained a dose of 2 mg while the other two achieved the target dose of 4.5 mg a day. All three patients had a significant decrease in itch, increased perception of suppleness of the skin, and improved quality of life.[25] Another series describes two patients with dermatomyositis-related itch who were treated with 5 mg naltrexone a day. Both experienced complete resolution of their symptoms—one within six weeks.[26] Additionally, LDN has been demonstrated to improve itch related to lichen planopilaris and psoriasis, as well as other symptoms of these conditions (see subsequent sections "Low-Dose Naltrexone and Lichen Planopilaris" and "Low-Dose Naltrexone and Psoriasis" for details and references).

In my personal clinical experience, I have seen clear benefits from using topical 1 percent naltrexone for localized neuropathic itch, including that related to prurigo nodularis and notalgia paresthetica. My experience with LDN for generalized itch of uncertain etiology has been mixed. I typically start at 50 mg a day, and if I don't see a benefit at four months, I convert to a low dose protocol. I definitely see an improvement in symptoms of itch when I use LDN to treat specific inflammatory skin conditions—in particular, psoriasis, lichen planopilaris, and atopic dermatitis.

Hailey-Hailey Disease

Hailey-Hailey disease—also known as familial benign pemphigus—is a rare blistering disorder in which epidermal keratinocytes are not able to maintain intercellular connections due to altered calcium levels. Hailey-Hailey is known to be due to a variety of mutations in the ATP2C1 gene. This gene encodes a protein that is responsible for maintaining appropriate intracellular calcium levels, which is essential for regulating cell growth and migration and intercellular adhesion. While Hailey-Hailey is an autosomal dominant disorder, novel mutations commonly occur.

Hailey-Hailey typically becomes clinically significant around or after puberty, but there are rare reports of the disease in prepubertal children.[27] Individuals affected with this condition experience flaccid blisters that lead to painful erosions and maceration, most commonly in the axillae, groin, inframammary areas, and lateral neck. Bacterial, fungal, and yeast infections of affected areas are common and tend to aggravate the condition. Other factors that exacerbate Hailey-Hailey include friction, heat, sweat, and UV radiation.[28]

Because Hailey-Hailey is so rare, literature focusing on treatment is limited. Patients and providers should emphasize minimizing exacerbating factors, managing inflammation, and preventing and appropriately treating secondary infections. Losing excess weight, wearing loose clothing, avoiding excessive heat, and avoiding sunburn can go a long way toward preventing flares. Diluted bleach baths (½ cup / 120 ml 6 percent sodium hypochlorite) or rinses (1 teaspoon bleach to 1 gallon / 4 liters of water) and antibacterial cleansers (4 percent chlorhexidine) are important for decreasing microbial colonization in the affected areas to prevent secondary infection. Topical steroids and topical calcineurin inhibitors can help manage inflammation, but need to be used carefully to avoid increasing microbial colonization. Topical antibiotics and antifungals are often necessary as well. Oral antibiotics and/or antifungals may be necessary once an infection has occurred.

Systemic medications that have been used with variable success include cyclosporine, methotrexate, acitretin, and oral tacrolimus. Interestingly, one case series describes three people with Hailey-Hailey who experienced rapid improvement over four weeks after starting oral treatment with 300 mg magnesium chloride daily. It is thought that this might help regulate the keratinocyte intracellular calcium levels, thus improving intercellular adhesion.[29]

Procedural options for managing perspiration include localized botulinum toxin, surgical excision of affected intertriginous areas, CO_2 laser ablation of affected areas, and electron beam radiation for ablation of sweat glands. These procedures are painful and can lead to permanent scarring.[30]

Low Dose Naltrexone and Hailey-Hailey Disease

Patients with Hailey-Hailey have been successfully treated with low dose naltrexone. The effectiveness of LDN for this condition is thought to be due to its anti-inflammatory activity, as well as its ability to stabilize intracellular calcium via TLR pathways.[31]

There are four case series of patients with Hailey-Hailey disease who were treated with LDN. The first case series includes three people with recalcitrant Hailey-Hailey. All medications were stopped, and the patients were given between 1.5 and 3 mg naltrexone a day. After three to four months of treatment, each patient achieved between 80 and 90 percent clinical and symptomatic improvement with no significant adverse effects.[32] The second case series includes three patients with long-standing Hailey-Hailey who were given between 3 mg and 4.5 mg naltrexone a day. All three experienced significant clearance of skin findings within two months of treatment. Treatment was then stopped, and all the patients relapsed. LDN was restarted, and the patients again cleared.[33] The third case series includes three patients with long-standing disease. Interestingly, in this series, only one patient was treated with the low dose protocol. This patient was given 4.5 mg a day and experienced clearance at 18 months. The second patient had complete resolution at two months with 12.5 mg per day (the higher dose was due to insurance coverage). After she cleared, she stopped naltrexone and experienced a flare of her disease. She restarted naltrexone at 4.5 mg a day, which again resulted in improvement. The third patient was treated with 50 mg a day due to concomitant brachioradial pruritus, and had no response.[34]

The largest case series includes 14 patients with Hailey-Hailey who were treated with naltrexone between November 2017 and November 2018. Their starting doses ranged from 1.5 mg to 6 mg. Five patients were maintained in the low dose range, and the other nine were escalated to between 25 mg and 50 mg a day. Only 2 of the 14 patients had sustained improvement. Interestingly, these patients were maintained at 3 mg and 4.5 mg a day. Six patients had initial improvement but then relapsed. Of these, only one was maintained in the optimal dose range at 3 mg a day with no dose escalations. The other five had their doses increase to between 6 mg and 12 mg a day. Of the six patients who had no improvement, two were started at 6 mg a day from the beginning, and the daily dose was increased to 50 mg in one case and 12 mg in the other. One of the non-responders was started at 1.5 mg and stayed at this dose, which is on the low end of effective doses for inflammatory and autoimmune conditions. The remaining three non-responders were started at 3 mg a day. One was maintained at that dose, one was increased to 12 mg a day, and the other was increased to 50 mg a day. Four people experienced side effects of nausea and dizziness, and two discontinued naltrexone because of these side effects. The follow-up time in this series varied between 15 and 54 weeks.[35] It isn't clear from the paper how long each patient was on the medication, how dose adjustments were determined, and how long each specific dose was maintained before it was escalated. While it is difficult to draw firm conclusions from this paper, it does support the hypothesis that higher doses of naltrexone are not as effective as the low dose regimens for this condition.

In addition to these four case series, there are a few case reports supporting the use of LDN in Hailey-Hailey. One report describes a woman with a 20-year history of recalcitrant Hailey-Hailey who achieved clinical clearance after taking 1.5 mg naltrexone daily for just 26 days.[36] Another demonstrated the effectiveness of LDN combined with oral magnesium,[37] and the last described a patient who cleared with LDN and then maintained clearance with a topical combination of ketamine and diphenhydramine.[38]

While I do not have clinical experience treating Hailey-Hailey disease with LDN, given the significant morbidity of this condition, the lack of consistently effective and safe treatment, the encouraging support for benefit, and the safety profile of LDN, there is enough evidence to support early treatment with LDN in doses of 1.5 mg to 4.5 mg a day in patients with Hailey-Hailey disease.

Lichen Planopilaris (LPP)

Lichen planopilaris (LPP) is a scarring hair loss condition most commonly seen in postmenopausal women.[39] In this condition, follicular inflammation leads to permanent scarring of the affected hair follicles. Clinically, perifollicular papules and erythema are present in the inflammatory stage. This is typically associated with symptoms of burning, itching, or tingling. As the disease progresses, the hair follicles become scarred, and hair is permanently lost. At this point symptoms typically resolve, and the affected areas become smooth and depressed due to the development of scar tissue. Lichen planopilaris shows up in a couple of typical patterns. The classic presentation consists of irregularly shaped areas of involvement, primarily on the crown, but can extend to involve other areas of the scalp as well. In late stages the scarred areas can coalesce into a network of interesting patterns of hair loss on the scalp. In frontal fibrosing alopecia (FFA), the affected hair follicles form a band along the frontal hairline. In late stages this type can result in the loss of up to a couple of inches of the frontal hairline. Eyebrow involvement is common, with eyelash involvement possible but relatively uncommon. The final presentation is called Graham-Little-Piccardi-Lasseur syndrome. This consists of patchy scarring hair loss on the scalp, nonscarring hair loss in the axillae and groin, and follicular lichen planus on the body and/or scalp. Follicular lichen planus consists of hyperkeratotic follicular-based papules, often with purple to brownish hyperpigmentation. Regardless of the clinical type, the course of LPP is very unpredictable. While LPP doesn't result in complete baldness, the hair loss may be dramatic and can cause significant social and emotional distress.[40]

The pathogenesis of LPP is not well understood. It does appear to be an autoimmune-related inflammatory disease that specifically targets the area of the hair follicle where follicular stem cells are found. Hormones appear to play a role, though how they impact this condition is unclear. LPP occurs most commonly in postmenopausal women, and treatment with anti-androgen medications can be helpful in some cases.[41] People with LPP have a significantly higher risk of developing thyroid disease, with hypothyroidism being the most commonly associated thyroid condition.[42] It is important to screen people with LPP for thyroid disease and manage appropriately. Unfortunately, the normalization of thyroid function does not impact the course of this disease.

Treatment of LPP can be quite challenging. LPP has a tendency to burn out on its own over several months or years. However, the course of the disease often fluctuates, and the final outcome is unpredictable. Additionally, patients need to understand that once follicular scarring has occurred, there is nothing that can enable hair to regrow in the affected area. The goals for treatment should focus on managing symptoms and slowing or stopping the inflammatory process in order to minimize the progression of permanent scarring.

Initial treatment of LPP often includes steroids, either applied topically, injected into the affected areas, or both. A high potency steroid is typically applied twice a day (BID) for up to four months. Based on limited data, this appears to help 50 to 60 percent of people.[43] Intralesional steroids can also be helpful. Triamcinolone acetonide is injected intradermally to the affected area(s) every four to six weeks at concentrations of either 5 mg/ml or 10 mg/ml. Dermal atrophy is the main risk associated with steroid use, and a good reason to stick to lower concentrations, especially along the frontal hairline.[44]

When these measures are not helpful within three to four months, oral medications are often considered. Oral steroids can be used to control a rapidly progressing disease. Case reports have shown mixed results, and the benefits and risks need to be carefully weighed with the patient when considering this option.[45] Hydroxychloroquine at a dose of 200 mg twice a day is commonly used in the setting of LPP due to its immunomodulating activity. It appears that somewhere around 15 to 25 percent of people have a good response within four months.[46] Other systemic medications that have been used with limited success include cyclosporine, mycophenolate, methotrexate, retinoids, rituximab, pioglitazone, and anti-androgens, including finasteride, dutasteride, and minoxidil.

Low Dose Naltrexone and Lichen Planopilaris

There is one case series that looks at LDN and LPP, and it includes four patients with refractory LPP. These patients were given 3 mg naltrexone a day. All four experienced reduction in itch as well as decreased clinical evidence of active disease and decreased disease progression. Benefits were seen within the first two months, and the medication was well tolerated with no adverse events.[47]

I have used LDN for several patients with LPP—mostly in combination with topical or intralesional steroids and/or hydroxychloroquine. I have not seen dramatic results regarding the resolution of clinical evidence of active inflammation, but many patients report fewer symptoms of itching, burning, and stinging while on LDN. This suggests that it is having an impact on the inflammatory process. The fact that LDN takes several months to work and that this condition is self-limited makes it very difficult to evaluate the effect of any treatment, including LDN.

Psoriasis

Psoriasis is a systemic inflammatory condition that affects about 3 percent of Americans. It can be associated with psoriatic arthritis, metabolic syndrome, obesity, diabetes, cardiovascular disease, and depression.[48] The pathogenesis of psoriasis is multifactorial, including genetic and environmental factors. Up to 40 percent of people with psoriasis have a family history of psoriasis, and several genes have been identified as playing a role in the development of this condition.[49] Environmental factors also play a significant role. Smoking, alcohol consumption, obesity, and stress have all been associated with psoriasis and psoriatic flares. Drugs—including lithium, beta-blockers, antimalarials, and TNF-alpha inhibitors—can trigger psoriasis. Finally, infections are known to play a role in psoriasis. Streptococcal infections are a common trigger for guttate psoriasis, and HIV is known to trigger and/or exacerbate psoriasis.

The current understanding of the mechanisms of this disease is that psoriasis is a disorder of immune regulation and abnormal inflammation. Altered epidermal keratinocyte differentiation is seen, along with keratinocyte hyperproliferation and decreased epidermal transit time (the normal transit time from the basal layer to the topmost layer is decreased from about 27 days to 3 or 4 days). These abnormalities can be attributed to abnormal intracellular calcium fluctuations. Normalization of calcium levels within the cell is one way to potentially impact this condition.[50] Additionally, a number of inflammatory cytokines are known to be elevated in psoriasis, including TNF alpha, interferon alpha, and interleukins 1, 6, 17, and 23, as well as others.[51]

Clinically, psoriasis can present in several patterns. The most common are chronic plaque psoriasis (also known as psoriasis vulgaris) and guttate psoriasis. Pustular psoriasis and erythrodermic psoriasis are more severe but less common presentations. Both chronic plaque psoriasis and guttate psoriasis appear as sharply demarcated erythematous plaques with a silvery scale. In chronic plaque psoriasis, the plaques tend to be large and thick. They commonly affect the scalp, elbows, knees, umbilicus, and gluteal cleft, but can affect any cutaneous surface. Inverse psoriasis is a subtype where the intertriginous areas are preferentially affected. Guttate psoriasis has a similar presentation, but plaques tend to be smaller and more diffusely distributed. This type often occurs after an upper respiratory illness, especially strep throat. Pustular psoriasis presents with superficial pustules and scale on an erythematous base. Erythrodermic psoriasis consists of widespread erythema with scale covering most of the body surface area. Both of these variants can have an abrupt onset and can be associated with systemic manifestations including malaise; fever; chills; kidney, liver, respiratory and cardiovascular dysfunction; electrolyte abnormalities; fluid loss; proteinuria; and infection. Both types need to be addressed promptly, and patients may require hospitalization to manage the systemic complications.

Psoriatic arthritis is most commonly seen in the setting of cutaneous psoriasis, but can occur alone. Unlike many other forms of autoimmune-related arthritis, psoriatic arthritis is a progressively destructive condition that can lead to permanent joint damage and warrants more aggressive treatment. Because there are many different types of arthritis, appropriate imaging of affected joints and involvement of a rheumatologist can be helpful.[52]

Psoriasis is a chronic condition characterized by a fluctuating course. It is important to educate patients that there is no cure and to help them set realistic expectations. Patient preference and the degree of skin involvement that is acceptable for each patient are important to take into consideration when constructing a treatment plan. There are a number of therapeutic options for psoriasis, both topical and systemic. It is important for patients to understand that even if they do clear, it is likely that they will experience breakthrough flares, and they may need to adjust their treatment regimen.

Optimizing skin hydration is the first step in managing psoriasis. This is especially important for minimizing itch, and can help prevent/limit flares. Topical steroids are the first-line treatment for localized psoriasis. The specific steroid and concentration depends on the site being treated and the thickness of the plaque. Tachyphylaxis refers to decreased responsiveness to a medication over time, and is commonly seen with topical steroids in the setting of psoriasis. Intermittent medication holidays and/or combining steroids with other topical medications helps to avoid this phenomenon. The vitamin D analog calcipotriene has an antiproliferative effect on keratinocytes and is commonly used for psoriasis.[53] Other non-steroid options include tar and retinoids. Topical calcineurin inhibitors such as tacrolimus and pimecrolimus can be especially helpful for facial or intertriginous involvement.

Phototherapy offers an effective non-pharmacologic option for treating psoriasis. Narrow-band UVB treatment is known to have both antiproliferative and anti-inflammatory effects on the skin and is often very effective for managing psoriasis.[54] Treatments are given two to three times a week and are very well tolerated. The primary downsides include the challenge of locating a phototherapy unit and scheduling.

Severe or widely distributed psoriasis may require systemic immune-modulating medications, including methotrexate, oral retinoids, or cyclosporine. Additionally, an ever-growing number of biologic immune regulators have been created to address some of the specific inflammatory cytokines elevated in patients with psoriasis. These include the TNF-alpha inhibitors (etanercept, infliximab, adalimumab, certolizumab pegol), inter-leukin-17 (IL-17) inhibitors (secukinumab, ixekizumab, brodalumab), and IL-23 inhibitors (ustekinumab, guselkumab, tildrakizumab, risankizumab).

It is important to recognize that mood issues are commonly seen in patients with psoriasis—depression being the most prevalent. Quality of life is typically poor in many people who struggle with psoriasis, and it is important to involve psychologists, psychiatrists, and/or therapists to help patients cope with the psychosocial aspects of this condition.[55]

Low Dose Naltrexone and Psoriasis

While evidence for the effectiveness of LDN in the treatment of psoriasis is limited, LDN is a logical treatment because of the anti-inflammatory activity and its potential to regulate keratinocyte migration and differentiation. There are three case reports in the literature at this time. One report is of a 60-year-old woman with moderate diffuse plaque psoriasis involving 10 percent of her body surface area. She was treated with 4.5 mg LDN nightly. No other medications were used during this time. After three months, there was a significant improvement in her psoriatic lesions. By six months her body surface area involvement decreased to 1 percent, and her psoriasis area severity index (PASI) decreased from 7.2 to 0.9. LDN was well tolerated with no adverse effects.[56] In another report a 75-year-old male with guttate psoriasis was successfully treated with 4.5 mg LDN daily. After four weeks his lesions decreased in number and severity, and his itching was significantly decreased. LDN was well tolerated, with the only reported side effect being dry skin.[57] Finally there is a report of a 38-year-old female whose psoriasis had been adequately controlled with methotrexate. She stopped taking the medication due to side effects and experienced rapid progression to erythrodermic psoriasis. She developed widespread psoriatic plaques with edema, weeping, chills, and significant itching. She did not want to take traditional medications, so LDN was started at 4.5 mg a day, along with hydroxyzine every 12 hours to help manage her pruritus and a colloidal oatmeal moisturizer. Hydroxyzine was stopped on day 9. By day 10 her edema improved and her itching subsided. By day 20 her edema and erythema continued to improve. At three months she was completely clear and remained in remission at six months.[58]

My personal experience in treating psoriasis with LDN has been very positive. My most remarkable example is of an elderly woman who had 75 percent body surface area covered with thick psoriatic plaque. She had a history of two different solid organ cancers, and was therefore not a candidate for systemic immunosuppressive therapy or the newer biologic immunomodulatory medications. Topicals were not a reasonable option given the significant skin involvement, and phototherapy hadn't helped her enough in the past. She was started on 1.5 mg LDN at night, which we increased over three weeks to 4.5 mg nightly. Within four months the plaques were gone and she had only macular erythema, which completely resolved by six months. She has remained clear for over two years and tolerates the LDN well with no side effects. This patient's story is exceptional. In my experience, it is not common to see this degree of clearance in such a short period of time. Often, doses need to be carefully adjusted and expectations managed. I do find that LDN helps the significant majority of my patients with psoriasis. This does not mean that they clear completely. Sometimes people notice that they don't flare as much in the winter, that their flares are not as bad when they do happen, or that their skin is easier to manage with topical therapies. Many of my patients report that they feel better, and that their stress, anxiety, and/or depression are not as significant a problem for them. This reduction of stress definitely has a positive impact on their skin disease as well. I counsel patients that LDN is a slow-acting medication, and suggest that they commit to using it for a year before making a judgment about its effectiveness. I also let them know that careful dose adjustments may be needed to obtain maximum benefit from this medication.

Conclusion

Clearly, data regarding the effectiveness of LDN for the treatment of dermatologic conditions is limited. Given the known mechanisms of action, topical or systemic LDN should be helpful in a wide variety of inflammatory and autoimmune skin diseases. Along with the dermatologic conditions discussed above, I have used LDN successfully to treat alopecia areata,

DR. BODEMER'S DOSING PEARLS

For patients with autoimmune and inflammatory skin disorders:

- 1.5 mg before bed for one week.
- 3 mg before bed for one week.
- 4.5 mg before bed thereafter.
- Assess progress after six months. If desired control has not been achieved, decrease back down to 3 mg a day and slowly increase by 0.5 mg increments every two to four months back up to 4.5.

For patients with anxiety and/or depression:

- 0.5 mg nightly for one to two weeks.
- 0.5 mg BID for one to two weeks.
- 0.5 mg in the morning and 1 mg at night for one to two weeks.
- 1 mg BID thereafter.
- If there are concomitant inflammatory skin conditions, keep the patient at 1 mg BID for four months, then slowly increase by 0.5 mg increments for a total dose closer to 3 to 4.5 mg.

For patients with thyroid abnormalities or for patients who are on thyroid replacement medication:

- 0.5 mg before bed for one week.
- 1.0 mg before bed for one week.
- 1.5 mg before bed for one week.
- Recheck thyroid function at three months, and then continue to increase by 0.5 mg every two weeks up to between 3 and 4.5 mg a day.
- Recheck thyroid stimulating hormone (TSH) every three months until a stable dose is achieved.
- Counsel patients to watch for symptoms of hyperthyroidism, including palpitations, anxiousness, difficulty sleeping, increased sweating, shortness of breath, weight loss, and tremor.

vitiligo, and localized morphea. I also use LDN for people with a history of melanoma to potentially prevent the development of new melanomas and to limit recurrence/metastasis. Additionally, there is promising data indicating that LDN will likely be effective for treating chronic wounds and diabetes-related skin disorders.[59] Due to the safety and low side effect profile, LDN could be considered as an initial option—especially for people who either can't use standard medications or want to avoid the toxicity of some of the drugs commonly used for chronic skin conditions.

When deciding on a treatment plan that includes LDN, it is important to screen for thyroid disease and opioid use (prescription and recreational). It is also important to take into account the patient's other health issues—if they have fibromyalgia, inflammatory bowel disease, other autoimmune conditions, or depression/anxiety, LDN is an especially good option. Hopefully, as LDN becomes more widely understood and accepted, more and better data will be collected regarding its use in treating disorders of the skin.

– FIVE –

Parkinson's Disease

KIRSTEN SINGLER, NMD

Parkinson's disease (PD) is one of the most common neuromuscular disorders—a broad category of diseases that all share dysfunction of the nerve and muscle systems of the body. This category includes diseases such as multiple sclerosis (MS), polymyositis, hereditary spastic paraplegia, Lambert-Eaton syndrome, muscular dystrophy, amyotrophic lateral sclerosis (ALS), and other disease processes that vary in etiology and mechanism. Most of the diseases in this category are not well understood, and their causes still unknown. Some have a genetic component, while others are thought to be caused by an autoimmune response, virus, toxic exposure, or tumor. While a few of these conditions manifest in childhood, many—such as ALS, MS, and Parkinson's—develop in adulthood. Symptoms usually include weakness in the muscles, diminished motor function, numbness, pain, tingling, spasm, muscle rigidity, muscle wasting, and tremor. Often, treatment includes immune suppressants, antispasmodics, antidepressants, and pain medication. Though the standard of care can relieve some of the symptoms and stall progression, most conditions in this category are considered irreversible. Frequently, patients and their caretakers go in search of alternative and/or conjunctive care in the hope of improving quality of life.

Such was the case when I met Anna, who at the time was in her 70s and had been diagnosed with and treated for Parkinson's. At our initial meeting, Anna entered in a wheelchair pushed by her caretaker, as she could not walk independently despite her strict compliance with the medications prescribed by her neurologist. Her guardian did all the talking during the consultation because Anna was almost mute. Her voice was inaudible— softer than a whisper. She could not frown or smile, as she had no control over her facial muscles. Simply put, 10 years of analgesics and Sinemet had not adequately managed her symptoms. Her family wanted to explore adjunctive treatments in the hope of improving any of her numerous symptoms. They had been researching integrative medicine and, though skeptical, wanted to learn more.

Functional medicine is complex, involving the treatment of the whole person. It often requires changes in lifestyle and food habits, as well as the patient's willingness to try new therapies and be an active participant in their healing. The process of healing can be arduous, especially when facing a progressed chronic illness. Since Anna was significantly debilitated, she would need the help of her children to incorporate new therapies and make adjustments to her habits at home. I explained to Anna's caregivers that compared with allopathic care, which focuses singularly on the pathology, complementary medicine aims to evaluate and treat the entirety of the person. A good analogy to understand this would be to think of a person's health as an entire forest; allopathic care focuses on just one tree, while the focus of functional medicine is the whole forest. Functional doctors take inventory of every impediment to the patient's health and address each area in their treatment plan. Furthermore, Parkinson's disease is a complicated disorder with multiple overlapping causative factors such as toxic exposure, metabolic hindrance to detoxification and mitochondrial function, inflammation, and gastrointestinal and immune dysfunction. Each of these areas would need to be additionally evaluated to gain leverage in Anna's therapy. Intent on improving Anna's quality of life, her children agreed to participate by making changes at home and committed to be active partners in her care.

Parkinson's Etiology and Mechanism

Parkinson's disease was named for James Parkinson, who first identified the condition in Western medical literature in 1817. Though it wasn't until the 1950s that we began to understand the mechanism behind Parkinson's, the disease had been well documented in Ayurvedic and Chinese medical texts as early as 5,000 years ago.[1] Parkinson's disease affects the dopaminergic neurons in the midbrain's substantia nigra, which results in progressive symptoms including tremor, slowed movements, rigid limb movements, reduced facial expression, difficulty verbalizing, reduced sense of smell, digestive and urinary problems, fatigue, depression, pain, cognitive changes, vertigo, vision changes, uncontrollable repetitive motions, micrographia, and dementia. The disease progression is unique for every individual, but most patients experience paralysis of facial expression—or rigidity—and tremors. Although we can identify the location and basic pathologic presentation of the disease, we still know little about its pathogenesis and how to reverse it. There is no single determinant of Parkinson's; rather, it is predominantly considered to be an oxidative and immune-mediated culmination of multitudinous agents that cause degeneration of the nigral neurons in the brain. Research implicates many factors, from inherited genetic mutation, to exposure to a toxic chemical or virus, to bacterial imbalances.[2] Despite these varied triggers, Parkinson's fundamentally consists of the presence of pathologic, misfolded alpha-synuclein proteins that make up Lewy body aggregates, nigral cell damage, and inhibited dopamine production by the neurons in the substantia nigra.[3]

In 1996 genetic mapping allowed us to identify more than 15 genetic mutations associated with Parkinson's, including mutations of the SNCA, PRKN, PINK1, DJ-1, LRRK2, G2019S, GBA, MAPT, mtDNA, and iPD genes. These mutations impact mitochondrial, antioxidant, and immune function.[4] The first mutation identified, SNCA mutation, is associated with an increase in alpha-synuclein protein, and though the function of this protein is not completely understood, it is found to be associated with Lewy body formation, neurodegeneration, and dementia. PRKN, on the other hand, is associated with mitochondrial maintenance, as well as the degradation and cleanup of unwanted proteins. Similarly, DJ-1 plays a role in neuroprotection of the mitochondria and the cell's ability to ameliorate to oxidative stress. DJ-1 is found in almost every cell of the body, but is notably found excessively oxidized in the neurons and glial cells of Parkinson's patients. Additionally, DJ-1 plays a role in the regulation of tyrosine hydroxylase, which converts tyrosine to L-DOPA in the brain.[5]

The LRRK2 gene is associated with 1 to 2 percent of Parkinson's diagnoses and, though believed to protect against pathogenic infection, has also been implicated in immune- and inflammation-based neuronal death. Notably, a case report of LRRK2-positive twins found that only one of the siblings had Parkinson's, thus highlighting the significance of epigenetics and the complexity of factors leading to the development of the disease.[6] Overall, the polymorphisms reduce the neuron's tolerance to cytotoxicity that may be caused by multiple mechanisms, including immune dysfunction, elevated levels of human leukocyte antigen, liposomal damage, excess free radical exposure, oxidation, accumulation of iron and copper, lysosomal dysfunction, granulin dysregulation of fatty acid metabolism, endocytic pathology, neuroinflammation, problems with phosphorylation, and microglial activation.[7] Though genetic polymorphisms do not predict Parkinson's, they help evaluate the risk associated with environmental exposure, predict the age of disease onset, and illuminate the mechanisms behind mitochondrial defects and the role of reactive oxygen species, oxidative damage, and abnormal protein aggregation.

Only 10 to 15 percent of Parkinson's diagnoses are associated with genetic mutations, so researchers continue to catalog possible causes for the predominance of diagnoses. It appears that anything that could inhibit mitochondrial function and increase inflammation may be implicated, and toxic exposure ranks highly as a possible trigger. Patient history and lab animal exposure reveal that the pathological process of Parkinson's has been induced with chemical toxicants. Famously, MPTP, a by-product of synthetic heroin, was noted to cause the onset of Parkinson's in case reports of illicit drug overdoses. In studying this substance in animal and in vitro specimens, researchers were able to identify mitochondrial damage as a leading factor in Parkinson's pathology.[8]

Further investigations identify other toxicants and harmful agents that cells cannot neutralize as potential triggers for Parkinson's. In the last 30 years, specific agents found in insecticides, chemical solvents, herbicides, piscicides, and medications have been linked to neuronal damage of the striatal cells.[9] Specific neurotoxins that are identified as causing nigrostriatal damage include 1-methyl-4-phenyl-1,2,3 (MPTP), 6-hydroxydopamine (6-OHDA), 2,4-dichlorophenoxyacetic acid (DDT), trichloroethylene, paraquat, rotenone, polychlorinated biphenyls (PCBs), organochlorine pesticide, hexachlorobenzene, perchloroethylene, organophosphates, gasoline fuels, and metals such as manganese, copper, and iron.[10]

Adding further complexity, an autopsy of a postmortem Parkinson's patient revealed low glutathione in the substantia nigra, which is theorized to be connected to excess oxidative stress either from an innate inadequate glutathione production or from disproportionate free radical exposure.[11] Demands for free radicals and glutathione can increase in the event of toxic exposure. In addition, the midbrain naturally produces several oxidants as by-products during normal function. Physiologically, the substantia nigra has high levels of iron, dopamine, and neuromelanin that convert into hazardous free radicals. Glutathione is the critical agent that absorbs and neutralizes these free radicals. Glutathione also plays a crucial role in the mitochondrial complex that preserves the viability of the neuron. Notably, the substantia nigra was the only part of the brain found to be deficient in glutathione, while other areas of the brain had comparably adequate levels. This suggests that Parkinson's may be due to localized excess free radical oxidation that leaves glutathione depleted.[12] Glutathione deficiency is also found in the substantia nigra of lab animals with induced Parkinson's. Finally, lab animals genetically engineered to have inhibited glutathione production were studied for inhibited mitochondrial complex I activity and increased neurotoxicity from chemical agents such as buthionine sulfoximine. The researchers concluded that elevated intracellular glutathione levels are protective to neurons—especially neurons exposed to higher oxidation and free radicals, such as those in the substantia nigra.[13]

The etiology of excess free radical oxidation and neuroinflammation had been unknown until 2014, when researchers at Columbia University Irving Medical Center (CUIMC) established that neurons are susceptible to immune T-cell attack.[14] Dr. Sulzer's team at CUIMC went on to find that immune cells could be taken from live PD patients, and their characteristics studied. The team noted that T cells of living Parkinson's patients would attack alpha-synuclein proteins, while non-Parkinson's T cells did not have an immune reaction to alpha-synuclein.[15] This phenomenon instigated theories that Parkinson's might be an autoimmune disorder of T cells and microglia stimulated by alpha-synuclein deposits.[16] German researchers at Universitätsklinikum Erlangen similarly found that Parkinson's patients had increased Th17 cells—T cells associated with autoimmune diseases—thought to be attacking the dopaminergic neurons.[17]

Additionally, researchers at Parkinson Disorders Research Laboratory in Iowa published details of their 2016 animal and human studies isolating an enzyme involved in immune activities—protein kinase C delta (PKCd)—and its role in Parkinson's. In their research, Gordon et al. established PKCd as being upregulated by misfolded alpha-synuclein protein. PKCd was identified as a mediator that increased inflammatory response via microglia and lipopolysaccharides (LPS). Blocking PKCd resulted in neuroprotection from agents that would otherwise stimulate Parkinson's damage to the dopamine neurons.[18] Further substantiating the immunopathologic nature of Parkinson's, researchers have consistently identified immune-mediated dysfunction involving glial cells, neuroinflammatory cytokines NF-kB and PKCd, alpha-synuclein misfolding, tumor necrosis factor alpha (TNF-a), and lipopolysaccharides, all of which play a significant role in inflammation-induced damage in the midbrain.[19]

More recently neuroscientists have begun to examine the role of gastrointestinal health as a principal component driving increased alpha-synuclein misfoldings and excessive immune activity. Parkinson's patients often present initially with gastrointestinal symptoms and dysfunction, and Lewy body pathology in submucosal neurons of the enteric nervous system. Researchers in Brazil and Italy have proposed intestinal microbial dysbiosis as a prime neuroinflammatory trigger and instigator of alpha-synuclein protein malfunction, while other researchers, such as those at Poznan University of Medical Sciences and Duke University Medical Center, have suggested that the dysbiosis-driven a-synucleinopathy is evidence that PD might be a prion disorder originating in the enteric nervous system.[20] Animal studies at the Universidad Andrés Bello in Chile showed that inflamed dysbiotic gastrointestinal mucosa generated Lewy bodies in the enteric nervous system and increased T-cell-mediated inflammation that started in the gut and advanced to the brain.[21] Animal studies performed at Michigan State University in 2018 revealed that alpha-synuclein pathology could be stimulated in the enteric nervous system, leading to inhibited gut motility.[22] Additional animal studies published in 2018 showed that reducing the T-cell inflammatory response reversed neurodegeneration associated with Parkinson's.[23]

Neuroscientists theorize that overstimulation of the immune system in the gut may be a critical determinant of proteinopathy and neuroglia dysfunction.[24] These discoveries have launched multitudinous new studies investigating promising therapies to help reduce the inflammatory, immune, and oxidative degeneration involved in Parkinson's, starting with digestive health.

Treating Parkinson's

When evaluating a patient with Parkinson's symptoms, functional practitioners consider the complexity and dynamism of the disease and will choose therapies based on the individual's unique clinical presentation and history. Therapies are designed to address each facet of the individual's state of health, including their exposure to environmental toxins, history of trauma, chronic stressors, constitution, familial predisposition, digestive integrity, essential organ function, efficiency and viability of detoxification pathways, comorbidities, vitality, and ability to heal. Therapies include gluta-thione supplementation, low dose naltrexone (LDN), acupuncture, detox-ification (depuration) protocols, nutritional changes, stress management, psycho-emotional therapies, botanical therapies, and nutraceutical inter-vention. Nutraceutical support may include probiotics, N-acetylcysteine (NAC), *Mucuna pruriens*, and other nutrient supplementation based on the individual's deficiencies. Glutathione is often used when a patient's symp-toms present after a toxic exposure, or when mitochondrial dysfunction is suspected. LDN helps to reduce inflammation, chronic fatigue, impaired gut motility, and pain. Acupuncture reduces pain and improves energy, mood, sleep, and digestive processes. Of the numerous functional therapies to choose from, glutathione and LDN have shown significant promise in research. The sections below examine the role of these two therapies in treating Parkinson's disease.

THE ROLE OF GLUTATHIONE IN PARKINSON'S TREATMENT

Glutathione is one of the most important antioxidants in the body. It affects multiple mechanisms in the Parkinson's pathological process. It protects tissues from damage induced by inflammation, neutralizes hydroxyl radi-cals, participates in phase I and II liver detoxification, is essential to mito-chondrial function and DNA maintenance, and assists with the excretion of both endogenous and xenobiotic cytotoxins. It also aids in preserving and enhancing the efficacy of dopamine in the midbrain.

Similarly, glutathione protects DNA from damage caused by reactive oxygen species.[25] Low levels of glutathione are tied to chronic chemical exposure, chronic illness, advanced aging, and neurodegenerative disor-ders. Glutathione is made in the cytosol from the amino acids cysteine, glycine, and glutamic acid, and then transferred into the mitochondria in high concentrations throughout the body.[26] If cells have excessive oxida-tive stress, inflammation, or xenobiotic concentration, cysteine will be liberated to increase the manufacturing of glutathione. Therapeutically, glutathione is administered via IV; alternatively, its amino acid precursor, N-acetylcysteine, is given as an oral supplement. Both NAC and glutathione have been used to attenuate neurotoxic damage from chemicals, improve mitochondrial function, protect dopamine neurons from oxidative damage, and protect DNA from damage due to reactive oxygen species and aging.[27]

The glutathione system has gained significant attention in the area of Parkinson's research because we have long identified glutathione deficiency in the substantia nigra as a key to Parkinson's pathogenesis, though this deficiency appears to be triggered by multiple destructive agents. Causes of glutathione deficiency associated with Parkinson's are natural aging, DNA degradation, excess free radicals, low antioxidant status, neuromelanin, excess iron, and exogenous toxicants.[28] Glutathione deficiency is specifically correlated with the severity of Parkinson's symptoms.

Glutathione's role as an antioxidant is especially crucial in the midbrain. Harmful reactive oxygen species (ROS) are natural by-products of energy production in the cell. They perform varied and complex functions such as cell signaling. They aid antimicrobial processes, but also harm lipids in the cell membrane and cause damage to mitochondrial DNA and RNA proteins.[29] While free radicals are unstable because they lack an electron, antioxidants such as glutathione can remain stable even after giving up an electron. Glutathione resides in the cell in high concentrations and is pumped into the mitochondria to mitigate damage from free radicals. Mitochondria aid in energy production, biosynthesis of hormones, nutrient metabolism, regulation of Ca^{2+}, cell homeostasis, autophagy, and gene expression. Imbalance of the cell's energy needs, production of ROS, and disturbance in the removal of free radicals result in damage to the mitochondrial DNA. These phenomena make up the natural aging process and form the basis for the mitochondrial theory of aging.[30] Considering that 96 percent of Parkinson's diagnoses occur after age 50, mitochondrial damage due to age is considered the most important risk factor for Parkinson's.[31] Moreover, similar mitochondrial dysfunction is identified in younger Parkinson's patients. In this demographic, diagnosis is often attributed to genetic etiology.[32]

With regard to glutathione's role in DNA protection, there are multiple relevant studies both in vitro and in vivo detailing how glutathione reduces the natural aging and degeneration of DNA. This is significant because DNA erosion is tied with aging as a top risk factor for neurodegenerative disorders.[33] When DNA cannot be repaired, the dopaminergic system and alpha-synuclein pathology grow more dysfunctional.[34] In vivo and human studies show that glutathione protects the activity of telomerase, which regulates DNA from damage due to chronic oxidative stress or other comorbid disease processes.[35] Also, as the main antioxidant in the cell, glutathione further protects mitochondrial DNA against free radical damage.[36] When glutathione is administered, it ameliorates this degenerative process. However, results depend on means of administration since oral glutathione has limited efficacy; sublingual and IV forms appear to have greater therapeutic value.[37]

In terms of how glutathione improves patient symptoms, there is increased interest in the glutathione complex reducing motor inhibition and dopaminergic damage. Small-scale studies and case reports continue to inundate the indexes of PubMed's archive, documenting the ameliorative effect that glutathione has on motor function in Parkinson's. Case studies made famous by neurologist Dr. David Perlmutter chronicle the therapeutic use of IV glutathione to improve motor function.[38] Other publications, such as a case report by published naturopaths Otto and Magerus, detail relief of Parkinson's rigidity and tremor when glutathione IV is added to the standard of care regime.[39] In these cases glutathione treatment was adjunctive, alleviating symptoms still present after standard of care had been exhausted. In contrast, previous research by neurologists at the University of Sassari documented that IV glutathione as a monotherapy reversed symptoms in untreated Parkinson's patients.[40]

Glutathione's precursor, NAC, has also been widely studied for its use in Parkinson's. It has been used historically to treat liver toxicity, acetaminophen overdose, cystic fibrosis, and human immunodeficiency virus. NAC recently garnered attention for its role in upregulating glutathione in cells, thereby increasing antioxidant response in the central nervous system and ameliorating mitochondrial neurotoxicity from environmental and endogenous contaminants. As discussed previously, mitochondrial damage and loss of nigrostriatal dopamine are associated with damaging metabolites within the cell, such as neuromelanin, metals, excessive oxidation, and exogenous chemical exposure.[41] In animal studies, administration of NAC mitigated neurotoxic damage to striatal neurons caused by many of the chemicals associated with Parkinson's, such as MPTP, 6-hydroxydopamine, rotenone, and other neurotoxicants.[42] Significantly increased brain glutathione levels were detected in multiple studies using magnetic resonance spectroscopy after IV administration of NAC to Parkinson's, Gaucher's disease, and hypoxic-ischemic encephalopathic patients.[43] Researchers at the University of Pittsburgh demonstrated that NAC independently protects astrocytes from the proteotoxic damage of alpha-synuclein.[44] Their findings assert that NAC's neuroprotective effects are not dependent solely on conversion to glutathione, although glutathione conversion may be an added benefit.

Further, reports from Spain's Hospital Universitario La Paz indicate that NAC used in vitro and in vivo reduces mitochondrial dysfunction and neurodegeneration in aging mice.[45] Another animal study from Beth Israel Deaconess Medical Center shows that oral NAC attenuates alpha-synuclein protein and preserves dopamine neurons, as compared with controls.[46] Recent research from Thomas Jefferson University saw improvement with both oral and IV NAC in Parkinson's patients' motor symptoms and dopamine transporter function.[47] NAC continues to be one of the least expensive and most researched supplements to decrease damaging agents in Parkinson's.

Lastly, glutathione deficiency is further implicated when evaluating Parkinson's risk associated with mitochondrial toxicants such as heavy metals and organophosphates. These chemicals are affiliated with glutathione depletion in the mitochondria. For example, mouse studies published in 2006 elucidate how rotenone poisoning inhibits complex I of the electron transport chain in the mitochondria, thus reducing glutathione and ultimately leading to cell death.[48] Glutathione works via the Nrf2 protein that governs phase II and III of the liver's detoxification pathways. The glutathione system significantly aids in the depuration and elimination of heavy metals and organic pollutants via the use of Nrf2 protein in phase II and III detoxification pathways.[49] It has shown to improve liver function, lower abnormal liver enzymes, and aid in the clearance of poisons.[50]

Parkinson's patients can be evaluated for heavy metals, iron accumulation, and pollutants via serum, urine, and hair analysis. When there is significant exposure limiting the patient's ability to heal, naturopathic physicians will incorporate glutathione IV with other therapies intended to relieve the toxic burden of the cells. Depending on the degree of exposure and the patient's constitution, age, and comorbidities, a functional practitioner will commonly add therapies such as sauna, specific diet protocols, and botanicals to further enhance detoxification. Phlebotomy may be used to decrease iron storage, and chelation therapy may be used for heavy metals. Identifying the cause of exposure and educating the patient to reduce the recurrence of exposure in their home, food, or environment is crucially important.

THE ROLE OF LDN IN PARKINSON'S TREATMENT

Another prominent feature of Parkinson's pathology is immune and inflammatory activity in both the peripheral and central nervous system. Numerous clinical, postmortem, and animal studies correlate pervasive inflammatory cytokines, microglial, and T-cell activity in the Parkinsonian midbrain with impaired dopaminergic neuron function. These studies identify viral, bacterial, and toxic catalysts that drive the inflammatory cascade of cytokines, alpha-synuclein proteins, and aberrant T-cell activity that crosses the blood-brain barrier and induces destructive microgliosis in the midbrain.[51] The high levels of inflammatory cytokines are tied to nonmotor Parkinson's symptoms such as pain, constipation, and dementia, while elevated immune microglial and T-cell levels are associated with degeneration of the midbrain and motor system symptoms.[52]

Some of the key pro-inflammatory agents found in the midbrain of postmortem patients and animals are alpha-synuclein, tumor necrosis factor alpha (TNF-a), lipopolysaccharide, interleukin-6 (IL-6), protein kinase C delta (PKCd), activated microglia, and T cells. Additionally, IL-1B and IL-6 are elevated in Parkinson's cerebrospinal fluid as compared with that of non-Parkinsonian controls.[53] Significantly, alpha-synuclein, TNF-a, interferon gamma (IFN-y), IL-6, and glial activation markers (GFAP and Sox10) are found in the ascending colon. Scientists currently hypothesize that enteric inflammation is the possible root of the neuroinflammatory cascade, because CD4+ T cells, colonic cytokines, and Lewy bodies act on central nervous endothelial cells, causing permeability and extravasation of the blood-brain barrier.[54] In fact, early involvement of inflammation in the gut, CD4+ T cells, and constipation are hallmarks that appear years before severe motor impairment.[55]

Other autoimmune conditions, such as MS, are also linked to elevated glial and T-cell activity. In MS, immune T cells attack the oligodendrocytes, while in Parkinson's, T-cell activity triggered by the a-synuclein protein damages neurons in the substantia nigra via excess ROS.[56] In both conditions there are high amounts of pro-inflammatory cytokines—such as TGF-B, IL-1B, IL-6, IFN-y, and IL-1—present in the central nervous system.[57] Researchers are able to slow the progression of dopaminergic damage when targeting the inflammatory mechanisms, reducing glial and T cell involvement in Parkinson-induced models.[58] Though the neuroinflammatory process is complex, researchers continue to expand on the details and inevitable treatments for these findings.

In animal studies, alterations in gut microbiota resulted in increased alpha-synuclein, driving an overactive immune response in both the submucosal myenteric plexus and the brain.[59] Additionally, researchers induced a similar gastrointestinal response when lab animals were given oral rotenone.[60] Other areas of research show viral or bacterial exposure triggering an inflammatory response, leading to immune and protein malfunctions.[61] Additionally, when Parkinson's-induced animals (via A53T a-synuclein mutation) were administered FK506—a T-cell immune-suppressive drug—dopamine neurons were preserved.[62] Other markers of immune dysfunction have been identified as MHC-coding proteins that are found to increase with disease severity and cause dopamine neurons to be susceptible to glial activation.[63]

Glial cells and their inflammatory cytokines are especially pertinent for examination since they have been found in high concentrations in the midbrain of Parkinson's patients.[64] Alpha-synuclein aggregates are found to stimulate microglial activation, leading to excessive inflammation and then neuron death. Other relevant microglial activators are neuromelanin, matrix metalloproteinase-3 (MMP3), fibrinogen or environmental lipo-polysaccharide toxins, MPTP, pesticides (rotenone, paraquat), proteasome, and heavy metals. Remarkably, when microglia are inhibited, dopamine neurons are preserved, and Parkinson's disease progression halts. Multiple studies show that Parkinson's-induced animals were successfully treated with NEMO-binding domain (NBD) peptide, which inhibits NF-kB, microglial activation, and halts inflammatory neuronal destruction.[65] Other animal studies performed on mice with microglial suppression showed similar dopaminergic protection, while agents that increased micogliosis exacerbated the destruction of dopamine neurons.[66] Current and ongoing research for new treatments to reverse Parkinson's are focused on reducing neurotoxic inflammation and immune dysregulation with immune-modulating therapies.[67]

Naltrexone has been used clinically at low doses to decrease inflammation and immune dysregulation. It is well documented that the mechanism of LDN regulates T-cell function and reduces glial activation and the associated neurotoxic inflammatory cascade, all of which are hallmarks of Parkinson's pathophysiology.[68] It has shown promise in treating inflammatory auto-immune conditions such as Crohn's disease, inflammatory bowel disease, Hashimoto's thyroiditis, fibromyalgia, lupus, rheumatoid arthritis, and multiple sclerosis by reducing toll-like receptor 4 and cytokine responses such as a toll-interleukin receptor, interferon beta, interferon gamma, and tumor necrosis factor.[69] Similar to Parkinson's disease, multiple sclerosis involves elevated microglial activation at the sites of lesions, excessive inflammation, oxidation, ROS, and deterioration of neuronal tissue (demyelinated plaques in the white and gray matter).[70] LDN has been repeatedly studied as a treatment for mitigating microglial inflammation and symptom reduction in MS, suggesting promise for related Parkinson's symptoms.[71] In studies of Parkinson's-induced rats, naloxone was shown to decrease microglial free radicals and pro-inflammatory agents, thereby protecting the dopaminergic neurons.[72] In vitro naloxone-treated midbrain glial cultures showed that naloxone bound to Nox2 as a mechanism to prevent microglial and superoxide neurodegeneration.[73] Small studies and case reports published on the clinical application of LDN reveal promising results. Thomas Guttuso et al. published findings that LDN brought symptomatic relief to Parkinson's patients' chronic fatigue.[74] Large-scale studies on the uses of this medication for Parkinson's are lacking, but considering the neurological anti-inflammatory effect, it may be a promising area of research.

Neurologist Dr. Bernard Bihari was the main pioneer of therapeutic LDN. He reported that he had overseen seven Parkinson's patients whose disease progression had halted or regressed upon LDN treatment. Dr. Bihari proposed that LDN affects a different player in chronic disease: endorphins. He noted phenomenon in his practice whereby patients would develop chronic illness after a severe stressor, such as the death of a loved one. Trained in neurology, brain physiology, and psychology, Dr. Bihari had a unique background from which to understand the physiological effects of endorphins. He posited that those significant stress events lowered the patient's endorphins, making them more susceptible to the disease process.[75] Subsequent research substantiates the hypothesis that endorphins play a significant role in reducing inflammation and immune dysfunction in Parkinson's and many other chronic conditions.[76] Endorphins are neuropeptide hormones whose levels elevate, according to studies, when we participate in pleasurable activities such as exercise, dancing, singing, laughing, meditation, fasting, intimacy, yoga, tai chi, and acupuncture.[77] Research has shown that the anti-inflammatory effects of endorphins have the capacity to reduce symptoms associated with autoimmune conditions and chronic illness.[78]

Endorphin decline may play a significant role in the chronic pain Parkinson's patients suffer. Studies show Parkinson's patients have low levels of endorphins in plasma and cerebrospinal fluid.[79] In terms of affecting endorphins, LDN is particularly famous for aiding beta-endorphin production, thereby reducing chronic pain in conditions such as fibromyalgia, rheumatoid arthritis, and complex regional pain syndrome.[80] Other therapeutic considerations for increasing endorphins and stabilizing Parkinson's disease progression include activities such as yoga, tai chi, acupuncture, dance, and exercise, all of which have been shown to improve Parkinson's outcomes, ease symptoms, and/or reverse changes on brain MRIs to some extent.[81]

Lastly, there has been significant research inquiry into the role of inflammatory bowel in Parkinson's pathogenesis. Bowel disorder is commonly accepted as one of the main symptomatic manifestations of Parkinson's disease, as neuromuscular inhibition causes slowing of bowel transit, which then exacerbates a host of other dysbiotic sequelae. But only recently have researchers begun to posit that inflammation and changes to the gut microbiome may be original contributors to the formation of abnormal alpha-synuclein protein replication, autoimmune-like dysfunction, and neuroinflammatory processes.[82] In 2014 neurologists and gastroenterologists teamed up at the University of Malaya to evaluate small intestinal bacterial overgrowth (SIBO) in PD patients. They found that almost 25 percent of the participants tested positive for SIBO. These patients were found to have more severe motor dysfunction than non-SIBO patients.[83]

Similarly, in 2016 researchers at Xinxiang Medical University diagnosed SIBO in 30 percent of their Parkinson's patients. Additionally, the SIBO diagnosis was associated with more progressed motor symptoms than non-SIBO patients.[84] These studies have spurred a plethora of human and animal research examining the gut-brain connection and treatments to reduce alimentary inflammation via diet modification, prokinetics, probiotics, laxatives, fecal transplants, and antibiotics.[85] All have shown improvement in disease presentation through regulation and improvement of gut function. In terms of LDN's use as both a prokinetic and anti-inflammatory medication, this may be another means by which LDN can mediate Parkinsonian dysbiosis and its inflammatory/immune cascade. A noteworthy study published in 2018 by Mitchell et al. found that LDN improved clinical symptoms of 74.5 percent of patients suffering from inflammatory bowel disease (IBD). The authors conclude that LDN is a safe and effective treatment for IBD.[86]

Case Study

My notes from Anna's initial intake list her symptoms: "urinary incontinence, freezing paralyzed motion, diminished voice, bradykinesia, unable to drive her scooter in her house, crashes scooter due to slow reflexes, burning feet at night, tight, painful leg muscles that wake her at night, inability to perform activities of daily living, cannot cook or drive herself, inability to walk most days, shuffled gait, inability to move through doorway or turn corners, arms stationary without swing when trying to walk." She had a significant history of breast cancer and hypothyroidism, and her husband was recently deceased. We conservatively assessed basic labs for homocysteine, methyl tetrahydrofolate reductase (MTHFR), thyroid stimulating hormone (TSH), complete blood count (CBC), comprehensive metabolic panel (CMP), ferritin, iron, B_{12}, A1C, erythrocyte sedimentation rate (ESR), and C-reactive protein (CRP). Typically, functional doctors will run additional genetic, heavy metal, organic acid, and chemical testing for environmental and microbial exposure. In this case, her family desired a minimalistic approach, requesting that we run the smallest number of labs possible. Her lab findings showed elevated homocysteine, hypothyroid, iron-deficiency anemia, and positive methyl tetrahydrofolate reductase polymorphism. Her breast cancer treatment included Faslodex, tamoxifen, CHOP, and Taxol. This history, together with MTHFR polymorphism, were likely the most notable stressors to her long-term health, because MTHFR is tied to reduced glutathione production and low tolerance for medications. Additionally, her sleep was poor due to pain, she frequently skipped meals, and she was not getting exercise.

We started with a modest plan of LDN 3.0 mg per night, IV glutathione per the work of neurologist Dr. David Perlmutter, the dopamine-boosting botanical *Mucuna pruriens*, and whole-food-based diet modification.[87] Because Anna was frail and her condition so progressed, we proceeded cautiously, incorporating one new therapy at a time and watching for an adverse reaction. The frequency and concentration of the glutathione IV were increased slowly each week. After four weeks of treatment, we followed up to review the efficacy of the plan. I was pleasantly surprised to hear Anna's own voice reporting her improvements. Though her voice was audible, her facial expressions were still diminished, and her gait was not yet prominently changed. But she was feeling better, and her daughter happily reported that after the first IV, she had been able to walk independently for two days. Anna and her family were encouraged by the small but remarkable changes that had already occurred.

Together with Anna's children, we planned that she would increase the frequency of her glutathione IVs to twice a week if possible, but at least once a week, and monitor her progress every two weeks. She continued her Sinemet and let her neurologist know she was seeking adjunctive care. Over the following six months, I watched as Anna made remarkable strides. Her voice became stronger, her facial expressions returned, and she smiled and laughed. Other symptoms gradually lessened. Her gait improved, her energy increased, and her incontinence decreased. At each visit I monitored her gait fluidity. Though she moved slowly and shuffled around corners, she moved smoothly down the hallway. She traded the wheelchair for a walker, and then traded the walker for gentle arm support when navigating around corners. After three months she had improved enough to spend an afternoon with her daughter, walking around without assistance while shopping, lunching, and getting her hair done. As she began to feel better, we continued to make small but impactful changes to her therapy plan.

In Anna's case, her symptoms and diagnosis presented after two enormous stressors: her husband's passing and her chemotherapy treatment for breast cancer. These two stressors were likely profound obstacles that ultimately inhibited her mitochondrial function and impaired her body's ability to repair the damage, paving the way for unrestrained inflammatory degeneration to take its toll. We addressed the potential mitochondrial damage from toxic exposure with glutathione IV, and added LDN to help reduce neuropathy and normalize gastrointestinal function. We followed those measures with acupuncture to help relieve her urinary incontinence, increase endorphins, and improve her mood and vitality. Once she was feeling better, we set small, weekly goals to improve her nutrition and cultivate an elemental diet. We also set goals for her to interact socially with her children and grandchildren. Over time we added oral NAC, iron, and *Mucuna pruriens*. With this protocol Anna gradually regained the ability to walk with the support of another person holding her hand, and could rise independently from a seated position, talk, laugh, and gesture freely. Her urinary incontinence decreased, her sleep improved, and she reported less pain. She was able to make a simple meal for herself at home and resume driving her scooter. Anna's response to treatment was remarkable, and the brightness of her personality that returned was a blessing to witness.

Conclusion

In summary, Parkinson's is a complex disorder that involves multiple, overlapping areas of dysfunction, making it difficult to pin down a single cause. It may be that, like other chronic illnesses, there is no one reductionist cure, but rather multiple avenues of treatment that must be specifically tailored to the patient's history and constitution. Parkinson's research demonstrates that even though the condition involves an obvious deficit in the midbrain, the function of the entire body is implicated. I am a naturopathic doctor, and treating the entire person is fundamental to my training. Functional doctors understand that any condition has the potential to improve if the health of the whole person is addressed. Typically, a thorough intake will reveal important obstacles that have inhibited the healing process, and a unique protocol can be created for each patient. Naturopaths rarely standardize their therapies in cookie-cutter formulas. Rather, patient plans are comprehensive and unique; what works for one patient might not be what the next one needs. Functional practitioners explore and treat the complex, dynamic, and overlapping nature of our physiology. This holistic approach may be the additional key to helping us understand and remediate unsolved conditions like Parkinson's.

SIX

Pediatrics

VIVIAN F. DeNISE,
DO, ABAARM, FAARFM

While advancements in most branches of medicine appear to be progressing at warp speed, progress in the field of pediatric neuro-cognitive disease seems to be at a prolonged, painful standstill. This leaves pediatricians and parents, the trusted caregivers of our children, helpless and hopeless. In fact, for conditions such as autism, anxiety, depression, pediatric acute-onset neuropsychiatric syndrome (PANS), pediatric auto-immune neuropsychiatric disorder associated with streptococcal infections (PANDAS), attention deficit hyperactivity disorder (ADHD), and many others, treatments are either limited or nonexistent. Currently, 7.1 percent of all children (4.4 million children) between the ages of 3 and 17 have been diagnosed with anxiety, and 3.2 percent with depression.[1] Historically our only solution had been to medicate affected children with drugs that have myriad severe side effects on their developing minds and bodies with little return. However, LDN offers an underutilized tool to blaze new frontiers with such challenging conditions. In this chapter I will share my experiences with the use of LDN in autism, anxiety, PANS/PANDAS, and juvenile chronic fatigue syndrome (CFS).

Autism Spectrum Disorder

In the past, pervasive developmental disorders that are now under the umbrella of autism spectrum disorder (ASD) were divided into autism, pervasive developmental disorder not otherwise specified (PDD-NOS), Asperger's, Rett syndrome, and childhood disintegrative disorder, classifications based on severity and age of onset of symptoms. The hallmark of

the disorder is impaired social communication and interaction with repetitive behaviors. Persons diagnosed with ASD under the *Diagnostic and
Statistical Manual of Mental Disorders,* fifth edition (DSM-5), must meet
all three criteria under the social communication / interaction domain
(deficits in social-emotional reciprocity; deficits in nonverbal communica-
tive behaviors; and deficits in developing, understanding, and maintaining
relationships) and at least two of the four criteria under the restrictive/
repetitive behavior domain (repetitive speech or motor movements, insistence on sameness, restricted interests, and unusual response to sensory
input).[2] These disturbances are not better explained by intellectual disability or global developmental delay.[3] Currently, 1 in 59 children in the United
States is diagnosed with autism, with boys four times more likely to be
diagnosed than girls.[4]

Severity is categorized into three different levels: requiring support,
requiring substantial support, and requiring very substantial support.[5]
According to the DSM-5, "the best prognostic factors for individual
outcome within the autism spectrum disorder is the presence or absence
of associated intellectual disability, language impairment, and additional
mental health problems."[6]

A BRIEF OVERVIEW OF HOW WE SPEAK

The brain has many different parts, but the largest part is the cerebrum.
The cerebrum is divided into two sides or hemispheres, the left and right.
In most people (66 percent) speech is controlled by the left side. In the
other 33 percent—usually left-handed people—speech is controlled by
the right side. Each hemisphere is further divided into lobes: the frontal,
temporal, parietal, and occipital. Speech is mainly dictated from the frontal
and temporal lobes. Each lobe is further subdivided. Within the left frontal
cerebrum is an area called Broca's area, which is responsible for turning
thoughts and ideas into actual words by sending signals to the motor
cortex, which controls movements of the mouth, forming the words. The
second area in the cerebrum is Wernicke's area, located in the temporal
lobe right behind the ear. This area is responsible for understanding speech
and producing the correct words and written language. These two areas
are bridged by the arcuate fasciculus. This structure allows communication
between the Broca's and Wernicke's areas, allowing us to form words, speak
clearly, and understand language.

Two other areas of the brain involved in speech are the cerebellum and the previously mentioned motor cortex, which is in the frontal lobe. These areas are responsible for the act of speaking. The motor cortex controls your mouth, tongue, and throat while the cerebellum controls voluntary movement of the mouth but also language processing. However, none of these areas would function without substances known as neurotransmitters.

Neurotransmitters are chemicals in the brain and peripheral nervous system that enable one nerve cell to "talk" and relay messages to the next, ultimately leading to an action. There are neurotransmitters that are excitatory, inhibitory, or sometimes both depending on which receptor site is present. Within different areas of the brain, certain neurotransmitters are more abundant and play a bigger role. In the cerebral cortex the major neurotransmitters are: serotonin, norepinephrine, dopamine, acetylcholine, and GABA. GABA, serotonin, norepinephrine and acetylcholine are distributed to all areas of the cerebral cortex, whereas dopamine is distributed to only the frontal and cingulate areas of the cerebellum.

GABA is the main neurotransmitter of the cerebellum. Its role in the body is to inhibit or reduce the activity of nerve cells. It is necessary to feel calm and relaxed, and is used by the majority of cortical neurons. In 2011 a study by Harada et al. found that children with ASD have a diminished concentration of GABA in the frontal cortex.[7] It is believed that a disruption of the GABAergic system is associated with most neurodevelopmental disorders. The term *GABAergic system* refers to the synapses involved in the synthesis or breakdown of GABA. In fact, disruption in the genes GABRA5, GABRB3, and GABRG3 found on chromosome 15q11-13 is associated with developmental delay, autism, and other clinical features observed in these contiguous gene syndromes in addition to the imprinting defects.[8]

Another neurotransmitter, serotonin, is found in the cerebellum and intestines. Often referred to as the "happy neurotransmitter," it regulates mood, social behavior, appetite, digestion, and sleep.

Norepinephrine is an excitatory neurotransmitter. It is responsible for attention, learning, and emotions, and is part of the fight or flight response. It is produced in the adrenal glands and in the central nervous system. Most of the medications for treating ADHD target norepinephrine.

Acetylcholine is the most abundant of all neurotransmitters. It is produced in the central and peripheral nervous systems. It plays a part in learning, memory formation, regulation of the endocrine system, and, lastly, REM sleep.

Dopamine is an excitatory neurotransmitter responsible for feelings of pleasure and satisfaction as well as muscle control and gastrointestinal motility. It is important for the formation of speech with movement of the tongue. The drug Ritalin, often prescribed for ADHD, works by boosting dopamine. When dopamine is increased, GABA is decreased.

We find the methyl tetrahydrofolate reductase (MTHFR) variant higher in children with autism.[9] This gene is responsible for converting inactive folic acid to active folic acid. If folic acid is given in the methylated (active) form, more can cross the blood-brain barrier, which aids in increasing the formation of neurotransmitters and therefore increasing verbal communication.

What does all this have to do with LDN? To recap, LDN blocks opioid receptors for approximately four hours. This causes an increased production of endogenous opioids (endorphins and enkephalins). This in turn causes an increase in dopamine release in the synaptic cleft. Children with ASD in particular benefit by acquiring increased muscle control and therefore increased speech formation.

CASE STUDY 1: JACK AND JOHN

Jack was three years old and John was four years old. Jack was diagnosed with significant speech and developmental delay, John with autism and had severe speech delay with almost no language.

Both children were found to be carnitine-deficient. Both were begun on L-carnitine at 100 mg/kg daily. They were started on LDN at 0.5 mg and titrated to 4.5 mg.

Jack responded almost immediately with an increase in verbal abilities and social interactions. His frustration markedly decreased, and he began to answer questions appropriately. John began to have language approximately one to two months after beginning therapy, speaking in short sentences. His social interactions also increased and he began to make eye contact as well as respond and follow directions. They both continue to make great strides in language and socialization.

CASE STUDY 2: RICHARD

Richard was a five-year-old boy diagnosed with autism. He had no language. His parents were very reluctant to begin LDN; however, when Richard was five, they decided it was worth a try. Richard was begun as usual on 0.5 mg and titrated up to 4.5 mg. He began to grow very agitated during the day and no longer slept. We decided to decrease the dose to 3 mg and reevaluate. Within one to two weeks he began to have single words, and within a month to six weeks he began speaking in sentences and asking for what he wanted.

Obsessive-Compulsive Disorder

Obsessive-compulsive disorder (OCD) is a severe, prevalent, and most often chronically debilitating disorder characterized by repetitive, ritualistic, and distressing thoughts, ideas, and behaviors over which a person typically has very little if any control.[10] Fifty percent of patients experience onset in childhood and adolescence, and 17 percent have autism as a comorbidity.[11] Selective serotonin reuptake inhibitors (SSRIs) are not always effective as a monotherapy, even in high doses. Eighty percent of serotonin is made in the gut. Often children with autism do not have great eating habits, and without a healthy gut, less serotonin is produced.[12] Hence, if a drug depends on the presence of serotonin, how can it be expected to work in patients with lesser amounts? When dopamine antagonists are added to SSRI treatments, there is a more positive treatment response.

CASE HISTORY

Noah came to see me at the age of 12 for severe anxiety, obsessive-compulsive disorder, and tic disorder. Incidentally, he had loose bowel movements. The tics were the most severe I have personally witnessed. He had just been hospitalized in our children's psychiatric department because his symptoms became unmanageable despite the usual anxiolytic medications. If he wasn't having tics, he was having obsessive thoughts and actions. Noah was unable to attend school. Subsequently his mother had to resign from her work, which led to financial strain on the family. We began a trial of LDN and titrated to 4.5 mg. He was also found to be positive (homozygous) for the C677t variant of the MTHFR gene and was started on methylated B vitamins. His gut issues were addressed using glutamine and a probiotic. I always recommend that probiotics contain at least three different organisms and a colony count of 10 billion colony-forming units (CFUs) for kids, and 20 billion for teens and adults. Finally, after several weeks Noah was able to return to school with a para, and the tics were almost nonexistent. However, at this point he was extremely fatigued and was not able to keep his focus in the afternoon. I prescribed CoQ10 at 100 mg and phosphatidylserine at 100 mg in the morning. He is now actively participating in school without a para, and without anxiety, tics, or obsessive-compulsive thoughts and actions.

Anxiety

Anxiety is the most common psychiatric disorder of childhood and adolescence. In fact, 7.1 percent of children aged 3 through 17 have been diagnosed, totaling 4.4 million in the United States.[13] Children show anxiety in many ways: school avoidance, aggression, shyness, fatigue, trouble sleeping, hypochondriasis (usually abdominal pain), depression, despondency, and bed-wetting, only to name a few. Approximately one in three children have a comorbid condition such as behavior problems or depression.[14] Anxiety is often accompanied with physical symptoms such as sweating, palpitations, chest pain, fatigue, headache, and shortness of breath. Fear and anxiety are part of normal development and are adaptive. Anxiety becomes unhealthy when it doesn't resolve within six months and sets off inappropriate or irrational behaviors.

Two major areas of the brain are responsible for anxiety: the amygdala, which is found deep within the brain, and the hippocampus. It is thought that a decrease in GABA or an increase in glutamate is responsible. We also know that serotonin, norepinephrine, and dopamine play important roles.

Some dietary factors to consider that lead to anxiety include:

Hypoglycemia: When blood sugar drops, one compensatory response of the body is to release cortisol. Cortisol produced in the adrenal glands stimulates the pancreas to release insulin. When insulin is released and doesn't have "food" to work on, the brain signals a person to eat so the blood sugar is raised. In addition, cortisol also has a compensatory response to release epinephrine and norepinephrine. When released it leads to the fight or flight response (anxiety). I always make sure that young children are allowed extra snacks and older ones eat lunch at all! Eating a healthy breakfast containing a healthy fat will result in satiety for longer. Additionally, it is extremely important to watch the sugar intake in the drinks that children are given. Other common names for sugar on food labels are dextrose, fructose, maltodextrin, xylose, and malt syrup.

Caffeine: People with anxiety are more sensitive to caffeine than people without anxiety.[15] Children typically consume caffeine in soda, chocolate, and both hot and iced tea. There was a time that caffeine was thought to be helpful for children with ADHD, but clearly this isn't the case.

Monosodium glutamate (MSG): Glutamate is a primary excitatory neurotransmitter and is the precursor to GABA. It is imperative to learning and memory. Monosodium glutamate is a derivative of glutamate and is a food enhancer added to fast food, canned vegetables, canned soups, and processed foods including meats. Per the FDA, the symptoms from ingesting this additive—including headache, flushing, sweating, facial pressure or tightness, numbness, tingling or burning in the face, neck, and other areas, heart palpitations, numbness, and weakness—have been coined the MSG symptom complex.[16]

Aspartame: Aspartame is an artificial sweetener found in more than 6,000 foods and beverages worldwide. In the body, aspartame is metabolized into aspartate + phenylalanine + methanol. Phenylalanine is a regulator of neurotransmitters, and aspartic acid is an excitatory neurotransmitter. Methanol is quickly metabolized to formaldehyde and exits the body in the urine.[17] Following ingestion of aspartame there is a decrease in dopamine and serotonin production. In addition, aspartame disrupts the blood-brain barrier, increasing its permeability and altering the concentration of catecholamines such as dopamine. Aspartame metabolites cause neurobehavioral changes. Aspartame is associated with increased irritability, migraines, depression, and weaker spatial orientation.[18]

Lack of sleep is also a predictor of anxiety in adolescents.[19] Sleep disturbances have been found to co-occur with several psychiatric disorders, including anxiety and depression.[20] In addition co-sleeping at least two to four times per week is common for one in three children with anxiety. The more severe the anxiety, the more frequent co-sleeping.[21]

Traditional therapies for anxiety usually include antidepressants that work on increasing serotonin, norepinephrine, and dopamine. Buspirone stimulates serotonin and dopamine receptors, and the benzodiazepines increase the availability of GABA.

Side effects of these and other anxiolytics include drowsiness to sedation and confusion. Weight gain is a common side effect that is problematic in children who are already anxious in social situations. They also create a dependence. In addition to gut dysfunction (nausea, diarrhea, or constipation), there is also the possibility of headache and sexual dysfunction. Blood pressure and arrythmias must be monitored even in children. If these aren't bad enough, there is also the potential for suicidal thoughts.

Functional treatments of anxiety include:

- L-theanine 200 mg, one to three times a day.
- Magnesium glycinate 200 mg, two to three times a day.
- B complex. Because all B vitamins are in a delicate balance, it is better to take a complex instead of individual B vitamins.
- Folic acid. Individuals with the MTHFR gene mutation need to take methylated folic acid.
- 5-HTP, 50 to 200 mg per day, usually taken at night.
- Making sure there is no yeast overgrowth or food allergy. Because it is believed that 80 to as much as 95 percent of serotonin is made in the gut, it is important to make sure it is in good working order.[22]
- LDN beginning at 0.5 and titrating to 4.5 mg, depending on the response of the patient.

CASE HISTORY

A 13-year-old young man with dyslexia and global learning deficiencies, as well as a known MTHFR gene mutation, was seen for severe anxiety and insomnia. He underwent multiple drug trials to no avail. He was started on LDN beginning at 0.5 mg titrating up to 4.5 mg, and methylated B vitamins. Within a week and a half his demeanor changed. He became happier, less anxious, and more social. He was less defiant, was less confrontational, and began to sleep. In addition his appetite was in better control. At one point he tried not taking the LDN, and disruptive behaviors emerged once again.

PANDAS

Imagine putting your child to sleep one night and waking up with a totally different child. One that is anxious, aggressive, having obsessive and/or compulsive thoughts or actions. One that suddenly is having severe separation anxiety, and quite possibly a tic. This is how a child with pediatric autoimmune neuropsychiatric disorder associated with streptococcal infections often presents.

PANDAS was first recognized in 1998 by Dr. Susan Swedo, who found children with an abrupt onset of behavioral abnormalities including tics and/or OCD associated with a recent group A beta hemolytic streptococcal infection (GABHS). PANDAS is thought to be an extreme autoimmune response to GABHS. Approximately 1 in 200 children are affected by PANDAS and PANS.[23] The average age of diagnosis is between 4 and 13 for PANDAS, but there is no age limit for PANS. The clinical course is relapsing and remitting for both. PANS can be caused by any infection. PANS is also differentiated by an abrupt, dramatic onset of obsessive-compulsive syndrome and/or severe restricted intake of food. There may be severe anxiety, usually in the form of separation anxiety. School performance dramatically and suddenly deteriorates. Daytime enuresis may occur in a child already toilet-trained. The tics may be in a choreiform movement (fine piano-like playing movements of the fingers when outstretched).* Diagnosis is one of exclusion. All other causes either neurological and medical must be ruled out first.

Childhood acute neuropsychiatric syndrome (CANS) is a newly described syndrome and linked to toxic exposure to phthalates, PCBs, and heavy metals. Other causes include autoimmune issues, trauma (concussions), and hypoxia.

THE PATHOPHYSIOLOGY

This disease process occurs through molecular mimicry: The body makes autoantibodies that attack the basal ganglia of the brain. Molecular mimicry is a very important part of any autoimmune disease. It's when the body mistakes normal tissue for the "enemy" because of some molecular similarity between it and a part of the bacteria or virus, or receptor, and attacks it. This causes inflammation, which leads to malfunction of the area—hence neuropsychiatric symptoms. In the case of PANS/PANDAS, the body mistakenly attacks the basal ganglia in the brain. The basal ganglia are a group of neurons located deep within the cerebrum. They are responsible for coordinating voluntary movement, habitual learning, and emotion.

---

* The choreiform movement must be differentiated from Sydenham's chorea. Sydenham's chorea occurs in rheumatic fever that is also caused by group A beta hemolytic strep. In this disease there is chorea, which is jerking, rigid movements of large muscle groups that are not repeated or rhythmic, often accompanied by athetosis, a writhing movement.

Habitual learning is repeating behavior so that it becomes routine and without thought. For example, if you drive to work every day taking the same path, most of the time you don't even think about the turns and just arrive at your destination. The basal ganglia typically are affected by three neurotransmitters: GABA, dopamine, and glutamate.

In the case of PANDAS, repeated streptococcus pyogenes (group a beta hemolytic streptococcus) infections activate inflammatory cytokines (IL-6 and TGF-B1). These cytokines in turn activate strep pyogenes specific Th17 cells, which increase capillary permeability in several areas of the brain, allowing for invasion of autoantibodies. There is also an immunoglobulin G (IgG) induced elevation leading to an increase in calmodulin-dependent protein kinase II (CaMKII).[24]

In addition, evidence strongly suggests that human anti-brain autoantibodies induced by streptococcus pyogenes infections target the dopamine receptors, lysoganglioside, and tubulin, as well as activation of CaMKII.[25] In another study PANDAS patients were divided into two groups, one without choreiform movement and one with it. In the group without choreiform movement, there was elevation in antibodies against D2R, but in both groups there was an elevation in CaMKII, therefore making it a biomarker that needs to be investigated more.[26]

Diagnosis of PANDAS is made with a positive strep culture or Cunningham Panel. If there isn't a positive strep culture but there is a high index of suspicion, it is prudent to follow the ASO and DNase titers. ASO titers usually rise one to four weeks after the infection, and DNase will rise six to eight weeks after the infection. If there is a subsequent flare (a resurgence or peaking of symptoms), strep does not have to be a culprit; any infection can cause it.

The diagnosis for PANS is more challenging, as any infection can be the cause. Titers for Lyme and the Lyme co-infections such as babesiosis, ehrlichiosis, anaplasmosis, and bartonellosis should be obtained. Mycoplasma is also often a culprit, as well as viral illnesses including mononucleosis, Epstein-Barr, and influenza. Until this year respiratory syncytial virus (RSV) was usually confined to infants and young children, but this year I had two cases in adolescents.

TREATMENT

The following is not intended to be a thorough review but rather an overview. For patients or physicians who want a more in-depth review of treatments, see the website for the PANDAS Physicians Network (www.pandasppn.org) or the PANS Research Consortium.

Use of various treatments depend on the severity of the patient. Sometimes, if a case is mild, a watch and wait approach with psychological support is called for. Most physicians start with an antibiotic, awaiting the results of the blood tests. If a patient does not respond to treatment or has a high relapse rate, it is prudent to test all members of the family for group A strep. Even if the patient does not have it, being exposed via household contact may be enough to spark symptoms.

The following recommendations are based on those of the PANDAS Physicians Network:

Patients should undergo a thorough physical as well as psychological evaluation. Baseline studies such as EKG, EEG, blood chemistries, and brain MRI should be included. Emotional support for patients and their families are just as important as medical treatment, and must be started immediately. Cognitive behavioral therapy seems to be the most effective for all concerned.[27]

Depending on the severity, OCD, ADHD, aggression, depression, separation anxiety, and sudden weight loss or loss of appetite can be and should be pharmacologically addressed if needed. If there is any indication the patient is suicidal, or behavior is severe, then hospitalization is warranted.

School support is essential; however, school authorities are often unaware of this illness or are skeptical. A school's acknowledgment and understanding is imperative to the well-being of the student, as sometimes teachers and staff witness the onset before anyone else. Provisions must be made either through a 504 Plan (other health impaired) or an Individualized Education Program (IEP). For example, if a child is having a sudden deterioration in handwriting, the use of a scribe would be beneficial, as would allowing the patient to submit work that is typed. Sometimes assignments can be completed late or not at all without negative impact on the child's grades. It is up to the patient's support team to assure these needs be met.

Antibiotics

Antibiotics can be used at the onset of both PANS and PANDAS cases. Initially, the penicillins (including Augmentin), and cephalosporins are used. In my opinion Augmentin is a superior choice because it contains clavulanic acid. In recent literature it was found to have excellent penetration of the blood-brain barrier. Additionally, it has been found to have antidepressant effects as well as decreasing anxiety due to a dopamine release. It also has been implicated in inhibiting neurotoxins, which leads to neuronal survival.[28] Most clinicians treat for three weeks, and then reevaluate. If the patient responds, then the treatment may continue another two to four weeks.

If the patient is allergic or does not respond to the treatment within the first two weeks, then azithromycin or clarithromycin may be used. However, it is important to be aware of patients that have a prolonged QT interval, hence the need for an initial EKG. It is also contraindicated in patients already on medications that prolong the QT interval, such as SSRIs, antipsychotic medications, and psychoactive medications. After the initial course of treatment, the patient should be recultured two to seven days post-treatment. If this culture is positive, then the patient needs to be retreated. The clinician and family must be on the watch for household or close contacts that may be affected as well.

Long-term streptococcal prophylaxis is usually reserved for the most severely affected patients or those that have recurrent group A strep infection that experience multiple neuropsychiatric complications.

Mycoplasma pneumonia is tested by obtaining IgG and IgM titers. Mycoplasma infections are associated with many neurologic diseases including transverse myelitis and Tourette's. IgG titers will remain elevated, so it is better to watch the IgM titer.

Lyme borreliosis as well as the co-infections (Anaplasma, Babesia, et cetera) are treated with macrolides. The current recommendations are that even children under eight years of age should be treated with macrolides. It was once thought that the use of macrolides had an adverse effect on teeth if given prior to eight years of age, but that is no longer believed.

Non-Steroidal Anti-Inflammatories

These are used in cases that are mild to moderate in which symptoms last more than two weeks, and especially if they worsen. Treatment is usually six weeks or as tolerated.

Steroids

For mild to moderate cases, corticosteroids can be extremely helpful, especially in the first three days. Treatment is considered a short "burst," as it is only given for five days. If the patient relapses once the steroids are stopped, they can be restarted and then perhaps either given another burst or a longer course to be tapered gradually. Side effects to be aware of include worsening of obsessive-compulsive behavior, anxiety, rage, agitation, depression, emotional lability, or insomnia.

For moderate to severe cases, IV methylprednisolone can be given for three to five days. If a good response is received initially and then wanes, intravenous immunoglobulin (IVIg) may be added. IVIg can also be given alone for one to three days.

For severe cases, TPE (plasmapheresis) in five single doses for 7 to 10 days provides optimal results.[29] Possible side effects secondary to hypogammaglobulinemia may be alleviated with IVIg being given alongside and/or a brief burst of corticosteroids.

Tonsillectomy

The tonsils of patients with PANDAS have elevated levels of a substance called Th17. In animal research this substance has been shown to be an agent that opens the blood-brain barrier, therefore letting the antibodies penetrate this barrier in targeted areas of the brain.

Serotonin Selective Reuptake Inhibitors

Serotonin selective reuptake inhibitors (SSRIs) may be useful in the treatment of PANS/PANDAS as a treatment for obsessive compulsive behavior, anxiety, and depression.

Group A strep produces inflammatory cytokines in the brain, which can be suppressed by SSRIs. SSRIs are begun at a quarter of the regular dose and increased gradually. Additionally, if the patient does not have a healthy gut, SSRIs may not work, as 80 percent of the serotonin in the body is produced in the gut by good bacteria.

Note that black box warnings are associated with the use of SSRIs. These warnings include an increased risk of suicidal thoughts and behaviors. If these symptoms occur the drugs must be withdrawn immediately but gradually and the patient carefully observed or hospitalized.

Antifungals

It is prudent that patients on prolonged use of antibiotics be monitored for yeast infections either in the mouth (thrush) or vaginally as well as on other mucosal surfaces such as the rectum and the penis. If so, the yeast infection—like any infection—must be dealt with quickly.

Antihistamines

Histamine is an excitatory neurotransmitter that assists in controlling the sleep-wake cycle, as well as energy and motivation. There are two kinds of antihistamines. Both kinds are anti-inflammatory as well as being immune modulators. They are H_1 blockers, which are your typical allergy medications such as diphenhydramine, fexofenadine, and so forth. H_2 blockers work in the stomach and go by names such as cimetidine and ranitidine.

In some people antihistamines have what's known as an idiosyncratic reaction. That is, instead of being sedating (which can be beneficial in a patient experiencing insomnia), the medication causes the patient to become agitated.

Low Dose Naltrexone

Usually I begin patients at 0.5 mg at bedtime and increase by 0.5 mg weekly until I reach a dose in which we see a change, sometimes needing to go up to 4.5 mg to get a desired response. LDN increases endogenous enkephalins and endorphins, which leads to enhancement of the immune function of the body. LDN inhibits pro-inflammatory cytokines by regulation of T regular cells—a type of T cell that acts to suppress immune response therefore maintaining homeostasis, as well as inhibiting T-cell and cytokine proliferation—and production of IL-10 and TGF-B, which downregulate Th17. Th17 is the substance that increases the permeability of the vasculature in the brain and allows antibodies to penetrate and attack the basal ganglia.

CASE HISTORY

Jane was a 19-year-old college student. During her first year she began experiencing panic attacks and wanted to leave college despite doing well academically. She came home on a school holiday, and after completing a thorough workup it was determined she was MTHFR-positive, and positive for mycoplasma pneumoniae IgG as well as IgM. A diagnosis of PANS was made, and she was begun on Augmentin for a three-week course. After one week her anxiety and panic attacks seemed to decrease to a manageable level. We decided to continue the Augmentin for another three weeks. After the vacation she was ready to return to school, almost excited. A few short weeks later, the anxiety and panic attacks returned. She began LDN at 1 mg and titrated up quickly to 4.5 mg. The panic attacks once again subsided and remain very manageable.

Juvenile Chronic Fatigue Syndrome

Most people associate fibromyalgia and chronic fatigue syndrome with adult patients. However, children and adolescents experience CFS more frequently than expected, and its prevalence is rising. According to the Mayo Clinic, 2 to 6 percent of schoolchildren are affected. Most are adolescent females between the ages of 13 and 15, but I have diagnosed it in male children.[30]

There may be no single reason a child acquires this illness, although a frequent cause of juvenile chronic fatigue syndrome is psychological stress due to bullying, family disruption, death of a parent or sibling, academic stress, overscheduling of after-school activities, and social media. Another cause is physical stress such as accidents, concussion, overtraining or -exercising, mitochondrial dysfunction, surgery, or infections.

In addition, the MTHFR gene variant, which inhibits the way the body processes folic acid, can also be one of the causes leading to chronic fatigue, as active folic acid is an essential building block of adenosine triphosphate (ATP) synthesis. ATP is essential to produce energy in cells, and therefore to the patient's energy level. If the patient does not have enough active folic acid, then ATP will be lacking and overall energy will be low. There also seems to be a genetic predisposition, as CFS often affects multiple family members.

SYMPTOMS

Patients with juvenile chronic fatigue syndrome experience widespread pain (usually a dull ache) for a duration greater than six months, and at least four of the following symptoms. Pain must be felt on both sides and both above and below the diaphragm. Headaches are usually severe and frequent. Patients experience sleep disturbance, having difficulty both falling and staying asleep. Even if the patient can sleep, they often report severe fatigue. When sleep is disrupted, sleep apnea and restless legs syndrome are often reported. In addition, patients experience abdominal pain and cognitive impairment; ADHD, anxiety, and depression are often present as well.

DIAGNOSIS

In 1985 Dr. Muhammad Yunus and Dr. Alfonse Masi published a clinical study in *Arthritis and Rheumatology* that developed a criterion to diagnose fibromyalgia in the pediatric population. All major criteria and at least 3 of the 10 minor criteria must be met.[31]

Major criteria include generalized musculoskeletal aching in at least three sites for greater than three months, and four to five tender points. There is an absence of underlying conditions such as rheumatoid arthritis, Lyme disease, mono, et cetera. The patient must have normal test results.

Minor criteria can include chronic anxiety or tension, fatigue, poor sleep, chronic headaches, irritable bowel syndrome, subjective soft tissue swelling and numbness, and pain on activity, affected by weather or accentuated with stress and anxiety.[32]

While there are no definitive blood tests, in integrative medicine the following are often performed to rule out other disorders such as a complete blood count (CBC), erythrocyte sedimentation rate (ESR), and thyroid studies: serum ammonia, lactic acid, serum magnesium, carnitine, CoQ10 levels, and MTHFR.

TREATMENT

Treatment for juvenile chronic fatigue syndrome includes cognitive behavioral therapy and medications to control pain and lessen anxiety and depression, as per individual patient needs. The following are guidelines for patients diagnosed with juvenile CFS; however, each patient should have bloodwork done and an individualized plan created based on their test results:

- Magnesium glycinate 200 mg, two to three times a day if a deficiency is determined.
- L-theanine 200 mg, two to three times a day for anxiety and at bedtime for sleep.
- Melatonin 1 mg at bedtime for sleep.
- Carnitine 500 mg daily.
- CoQ10 60 to 100 mg daily.
- Lactulose syrup if ammonia levels are high: 1 teaspoon one to two times a day until stools are loose to decrease ammonia.
- In the case of patients with the MTHFR gene variant, supplementing with methylated folic acid is essential.
- Low dose naltrexone. Pain receptors in the brain are stimulated by pro-inflammatory cytokines, which are also responsible for fatigue. By decreasing these substances, there is a decrease in pain and fatigue.[33] Once again, the therapeutic dose is different for each patient, but I find most fall within the range of 3 to 4.5 mg.

CASE HISTORY

Paul, a 10-year-old, came with the diagnosis of ADHD that was resistant to all medications. He was exhausted and would go to bed at seven or eight o'clock and wake up very early in the morning. When he went to sleep later, he still would wake up at the same time. Speaking with him revealed a bright 10-year-old who spoke frequently about being picked on by other children and teachers. The school situation got so difficult that the district agreed for him to change elementary schools. In my opinion he didn't have ADHD but in fact had severe anxiety and juvenile chronic fatigue syndrome. His morning cortisol level was low, and serum ammonia and lactic acid levels were high. He was begun on CoQ10, which was included in a compounded mitochondrial formula aimed at mitochondrial dysfunction. Paul admitted to feeling much better and was beginning to sleep. His anxiety persisted. He was begun on LDN. At first his mom did not feel it was working and stopped it. Several months later the mom asked to restart it, and we are waiting to see the results.

SEVEN

Women's Health

Olga L. Cortez, MD, OB-GYN, FACOG

As low dose naltrexone finds its place among other therapies in the treatment of autoimmune disorders, it has now also made a contribution to women's health. A worthy question, then, is, "If you have a medication that reverses autoimmune disorders and decreases inflammation in chronic infections, how can this then be translated to the treatment of pelvic problems that are not autoimmune in nature?" The two main diagnoses that we will be addressing in this chapter— endometriosis and polycystic ovarian syndrome—have now been shown to have an inflammatory component. Seen in this light, these conditions can understandably be treated with LDN as an adjunct to traditional medical therapies.

Endometriosis

Endometriosis is defined by the American College of Obstetricians and Gynecologists (ACOG) as "a condition in which the type of tissue that forms the lining of the uterus (the endometrium) is found outside the uterus."[1] This typically causes significant pelvic pain during menstruation, and eventually extends to pelvic pain outside of menstruation. Traditionally, endometriosis has been treated either hormonally (with birth control pills, progestin IUDs, or gonadotropin-releasing hormone agonists), or surgically (the more conservative procedure being laparoscopy, and the more definitive, hysterectomy). So why try a pill that is used to treat autoimmune disorders?

A PubMed search of "endometriosis and autoimmune" returns a list of entries dating back to the 1980s. A 1987 article in the journal *Obstetrics and Gynecology* shows that abnormal polyclonal B-cell activation, a characteristic of autoimmune disorders, is associated with endometriosis.[2] Many experts agree that there is a definite inflammatory component to endometriosis. To treat endometriosis as though it were purely an autoimmune disorder, though, would be a disservice to the patient, as it is a multifactorial disease. Endometriosis requires a multifaceted treatment approach, but LDN can be a significant component of the regimen.

The following are some case studies from my private practice demonstrating LDN's effect on endometriosis patients.

CASE #1

The patient is a 23-year-old Caucasian female who presented with a long-standing history of pelvic pain and recurrent bladder infections. She had been on birth control pills for the past few years, which brought her some pain relief. Her pelvic sonogram was normal, but she felt like she had a persistent bladder infection. A urologist treated the patient for presumed interstitial cystitis. None of the treatment options offered by her urologist helped the patient.

When she presented at my practice, given that the patient did not have a definitive diagnosis, she opted to have a diagnostic laparoscopy. Endometriosis was discovered and excised. The patient had a Mirena IUD inserted one month later for continued endometriosis control. Two months later the patient reported a return of her pelvic pain and dysuria. The urine culture obtained was negative. She was placed on Elavil by her urologist. Over the next three years, the patient was seen by a pain management specialist. She then had her IUD removed for fertility reasons, and became pregnant a few months later. After a normal pregnancy, the patient underwent a primary cesarean section for failure to progress while in labor. The patient breastfed for the next several months.

A year after her delivery, the patient experienced a return of her pelvic pain and unexpected weight gain. A second pelvic sonogram was normal. Given her failure to respond to traditional therapies in the past, the patient was offered a trial of low dose naltrexone, which she accepted.

The patient started on LDN at a dose of 1 mg once daily, and slowly titrated up. Three months after starting LDN, her pain was significantly reduced. She had occasional bladder pain.

The patient has now been on LDN for over two years with good control of her pelvic pain. Her current dose is 8 mg once daily.

CASE #2

The patient is a 39-year-old Hispanic female who presented with a long-standing history of pelvic pain from endometriosis. She had nausea and emesis with each period. The patient had tried birth control pills and pain medication in the past, neither of which helped her pain significantly. She also had a laparoscopy for endometriosis excision and ovarian cyst removal. Her pelvic pain returned a few months after surgery.

The patient had a hysterosalpingogram as part of a fertility workup a few years ago. She was informed that one of her fallopian tubes was completely closed, and the other mostly closed. A recent pelvic sonogram was normal.

After initial lab tests with our office, the patient was discovered to have Hashimoto's thyroiditis. She was therefore offered low dose naltrexone, starting at 0.5 mg daily. We increased her daily dose by 0.5 mg each week, until she was taking 4.5 mg daily. Three months later the patient reported that her menstrual cycles were no longer painful. Six months later the patient requested a repeat hysterosalpingogram. Her hysterosalpingogram is now normal, with bilateral patent fallopian tubes.

CASE #3

The patient is a 36-year-old Caucasian female with two prior pregnancies and deliveries. She presented with a long-standing history of endometriosis. She had a Mirena IUD placed in 2010, after the birth of her last child. This worked well for pain management at that time. Her Mirena IUD was replaced with a new Mirena in 2015.

The patient presented in early 2018 with severe abdominal pain and abdominal bloating that only occurred on the 10th/11th of every month and again on the 23rd/24th of every month. She had no periods, as would be expected with a Mirena IUD. She had nightly nausea and emesis during her pain episodes. Three different gastroenterologists had seen the patient. She underwent an endoscopy and colonoscopy, both of which were normal. She then underwent a cholecystectomy, which was uneventful. She was told that her pain was possibly the result of IBS, but none of the medications prescribed by her gastroenterologist helped. Given the cyclic nature of her pain, we determined that it could be the result of her endometriosis, and her Mirena IUD was replaced for the second time.

At her two-month follow-up, the patient reported that the intensity of the pain had lessened but not completely resolved. The patient was then offered low dose naltrexone. We began at 1 mg once daily, increasing her daily dose each week by 1 mg. When she reached 4.5 mg per day, the patient did not have a resolution of her pelvic pain. We therefore instructed her to continue increasing her dose weekly until she reached 9 mg daily.

After three months on low dose naltrexone, the patient is now pain-free. Her GI symptoms have also resolved.

CASE #4

The patient is a 23-year-old Hispanic female with no prior pregnancies who presented to our office with severe pelvic pain, uncontrollable nausea, and vomiting during her periods. Her symptoms kept her at home while she was menstruating. At times, she also had pelvic pain before or after her periods. The patient had a pelvic sonogram, and the results were normal. We discussed the possibility that she had endometriosis that was not visible on the sonogram.

Lab work showed an elevated thyroglobulin antibody level of 1.0. The patient was therefore diagnosed with Hashimoto's thyroiditis. Low dose naltrexone was offered as a treatment option, which she accepted. She was started on 0.5 mg daily and increased her dose each week until she reached a dose of 4.5 mg daily.

Three months later the patient stated that the pelvic pain during her periods persisted but had improved. Her nausea was mild and unaccompanied by vomiting. Her thyroglobulin antibody level had increased, rather than decreased, to 1.6, so we therefore increased her dose to 9 mg daily.

After another three months her thyroglobulin antibody level was zero. She now has very mild pelvic pain with her periods, and no longer has any nausea or vomiting. She is very happy with these results.

Polycystic Ovarian Syndrome

Polycystic ovarian syndrome (PCOS) is defined by the American College of Obstetricians and Gynecologists as "a disorder characterized by hyperandrogenism, ovulatory dysfunction, and polycystic ovaries."[3] Patients with this condition can have a constellation of symptoms, including amenorrhea or menorrhagia, hirsutism, acne, insulin resistance, metabolic syndrome, and obesity. This condition is traditionally treated with combined hormonal contraception, progestin-only therapy, insulin-sensitizing agents (such as metformin), and lifestyle modifications (diet and exercise). Other therapies can be added depending on the patient's needs. For example, anti-androgenic medications such as spironolactone can be used for hirsut-ism or acne, while Clomid or letrozole can be used to induce ovulation in those patients wanting to conceive. The challenge in treating polycystic ovarian syndrome is that its etiology is largely unknown.

There are studies available showing that naltrexone can work as an adjunct or in isolation as a treatment for PCOS and related complications. For example, a 1997 study showed that "ovulation can be induced success-fully using naltrexone alone or naltrexone in combination with an anti-oestrogen in clomiphene citrate resistant anovulatory patients."[4]

Low dose naltrexone is safe to use with hormonal contraception, insulin-sensitizing agents, anti-androgenic agents, or medications for ovulation induction.

The following are some case studies demonstrating LDN's effect on PCOS patients.

CASE #5

The patient is a 28-year-old female who had been diagnosed with PCOS 10 years prior to visiting my office. She had been previously treated with birth control pills and had a laparoscopic ovarian cystectomy. The patient did not like birth control, as it caused her to have mood swings and intermenstrual bleeding. She also had recurrent bladder infections that she was attempting to address with a urologist. When she presented to our office, she was not on any birth control and had a pelvic sonogram consistent with PCOS.

The patient was diagnosed with Hashimoto's thyroiditis at this time, with a thyroglobulin antibody level of 2.1. She was offered low dose naltrexone as a treatment option. She began LDN at a dose of 0.5 mg daily, and slowly titrated up until she reached 4.5 mg daily. Three months later her thyro-globulin antibody level was zero and has remained there for over a year. The patient also developed normal monthly menstruation cycles and has only had two bladder infections in the past 12 months, since starting LDN.

CASE #6

The patient is a 24-year-old female who stopped birth control after several years of use, as she desired a pregnancy. Nine months after ending her birth control, she presented to our office with pelvic pain and irregular periods and was found to have PCOS. After discussing treatment options, the patient decided to try Clomid for ovulation induction in the fall 2018. After she failed to conceive on Clomid, the patient tried a gluten-free, dairy-free, sugar-free diet. She still did not conceive, but did lose approximately 15 pounds (6.8 kg). The duration between her periods was still elongated at this point—33 to 47 days. By April 2019 her anti-Müllerian hormone (AMH) level was 7.75 (greater than 6 is indicative of PCOS). The patient then opted to try low dose naltrexone. She was started on 2.25 mg daily and titrated to 9 mg daily. By October 2019 her AMH had declined to 4.32. She now has normal monthly cycles without the use of Clomid.

CASE #7

The patient is a 27-year-old female with a known history of Hashimoto's thyroiditis who presented to our office with an inability to conceive after eight months of attempting. On a pelvic sonogram, the patient was found to have multiple bilateral peripheral follicles consistent with PCOS. Her AMH at this time was 10.2. She had been making dietary changes and supplementing to decrease her thyroid antibody number. Given her eagerness to conceive, she agreed to try LDN. Even though we were treating her PCOS, we began her dose at 0.5 mg daily due to her Hashimoto's thyroiditis, increasing the dose weekly until she reached a dose of 4.5 mg daily. After nine months, the patient had a spontaneous miscarriage.

She then became disillusioned with the process and stopped LDN. After almost a year of not conceiving under the oversight of a reproductive endocrinologist, she agreed to restart LDN. At this point she could no longer tolerate LDN tablets due to side effects. We therefore switched her to LDN cream. We again started at 0.5 mg daily and increased the dose weekly until she reached a dose of 4.5 mg daily.

The patient now has normal monthly menstrual cycles and a thyroid peroxidase (TPO) antibody level lower than she has ever had. During this time, she has also eliminated caffeine, gluten, and artificial sweeteners from her diet.

Hormonal Changes

As we have treated patients for various conditions over the past few years using LDN in conjunction with other medications, we have often seen changes in our patients' hormone levels in their bloodwork. In some cases, these changes are clinically significant to the patient. While research in this area is lacking, a case study from my private practice demonstrates the potential for this outcome.

CASE #8

The patient is a 37-year-old Hispanic female with no prior pregnancies who had never used contraception and wanted to conceive. She stated that she menstruates once a month. Her period normally lasts 10 days. The first four days of her cycle consist of heavy bleeding with passing of blood clots vaginally. Her sonogram showed a 5 cm intramural fibroid, but was otherwise normal. She added that her menstrual cycles were very painful. Her initial blood lab work showed the following:

- Follicle-stimulating hormone (FSH): 16.6
- Estradiol: 58.8
- Testosterone: 3
- Progesterone: 3.0
- AMH: 0.306

Given her desire for fertility, a hysterosalpingogram was performed and was found to be normal. Treatment options were discussed at this point. The patient decided that she would like to try low dose naltrexone. The patient started at 2.25 mg daily and increased her dose to 4.5 mg daily. (She was instructed to increase her LDN dose past that but chose to stop at 4.5 mg daily.) After three months she reported that her periods were no longer painful. Her three-month follow-up bloodwork showed the following:

- FSH: 6.8
- Estradiol: 90.0
- Testosterone: 9
- Progesterone: 0.3 (while menstruating)
- AMH: 0.535

Her estrogen had increased with the corresponding decrease in FSH, her testosterone had increased slightly, and, more important, her AMH had increased after just three months. She was instructed to increase her dose of low dose naltrexone to 9 mg daily and follow up again in three to six months. Her next set of labs were as follows:

- FSH: 5.4
- Estradiol: 559.4
- Testosterone: 7
- Progesterone: 6.6
- AMH: 0.488

Again, her estrogen levels had improved, but there was no improvement in her testosterone or AMH levels.

This case brings up an important point. Typically, with a patient such as this, we would do a further workup (comprehensive stool study, food intolerance testing, testing for chronic infection, et cetera). However, the patient was self-pay and on limited funds, and so could not afford any further testing to determine the underlying source of inflammation. In the end, although low dose naltrexone can be used to decrease overall inflammation, if a patient has a source of inflammation that is not being addressed, it is less likely it will improve in the long term.

Fertility Changes

Infertility is a complex condition with multiple contributing factors. Although LDN cannot be classified as an infertility medication, it has been shown to help improve fertility. A 1993 study showed that naltrexone at a dose of 25 to 150 mg per day was found to cause a "complete normalization of the menstrual cycle in 49 of 66 patients." In addition, "of the 16 patients in the study also receiving infertility treatments, 18 pregnancies were achieved."[5]

CASE #9

The patient is a 38-year-old Hispanic female with two children, ages 21 and 17. She has used no form of contraception since delivering her 17-year-old. The patient has a long-standing history of PCOS and has had difficulty losing weight. Her periods are irregular, occurring every two to four months. The patient cannot tolerate birth control pills due to hypertension. She declines other forms of contraception that are progestin alone. She has been on metformin for several years as she works on losing weight with no success.

The patient's primary care physician discovered that she had an elevated uric acid level. The patient was then offered low dose naltrexone as a possible treatment option. Over the next year her weight dropped from 250 pounds (113.4 kg) to 215 pounds (97.5 kg) with no change in her diet or exercise routine. During this time she also developed normal monthly menstrual cycles, and her uric acid level dropped from 8.3 to 6.3. At age 39 she had an unplanned pregnancy. She continues to have normal monthly periods while on LDN.

Dosing Regimen

Below I will list the protocols that we have developed at our clinic, Cross Roads Hormonal Health and Wellness, after working with LDN since 2016. We instruct our patients that they may take LDN morning or night.

0.5 MG PROTOCOL

For this protocol we have the patient start at 0.5 mg once daily and increase the daily dose by 0.5 mg each week until they reach the goal of 4.5 mg daily.

This protocol is typically reserved for Hashimoto's thyroiditis patients, or any patient who might be prone to side effects with medications. We find that one week is enough time for most patients to adjust to a given dose, but this titration can be slowed down as needed. I have had patients stay on a given dose for one to three months before they are able to tolerate an increase. Dosing regimens should be tailored to the patient. If a patient feels great at 2 mg daily but has headaches or fatigue at 2.5 mg daily, then return to the 2 mg daily dose. The patient could stay at that dose for at least a month before you attempt to increase the dose again.

1 MG PROTOCOL

For this protocol, we have the patient start at 1 mg once daily and increase the daily dose by 1 mg each week until they reach the goal of 4.5 mg daily.

This dosing regimen is used for non-Hashimoto's autoimmune disorder patients who are not prone to side effects. This is currently the most infrequently used protocol of the three that we use in our clinic.

2.25 MG PROTOCOL

For this protocol, we have the patient start at 2.25 mg once daily and increase the daily dose by 2.25 mg each week until they reach the goal of 9 mg daily.

This is the most commonly used protocol for our gynecologic patients. Again, the titration should be tailored to the patient. If the patient cannot tolerate beginning at 2.25 mg, then we convert the patient to either the 1 mg protocol or the 0.5 mg protocol and titrate the dose on a slower schedule.

Unlike the other two protocols, this protocol will work the patient up to a dose of 9 mg per day. In our experience, many gynecologic conditions require a higher dose of LDN before we see an effect on the inflammatory component of the condition.

DIFFERENT COMPOUNDED FORMULATIONS

In our office we start all patients on LDN tablets, not capsules. We find that the patient's risk of incurring side effects is higher with capsules. The most common side effects that we hear about from patients taking capsules are headaches, worsening fatigue, and swelling. If a patient wishes to transition to capsules, we wait until they have reached their dosage goal and warn them that they may experience side effects with the capsules that they did not have with the tablets.

If a patient cannot tolerate LDN tablets, even at the 0.5 mg dose, then we convert them to a transdermal LDN cream. We then titrate up the cream dosage as we would a tablet dosage, using the above protocols. In our practice, we do not attempt to convert a patient using LDN cream to an oral formulation, as they're not likely to have developed a tolerance for the oral tablet.

DOSING FOR GYNECOLOGIC CONDITION WITH HASHIMOTO'S THYROIDITIS

For patients with this comorbidity, we always follow the 0.5 mg protocol and monitor them once they have reached the desired dose of 4.5 mg daily. Keep in mind that many gynecologic conditions do not improve at 4.5 mg daily. We usually need to continue titrating the dose until it is closer to 9 mg daily, depending on what the patient can tolerate.

DOSING FOR GYNECOLOGIC CONDITION WITH NON-HASHIMOTO'S THYROIDITIS AUTOIMMUNE DISORDER

With these patients, we err on the side of caution and use the 1 mg protocol. The 2.25 mg protocol is another option, but may be too much, too fast for this population of patients. Again, we work up to an intended dose of 4.5 mg daily, with the knowledge that the patient may need to continue increasing their dose to 9 mg daily in order to see an improvement in their gynecologic symptoms.

Conclusion

Low dose naltrexone has been shown repeatedly to be safe and effective for patients battling health conditions with inflammatory components, including PCOS and endometriosis. As we are looking to expand our treatment options in the field of women's health care, further research involving low dose naltrexone could lead to exciting possibilities.

EIGHT

Traumatic Brain Injury

Sarah J. Zielsdorf, MD, MS

Medicine is fraught with many misconceptions about head injuries, though our knowledge is rapidly expanding with new research that is leading to dramatic paradigm shifts in treatment. Traumatic brain injury (TBI) is defined as any brain pathology—including the alteration of brain function—attributed to an external, mechanical force. In recent years TBI classification has been subdivided. The most frequently occurring form of TBI is mild traumatic brain injury (mTBI), which the American Congress of Rehabilitation Medicine (ACRM) defines as an acute brain injury resulting from mechanical energy to the head from external physical forces, with any of the following symptoms: loss of consciousness (LOC) not exceeding 30 minutes, post-traumatic amnesia (PTA) for no more than 24 hours, a score of greater than or equal to 13 on the Glasgow Coma Scale (GCS) 30 minutes after injury (or upon presentation), a period (duration unspecified) of confusion/disorientation, or other transient neurologic abnormalities such as focal signs or seizures.[1]

Mild TBI has been further divided into subcategories of "complicated" and "uncomplicated." These categories are determined by the presence or absence of computed tomography (CT) abnormalities. Up to 10 percent of emergency department patients who exhibit imaging abnormalities (subarachnoid hemorrhage, intracranial contusions, or small extra-axial hematomas) have complicated mTBIs. A GCS of 13 to 15 is considered a minor injury, 9 to 12 is considered moderate, and 8 or less, severe.[2] While most TBI clinical trials utilize the GCS as their primary selection criterion for inclusion, this rating system does not provide specific information about the pathophysiologic mechanisms responsible for neurological deficits. Because most mTBI patients' injuries are not visible on imaging studies such as CT scans, the diversity and complexity of TBI presentation is an extremely significant challenge in finding effective and targeted therapeutic interventions. Thus an enhanced classification strategy may enable the validation of specific treatment strategies. It has been proposed that patients in clinical trials should be selected using a new TBI classification based on the pathoanatomic features of the individual brain injury, as these features likely share common cellular and tissue pathophysiologic mechanisms. This multidimensional approach would seek to establish a "targeted injury type."[3] In doing so, clinicians would have additional specific and objective criteria to classify TBI patients.

Burden of Disease

The economic cost of TBIs worldwide is nearly impossible to calculate given that the majority of mild TBIs go untreated. A 2009 study estimated the total cost of TBI—including fatal cases, those involving hospitalization, and those that were untreated—to be more than $221 billion in the United States alone. The emerging epidemic of TBI predominantly targets the able-bodied male workforce, and is predicted to become one of the leading causes of death worldwide.[4] Up to 90 percent of TBI cases are classified as mild, yet up to 25 percent of TBI patients will not fully recover. These individuals suffer from chronic neurocognitive impairments. Historically the main TBI pathology was undetectable through imaging. But now metabolic imaging techniques offer us a view of the diffuse brain inflammation, and thus potential for neurodegeneration, that occurs in TBI patients.

There are an estimated 5.3 million individuals in the United States living with long-term TBI-related disability. Special populations at greater risk for incurring TBI include military service members and athletes who participate in contact sports. Alcohol use is another risk factor for TBI. Recurrent TBIs are extremely common—up to 13.2 percent of sport-mediated head injuries are recurrent. Nearly 90 percent of military personnel who experience a TBI have a concomitant psychiatric diagnosis.[5] The most commonly reported post-TBI impairment is the development or worsening of psychiatric conditions, including depression, anxiety, and mood disorders. This can result in an overall decrease in quality of life and increase in long-term morbidity and mortality. In one study of 60 TBI patients followed over 30 years, nearly half of the patients suffering from a psychiatric disorder began experiencing symptoms only after their TBI.[6]

Concussion and Post-Concussion Syndrome— Do We Need New Terminology?

Concussion is an outdated, catchall term for head injury with persistent symptoms. There is no consensus regarding its definition, and the term has no association with pathology. The title of the paper "Concussion Is Confusing Us All" states it best. The vague term *concussion* leads to uncertainty of diagnosis, non-reproducible science, poor clinical guidelines, and potential errors in policy-making decisions. Neurologists, sports medicine professionals, and others are increasingly classifying the severity of TBI symptoms and then precisely diagnosing the underlying post-traumatic symptoms. The Mayo system classifies the severity of TBI symptoms based on the traditional measures of LOC duration, GCS score, and duration of post-traumatic amnesia. Neuroimaging incorporates measures of injury severity and separates the majority of patients with mild TBI into two groups, characterized as mild (probable) and symptomatic (possible) TBI. This highlights the heterogeneous nature of mTBI and its wide variety of possible neuropathologies.[7]

Similar to the term *concussion*, the term *post-concussion syndrome (PCS)* lacks specificity. The presence of acute post-injury symptoms, including headache, dizziness, light or noise sensitivity, double vision, or tinnitus, is associated with persistence of those symptoms. Additionally, early-onset post-concussion symptoms (one week to one month post-TBI) are consistently associated with and highly correlated with symptom persistence. A 2015 study of 103 mTBI patients found that 82 percent reported post-concussion symptoms one month post-injury. The findings showed that "being symptomatic at one month was a significant predictor of being symptomatic at one year, and depression was significantly related to PCS at both one month and one year."[8]

The clinical definition of PCS from the *Diagnostic and Statistical Manual of Mental Disorders*, fourth and fifth editions (DSM IV/V), and the International Classification of Diseases (ICD-10) is poorly defined. This reduces PCS to a persistent neurocognitive disorder after TBI, which serves to further hamper accurate risk stratification, identification, diagnosis, and management of patients. These vague definitions and classification systems exacerbate the difficult task at hand for clinicians and researchers to provide a standard of care for treatment. Furthermore, the variability of TBI presentation and the breadth of factors influencing prognosis determine whether or not a patient fully recovers from their initial brain trauma. For example, a cohort study of patients who had suffered mTBI found that 64 percent of those patients met the ICD-10 criteria for PCS three months after their injuries, whereas only 11 percent met the DSM-IV criteria.[9]

PCS is a heavily debated topic among experts—symptoms are highly variable in severity, duration, and onset, which makes quantifying the condition extremely challenging. Moreover, the symptoms are unspecific and overlap with those reported in patients without brain injuries, including patients with whiplash injuries, and even healthy individuals. Finally, patients who present with PCS symptoms are sometimes met with accusations of malingering, exaggeration, misattribution, and recall bias by clinicians, who may deny the existence of post-concussion symptoms.[10]

There is significant overlap between PCS symptoms and the hyperarousal aspect of post-traumatic stress disorder (PTSD), including irritability and difficulty concentrating and sleeping. Concomitant PTSD and PCS is most often reported among military personnel.[11] One prospective study of 534 adult TBI patients and 827 controls concluded that mTBI was a significant predictor for PTSD, but not for post-concussion symptoms. Further muddying the waters is the fact that nearly 50 percent of PCS patients were previously diagnosed with behavioral health conditions, including depression and anxiety. Females are more likely to report persistent post-TBI symptoms. Specifically, symptoms including high anxiety sensitivity, low resilience, and poor coping skills are the most significantly associated with the development of PCS. There is currently no validated model to predict patients at risk of persistent symptoms post-TBI in the first week after injury.[12]

Leaky Gut Equals Leaky Brain

I am disappointed that many of my colleagues (including gastroenterologists) have told my patients that their "leaky gut" did not exist. Far from being a fanciful diagnosis of the naturopathic/complementary/alternative practitioner, leaky gut refers to well-documented intestinal hyperpermeability. The intestinal mucosal barrier is made up of epithelial cells that are connected by tight junctions. These intestinal epithelial cells mediate the interaction between the mucosal immune system and the products received in the interior of the small intestine (luminal side), determining which molecules may cross the barrier. The bidirectional regulation of the gut by the immune system and the immune system by the epithelial cell layer is the basis for maintenance of homeostasis. When that homeostasis is disrupted, the increased intestinal permeability is thought to cause a chain reaction of chronic inflammation and illness.[13]

Another barrier, the blood-brain barrier (BBB), protects the brain from being overrun by enemies, whether foreign or domestic. It is both a gate-keeper and a filter, allowing beneficial proteins, nutrients, and messages to cross while blocking harmful molecules. An individual's gut flora (or microbiome) and the gut barrier, together with transport proteins, act at the interface of blood permeability barriers to help regulate the move-ment of large molecules between the digestive environment and the host. Lifestyle factors—including sleep, stress, antibiotic use, diet, and trauma—shape the individual's gut microbiome. Bacteria, viruses, fungi, and even protozoans and parasites make up a metabolically and hormonally active microbial ecosystem. This microbiome symbiotically associates with the gut-associated lymphoid tissue (GALT) in order to maintain a lock-in-key relationship between the digestive system and neural/cognitive functions. We now know that the gut influences the blood-brain barrier (BBB) through gastrointestinal (GI) derived hormone secretion, through cofactor produc-tion, and through signals known as cytokines, which can cause blood-brain barrier permeability, or a "leaky brain."[14]

A healthy BBB is paramount for optimal brain function and mental well-ness. With a leaky brain (hyperpermeable BBB), neuroinflammation results. This has been linked to myriad conditions, including but not limited to depression, anxiety, cognitive impairment, brain fog, headaches, migraines, chronic fatigue syndrome, attention deficit hyperactivity disorder (ADHD), schizophrenia, Alzheimer's disease, and Parkinson's disease.[15]

Many factors contribute to leaky brain, including chronic systemic inflammation, oxidative stress, autoimmune disease, chronic psychological stress, infections, poor diet (highly processed, high fat, nutrient-poor diet additives), disrupted sleep-wake cycles, excess alcohol, heavy metal expo-sure, and other environmental toxins.[16] Chronic peripheral inflammation is thought to be a root cause for the imbalances causing major psychiatric disorders, secondary to elevations in pro-inflammatory cytokines. Cells that usually clean up the waste produced by normal cellular functions are known as reactive oxygen species (ROS) or reactive nitrogen species (RNS). At normal levels these products are helpful to the cells lining the small vessels of the brain (endothelial capillaries). But at high levels for extended periods of time, ROS and RNS are inflammatory (called oxidative and nitrosative stress, respectively), and can cause mitochondrial dysfunction and BBB damage.[17]

Zonulin, Gluten, and Leaky Gut/Brain

The standard of care is that only patients with celiac disease should maintain a strict gluten-free diet. However, I recommend that all of my patients eat a nutrient-dense, unprocessed, and gluten-free diet—a recommendation for which I take a lot of criticism. I am highly concerned with maintaining the stability of both the gut barrier and the blood-brain barrier. Gluten—a group of proteins in wheat, rye, and barley cereal grains—has been shown to increase zonulin.[18] Zonulin is a protein that modulates the intercellular tight junctions. Therefore, disruption of zonulin increases the permeability of both the intestinal barrier and the BBB.[19] In the United States our wheat is often a hybridized strain, which is not recognized by our immune system and is also heavily sprayed with inflammatory herbicides, including glyphosate. Research is pointing to glyphosate as a contributor to the increasing incidence of celiac disease, as it is a potent microbiome disruptor and toxin.[20]

Papers discussing the association between increased zonulin production and gluten consumption still conclude that there is "not enough evidence to recommend removing gluten from the diet."[21] Despite that insistence, celiac disease has a strong body of research behind it, and clinical associations have been made between celiac disease and neurologic and psychiatric disorders. Well-known celiac-mediated conditions include cerebellar ataxia, peripheral neuropathy, epilepsy, dementia, and depression. Additionally, it is now thought that neurological symptoms may be the clinical presentation of extraintestinal gluten sensitivity. For example, case studies have shown that gluten sensitivity can cause visible changes to the white matter in the brain.[22]

We must understand that a person does not need to have intestinal pathology (enteropathy) to have either celiac- or non-celiac-disease-related symptoms. A highly controversial condition known as non-celiac gluten sensitivity (NCGS) is a common cause of neurologic syndromes (notably cerebellar ataxia). Non-celiac gluten sensitivity is evidenced by high levels of anti-gliadin antibodies, and gliadin is a protein found in gluten. Not only is there increased gut permeability with gliadin protein exposure, but the blood-brain barrier also becomes more permeable in response.

We recommend an elimination diet for patients who seem to be sensitive to gluten without genetic susceptibility or positive celiac disease testing. Gliadin proteins are resistant to digestion and can both induce a stress response and trigger innate immune system responses—perhaps these are reasons for gluten intolerance. Finally, monkey studies re-creating a Western diet, normal aging processes, and leaky gut pathology demonstrate gut barrier disruption without celiac disease.[23]

Studies on NCGS are mixed, and further research is necessary to assess the efficacy of a gluten-free diet and to address the underlying mechanisms of nervous system pathology in gluten sensitivity.[24]

The Microbiome and Gut-Brain Axis: A Two-Way Street

Not only does the microbiome dramatically impact the brain, but disruption to the blood-brain barrier impacts the microbiome, too, which leads to a vicious cycle. Researchers and clinicians have understood the connection between the physiological changes caused by surgery, systemic inflammation, and pathological changes in gut bacteria for decades. Trauma, burns, sepsis (systemic infection), and surgical injuries can result in a series of gut barrier changes, intestinal transit problems, nutrient malabsorption, and gut flora imbalances known as gut dysbiosis. Gut dysbiosis is a powerful trigger for a systemic inflammatory response. An overgrowth of opportunistic microbes may not usually be a problem, but an unstable microbiome coupled with injury more closely resembles an infectious state. The microbiome is disrupted within hours of injury; up to a 1,000-fold reduction in healthy species has been demonstrated in injured patients as compared with healthy controls. Septic patients' gut flora diversity actually diminishes to the extent that pathogens can flourish and trigger more severe disease states in the individual. The intestinal wall damage results in an inflamed mucosal barrier and altered metabolic environment, further favoring potentially dangerous bacteria (such as *Pseudomonas aeruginosa*, *Escherichia coli*, *Staphylococcus aureus*, and *Enterococcus* species).[25] This increased virulence correlated with sepsis-associated mortality in one study.

Gut bacteria may be the most important factor in the maintenance of the intestinal mucosal barrier, along with digestive enzymes and products from the pancreas and hepatobiliary system, the nervous system in the gut (enteric nervous system), and the central nervous system. A major connector of the bidirectional highway between the microbiome, gut, and brain is cranial nerve X, or the vagus nerve (called the wandering nerve because it the longest and innervates the organs in the chest and abdomen). Improving vagal nerve function strengthens the parasympathetic nervous system, which is responsible for mediating rest and digestion. It is the antidote for a person with a brain on fire due to neuroinflammation, or a person in fight or flight due to their sympathetic nervous system's response to a perceived threat.

The gut microbiome not only modulates the nervous system and immune system, but also targets hormones via neuroendocrine pathways and produces bacteria-derived metabolites. This microbiome-gut-brain axis influences neurotransmitter production and communication and abnormal behaviors associated with neuropsychiatric disorders. Therefore, modulation of this axis should be a priority for neuropsychiatric conditions. The human microbiome is nurtured or disrupted depending on many factors, including genetics, health status, mode of birth, and environment. Above all, one of the most critical modifiable factors throughout a lifetime is diet composition and nutritional status.[26] Specific gut flora composition can influence body composition and have far-reaching implications for metabolic health and disease development. For example, changes in the microbiome associated with obesity itself may contribute to changes in the endocrine, neurochemical, and pro-inflammatory state associated with obesity and its associated pathology.[27]

Pathophysiology of TBI

After brain injury, the tight junctions connecting the mucosal epithelial cells become dysfunctional and allow large macromolecules, such as food antigens, to cross into the bloodstream, activating the immune system. The mucosal lining can atrophy and die within minutes of brain injury. Similarly, the tight junctions of the blood-brain barrier disintegrate, and neuroinflammatory chemicals enter and wreak havoc. Brain injury often contributes to over- or underactivation of the immune system, which may lead to autoimmunity or immunocompromization, respectively. TBI can trigger autonomic dysfunction (activated sympathetic nervous system), disorders of visceral sensing and processing, and impaired gut motility.[28]

Immediately following TBI, there is an acute activation of the hypothalamic-pituitary-adrenal (HPA) axis due to the stress of the injury. This is evidenced by increased circulating plasma cortisol levels within one to two days of mTBI or moderate TBI. However, following severe TBI, baseline serum cortisol levels decrease in the one to three days following injury. Suppression of HPA axis activation could result in a worse outcome after more severe TBI, even though inflammatory responses may be blunted. Because many individuals do not seek any medical treatment after mTBI, it is likely that mild-injury-induced endocrine dysfunction occurs much more often than currently recognized. Screening for hormonal abnormalities of the endocrine system is not the standard of treatment for TBI, and these will often go undiagnosed. Furthermore, HPA axis suppression or dysfunction after TBI may occur on any level of the HPA axis—at the hypothalamic, pituitary, or gland level. The pituitary gland is highly susceptible to dysfunction and injury-induced pressure changes or bleeding after TBI. As the pituitary gland releases adrenocorticotropic hormone (ACTH) and stimulates cortisol synthesis by the adrenal glands, pituitary dysfunction often causes decreased release of ACTH and thus decreased production of cortisol. Diminished cortisol levels in post-TBI patients are associated with increased mortality. This HPA axis dysregulation is also a contributor to neuroinflammation. Together, these mechanisms are implicated in the development or worsening of psychiatric symptoms after TBI. Cortisol is a glucocorticoid steroid hormone that regulates motivation and emotion through the limbic system. Major depressive disorder is characterized by the same post-TBI changes of HPA axis hyperactivity and disrupted feedback inhibition. Decreased cortisol production leads to fatigue, weakness, weight loss, learning and memory deficits, impaired focus, and irritability—PCS symptoms.[29]

TBI involves two phases: primary and secondary injury. The mechanical forces of the injury itself cause primary injury. This includes axonal shearing, hemorrhaging, and contusion, and varies in severity from mild to moderate or severe. Secondary injury is the indirect phase caused by the prolonged inflammatory processes initiated by trauma, including swelling or changes in blood flow. Examples of secondary injury include neuronal damage and degeneration through molecular processes, including mitochondrial dysfunction, oxidative damage, and neuroinflammation. Persistent neuroinflammation is implicated in the development of post-injury neurodegenerative disease. Many cell types contribute to the neuroinflammatory response after TBI, but the most significant may be microglia. Microglial-mediated inflammation is associated with many symptoms after TBI, including motor deficits, mood disorders, and neurodegeneration.[30]

Role of Microglia

As the macrophages (cell eaters) of the central nervous system (CNS), microglia are the immune system's first line of defense. Even though microglia represent only 10 to 20 percent of the total cell population in the adult CNS, they are essential in defending the CNS throughout an individual's lifetime.[31] In an inactive or "resting" state, microglia actually change their morphology in a dynamic fashion, retracting motile processes in mere minutes. Researchers are working to understand how microglia develop after birth, and have shown that microglia are involved in adult neuronal plasticity and neuronal circuit function.[32]

In response to TBI, microglia migrate to the site of injury and eliminate cellular and molecular debris by engulfing it. These activated microglia release noxious chemicals, including pro-inflammatory cytokines and reactive oxygen and nitrogen species, and cause persistent neuro-excitation through the release of glutamate. This excitatory neurotransmitter causes more damage and precedes neurodegeneration. The role of microglia activation in TBI is more highly nuanced than previously described. Studies have shown that microglia are activated in different phenotypes, which correspond to neurotoxic (M1) or neuroprotective (M2) priming states. This is a sophisticated response, as microglia acquire different activation states to modulate these cellular functions. Upon activation of the M1 phenotype, microglia produce pro-inflammatory cytokines and neurotoxic molecules. These signals promote inflammation and cell death. In contrast, when microglia adopt the M2 phenotype, they trigger secretion of anti-inflammatory gene products and trophic factors, which facilitate repair and regeneration and restore homeostasis.[33]

There are currently no targeted pharmacologic agents used as standard of care to restore persistently activated microglia to their resting, inactive state. Once primed and active, they will continue to act in this pro-inflammatory way, eventually burning out and undergoing cell death. This is concerning, as it increases the risk of further neurodegeneration.

Low Dose Naltrexone as a Microglial Modifier

Low dose naltrexone is a powerful microglial modifier, and its use may help prevent TBI-related neurodegeneration and immune dysfunction. LDN has an antagonistic effect on non-opioid receptors, such as toll-like receptors (TLRs). TLRs are activated by different pathogen-associated molecular patterns (PAMPs), including components of bacteria, viruses, and fungi. LDN blocks TLR-4, and has more recently been found to inhibit TLRs 7/8 and 9.[34] TLR-4 is found on macrophages, including microglial cells. Chronic neuroinflammation post-TBI is responsible for the progression of brain injury. As the down-regulation of TLR-4 reduces inflammatory cytokines and modulate microglia, the use of LDN is potentially neuroprotective.[35]

Novel, Multidisciplinary Diagnostic and Treatment Approaches to TBI

In my clinic and others, we often assess patients for markers of inflammation, autoantibody production, and total toxic burden. We are also using novel panels looking at neural tissue autoantibodies, including markers that indicate increased risk of demyelination, blood-brain barrier disruption, optical and autonomic nervous system disorders, peripheral neuropathy, neuromuscular disorders, brain autoimmunity, brain inflammation, and infections (especially viral markers). Currently, the majority of TBI biomarker research focuses on severe TBI, with few studies specific to mTBI. Additional candidate biomarkers are needed. Innovative and unbiased methods of autoantibody identification complement more traditional approaches to aid in the discovery of novel mTBI biomarkers.[36] While initial brain insult involves acute and irreversible primary damage to tissue, the ensuing secondary brain injuries often progress slowly over months to years. This is incredibly important, as there is a latent period before autoantibody production is associated with end organ damage and clinical symptom detection. Therefore, there is a solid window of time to employ aggressive and comprehensive therapeutic interventions.[37]

The concept of neuroplasticity, whereby the brain can change continuously throughout a lifetime, is demonstrated most profoundly by "spontaneous recovery" that has been seen in some CNS injuries. We know now that many cellular players are behind the scenes orchestrating a dynamic series of responses to different signals over time. Injury-induced neuroplasticity is driven by microglia, which induce CNS responses. This brain modulation after injury by microglia has been called "plasticity of plasticity." This term wonderfully describes the ability of microglia to alter their morphology and gene expression in response to a disrupted environment or injury. Microglia and other CNS cells are finely tuned by extracellular and intracellular factors, such as the nature of the stimulus, the extracellular environment, and the underlying prior cellular function.[38]

DIET

One of the most high-yield anti-inflammatory therapies is the optimization of diet, including minimization of the omega-6 to omega-3 polyunsaturated fatty acid ratio. Our modern diets make it exceptionally difficult to eat enough omega-3s to offset the vast majority of even healthful foods that possess high omega-6 content. Omega-3 polyunsaturated fatty acid (ω-3 PUFA) plays a key role in human metabolism, and includes alpha-linolenic acid, eicosapentaenoic acid (EPA), and docosahexaenoic acid (DHA). Omega-3 fatty acids not only provide energy support through metabolism, but also regulate inflammatory responses and immune function. Moreover, they maintain internal organ function and optimize cell signaling. Several studies have shown that omega-3 fatty acids inhibit TBI-induced inflammatory responses, and that this inhibitory mechanism may be related to microglial activation.[39] Dosing should take into consideration the time elapsed since the injury. Acute injury may require more aggressive omega-3 therapy (EPA/DHA). New research is looking at specialized pro-resolving lipid mediators, or SPMs.

SPMs are derived from EPA or DHA, and include resolvins, protectins, lipoxins, and maresins. These novel substances reduce inflammation and heal damaged tissue, thus restoring tissue homeostasis. In our clinic we have been using a commercially available SPM preparation to treat physical injury with great success, especially for flares in rheumatologic/autoimmune conditions associated with joint pain and inflammation. The use of SPMs in conjunction with omega-3 fatty acids is an excellent strategy for quenching the fire of inflammation via favoring the expression of anti-inflammatory cytokines and pushing microglia toward the M2 (anti-inflammatory) primed state. Animal studies using SPMs have been favorable, showing that microglia express SPM (resolvin) receptors.[40]

Other dietary strategies for treating TBI include caloric restriction and a ketogenic diet. Caloric restriction is known to increase life span and insulin sensitivity across several species. It is one therapy to consider for neurodegenerative conditions, including TBIs. Ketogenic diets have proven promising for epilepsy, and also in pre-clinical models for Alzheimer's disease. The potential neuroprotective effects of a ketogenic diet include many possible mechanisms, via alterations in energy metabolism. Ketosis-mediated alternative energy usage is thought to increase resilience to neuron loss, improve resistance to metabolic stress, and stimulate energy production via mitochondrial biogenesis. Such a low-carbohydrate diet may increase the primary inhibitory neurotransmitter gamma-aminobutyric acid (GABA), which helps prevent neurons from firing. In addition, there may be protection from glutamate excitotoxicity (a major stimulatory neurotransmitter). Both of these modifications are helpful to a chronically inflamed brain. Finally, in animal studies a ketogenic diet has been shown to reduce chronic hypoglycemia, oxygen-glucose deprivation, and mitochondrial ROS.[41]

If recommending a high-fat, low-carbohydrate diet, it is important to take into account a patient's apolipoprotein E (ApoE) genotype. Patients with homozygous ApoE ε4/ε4 status may need to maintain a lower-fat diet than ApoE ε3 carriers.

Regardless of other dietary modifications undertaken to treat TBI, it is critical that patients avoid consumption of alcohol, as its neurotoxic properties are counterproductive to healing.

Aquaporins and TBI

In my clinic we often ask TBI patients with persistent symptoms to avoid corn, soybean, spinach leaf, and tomato aquaporins, in addition to the general anti-inflammatory diet recommendations. What is an aquaporin (AQP)? Every living thing requires water, though too much water can be fatal. Plants and animals move water in and out of cells via membrane channel proteins known as aquaporins. Plants happen to share similar amino acid sequences with human aquaporin-4 (AQP4), which is expressed abundantly by astrocytes, the starlike macroglia that link neuronal cells together. Thus, antibodies formed against dietary aquaporins may potentially cross-react with brain aquaporin, leading to blood-brain barrier permeability and setting the stage for neuro-autoimmunity and neurodegeneration. Astrocytes form a secondary layer of protection for the BBB in case of breach from a trauma such as a TBI. If there is a breach in the BBB, the endfeet of the astrocyte are exposed. The high concentration AQP4 in these endfeet means they are vulnerable to circulating food AQP antibodies. Studies have shown that the antibodies directed at corn, soy, spinach, or tomato AQPs, which circulate in the bloodstream during a breach of the

BBB, may attack AQP4, thereby destroying the secondary layer of protection for the brain. This is a model for a broken BBB, dysfunction of synaptic microenvironments, and neuro-autoimmunity.[42]

Additional Anti-Inflammatory and Antioxidant Supplements

The following dietary supplements have anti-inflammatory and antioxidant properties that can aid in supporting a highly catabolic (energy-consuming), inflamed state, such as that of TBI.[43]

Resveratrol: Protects/defends BBB, increases the brain's growth hormone, supports mitochondria.

Berberine: Resolves dysbiotic gut flora and stabilizes blood sugar; anti-inflammatory.

Activated B vitamins: Take if needed to lower homocysteine (marker of inflammation, indicates risk of neurodegeneration). Work with knowledgeable clinician on which forms to take (commonly B_6, B_9, and B_{12}).

Magnesium: Required cofactor for hundreds of reactions. Difficult to overdose. Magnesium glycinate and malate are better absorbed. Can use transdermal magnesium and Epsom salt baths.

NAC (N-acetylcysteine) and glutathione: Powerful antioxidants that support cellular detoxification.

Curcumin: One of the most powerful neuroprotective and anti-inflammatory compounds; reduces BBB permeability.

Vitamin D: Anti-inflammatory and immune system boosting; activates hundreds of genes required for normal organ function.

LIFESTYLE

Immediately following brain injury, it is crucial for the patient to observe a period of physical and cognitive rest, during which they refrain from elevating their blood pressure and heart rate and engaging in activities that exacerbate neurological symptoms or cause fatigue. The patient must work with their medical team to determine the proper rest period based on their individual clinical course. After the initial rest period, exercise is beneficial to healing. Exercise enhances the production of new mitochondria in the acute period, thus enhancing energy production.[44]

DEAL-BREAKERS IN TBI TREATMENT

The following conditions impair efforts to repair the blood-brain barrier, thereby limiting the extent to which TBI can be treated:

- Underlying infection.
- Anemia. If hemoglobin levels are low, not enough oxygen reaches the brain.
- Low blood pressure can result in poor circulation, including to the brain. "Cold hands, cold feet, cold brain." Lower blood pressure is not always better!
- Hyper- or hypoglycemia. Both conditions are inflammatory.
- Mold or mycotoxin exposure.

Stress Reduction

High stress elevates cortisol, which is a neuro-inflammatory hormone that negatively impacts the BBB. The following are options to help mitigate elevated stress response:

- Neurofeedback (an advanced form of guided meditation)
- Yoga
- Limbic system reset
- Myofascial release or other gentle bodywork
- Heart rate variability training (to balance the autonomic nervous system)

Optimizing Sleep-Wake Cycles: Cortisol and Melatonin

Sleep is one of the most poorly understood and underappreciated physiological states. Humans spend about one-third of their lives sleeping. Optimal sleep quality, quantity, and circadian rhythm are essential for health. Sleep is necessary for creation and retention of memory, learning and concentration, and neuronal communication. While poorly understood, sleep is suggested to act as a housekeeper for the removal of toxins in the brain, which accumulate during waking hours. Sleep affects nearly every cell in the body. It is essential for synthesis, regulation, and secretion of hormones and neurotransmitters. A lack of high-quality sleep increases the risk of all chronic illnesses, including but not limited to hypertension, cardiovascular disease, diabetes, depression, and obesity.[45] The following are solutions for optimizing sleep:

- If circadian rhythms are disrupted, consider a small dose of sustained-release melatonin one hour before bedtime (1 mg).
- The four-point saliva cortisol test determines the level of cortisol in the saliva at four points throughout the day. This can reveal adrenal dysfunction. The only recognized adrenal problems in allopathic medicine are adrenal insufficiency or hypercortisolism, both of which have extreme consequences. However, more subtle dysfunction in the normal daily cortisol curve can cause quite dramatic suffering for the patient.
- Cortisol and melatonin are inversely correlated. The normal diurnal cortisol pattern involves a cortisol spike within 30 minutes of awakening, known as the cortisol awakening response (CAR), followed by a stepwise decrease throughout the day and nadir at bedtime. If the circadian rhythm is upset due to chronic stress or other factors, then the patient may benefit from full-spectrum light in the morning and melatonin and blue-light-blocking glasses after sunset. Blue light suppresses the body's natural production of melatonin.
- Go to sleep at same time every night.
- No eating three hours prior to bed.
- Sleep in a cool, dark room.
- No screens in the bedroom.
- Abstain from caffeine or alcohol in the evening.
- No exercise in the evenings.
- Create a relaxing bedtime routine.
- Use mindfulness techniques to calm the sympathetic nervous system.
- Avoid lying in bed if you cannot fall asleep.
- If you snore, wake unrefreshed, or have restless legs, get a formal sleep study.

LDN IN CONJUNCTION WITH OTHER IMMUNE AND NEUROMODULATORY THERAPIES

Dr. Mark Cooper from the University of Washington coined the term *LDN+* to describe the use of multiple anti-inflammatory agents against neuroinflammatory injuries. Dr. Cooper describes endosomes as the cellular organs (organelles) that can serve as a storage site for toxic molecules—autoantibodies. The accumulation of these autoantibodies in the central and peripheral nervous systems can lead to severe neurological dysfunction. LDN is very promising for treating neuroinflammation and neuro-auto-immunity because it can cross the blood-brain barrier and accumulate in the tissues of the central nervous system, and can enter neuroinflammatory lesions. It often takes multiple combinations of therapies (LDN+) to gain function and enable possible symptom remission. Adding agents to LDN yields powerful results. Hyperbaric oxygen therapy (HBOT) has been used with LDN to help with TBI cases, as well as other cases of neuro-autoimmunity.[46] In animal models HBOT has been shown to reduce programmed cell death (apoptosis), increase production of growth factors, elevate antioxidant levels, and inhibit inflammatory cytokines.[47] TBI results in overall loss of blood flow to the entire brain, known as global hypoperfusion. Therefore, the most common symptom in TBI is cognitive impairment. If there is overall loss of oxygen to the tissues, regeneration cannot occur. Therefore, by increasing the oxygen level in blood and body tissues, HBOT can boost the natural cellular repair machinery.

A prospective, randomized, crossover-controlled trial of 56 mTBI patients with prolonged post-concussion syndrome examined those patients one to five years after injury. The trial included a HBOT protocol of 40 treatment sessions (five days a week for eight weeks), 60 minutes each, with 100 percent oxygen at 1.5 atmospheres absolute. Significant improvements were demonstrated in the cognitive function of both groups following HBOT, but no significant improvement was observed following the control period, during which no HBOT therapy took place. Single-photon emission computed tomography (SPECT) imaging following the 40 treatment sessions revealed elevated brain activity, which corresponded with the cognitive improvements experienced by the patients. This suggests that HBOT can induce neuroplasticity, leading to repair of chronically impaired brain functions and improved quality of life for mTBI patients with prolonged PCS at a late chronic stage.[48]

Finally, and most impressively, the lasting benefit of HBOT in TBI has been shown in a recent study testing mTBI patients with PCS and with or without PTSD. The study included 30 military personnel, aged 18 through 65, with one or more blast-induced mild to moderate traumatic brain injuries. Significant improvement occurred in 29 of the 30 subjects, as quantified via measures of neurological symptoms, IQ, memory, attention, dominant hand motor speed and dexterity, quality of life, general anxiety, PTSD, depression (including suicidal ideation), and psychoactive medication usage. Furthermore, at their six-month follow-up, the participants reported further symptomatic improvement. Compared with the controls, the subjects' initial SPECT imaging was significantly abnormal. Injury shown on the imaging significantly improved after 1 and 40 treatments, and became statistically indistinguishable from that of the controls in 75 percent of abnormal areas of the brain. Each outcome that was studied showed improvement: clinical medicine, neuropsychology, psychology, and SPECT imaging.[49]

Conclusion

My experience treating TBI patients who have suffered up to decades post-injury has taught me that the process of chronic inflammation and activation of downstream pathological effects is incredibly complex. TBI is a multidimensional disorder with highly variable presentation, severity, and duration. High-yield strategies to stop the neuroinflammatory cascade include a therapeutic diet that considers genetic and other risk factors, omega-3 fatty acid, and additional supplementation; correction of anemia, hypotension, and hyper- or hypoglycemia; reduction of chronic stress; adequate sleep; minimization of toxic exposure; and enhanced toxin metabolism/excretion. Brain rehabilitation strategies must always be tailored to the individual, but can generally include a combination of therapeutic agents to allow for a synergistic effect, symptom relief, and cellular repair. LDN remains a jewel in the crown of TBI management. In this summary I am hopeful that increased knowledge of this important immunomodulating and anti-inflammatory agent will be disseminated throughout the international medical community, and further research undertaken.

NINE

Dissociative Disorders

Wiebke Pape, MD

D issociative disorders are among the most common trauma-related disorders after post-traumatic stress disorders. *Dissociation*, as opposed to *association*, describes a lack of integration of relevant information, or the separation of normally related mental processes. As defined by the *Diagnostic and Statistical Manual of Mental Disorders*, fifth edition (DSM-5), "Dissociation is a disruption of and/or discontinuity in the normal, subjective integration of one or more aspects of psychological functioning, including—but not limited to—memory, identity, consciousness, perception, and motor control. In essence, aspects of psychological functioning that should be associated, coordinated, and/or linked are not."[1]

In an overwhelming traumatic situation, dissociation occurs as a part of the passive defensive response. It can be seen both as a pathological reaction and a protective mechanism, as dissociation makes it possible to keep traumatic memories from the conscious mind. The dissociative patient may experience amnesia around the traumatic event, or a feeling of detachment—the perception that the trauma did not happen to them (like, for example, the out-of-body-experience that often is reported by victims of car accidents). When an individual experiences repetitive and cumulative traumatization, especially during childhood, dissociative tendencies might enable them to disconnect from the traumatic events and form attachments, even to traumatizing or neglectful caregivers—a capacity that is crucial for survival. Another dissociative reaction to severe traumatization in childhood is the development of different personality states, some that are connected with traumatic memories and others that are settled in everyday life and often deny that the traumatization occurred.

The development of cognitive and social skills as though the trauma didn't happen is possible, but in adult life dissociative symptoms usually become a severe impairment.

The Structured Clinical Interview for DSM-IV Dissociative Disorders (SCID-D)—a standardized diagnostic tool—identifies five specific symptoms of dissociation:[2]

1. Amnesia or memory problems involving difficulty recalling personal information.
2. Depersonalization or a sense of detachment or disconnection from oneself. A common feeling associated with depersonalization is feeling like a stranger to oneself.
3. Derealization or a sense of disconnection from familiar people or one's surroundings.
4. Identity confusion or inner struggle about one's sense of self/identity.
5. Identity alteration or a sense of acting like a different person.

The *Diagnostic and Statistical Manual of Mental Disorders* (DSM-5), published by the American Psychiatric Association, defines three major dissociative disorders:[3]

1. Dissociative amnesia (see the definition above).
2. Depersonalization-derealization disorder (see the definition above).
3. Dissociative identity disorder (DID): "Disruption of identity in two or more distinct personality states . . . [with] marked discontinuity in the sense of self and sense of agency, accompanied by related alterations in effect, behaviour, consciousness, memory, perception, cognition, and/or sensory-motor functioning." People with DID typically also suffer from dissociative amnesia.

Dissociation research suggests differentiating two qualitatively distinct forms of dissociation: detachment and compartmentalization. *Detachment* refers to an alteration of perception—the feeling of disconnection and alienation concerning oneself or body (depersonalization) or surroundings (derealization). *Compartmentalization* describes a deficit of volitional control over normally controllable processes; the main symptom is dissociative amnesia (for instance, conversion symptoms, dissociative fugue, dissociative identity disorder).[4]

Another way to consider dissociative symptoms is to categorize them as positive (productive symptoms that indicate unintegrated traumatic material, such as intrusive memories, flashbacks, trauma-associated pain, hearing voices) or negative (symptoms that result in the disruption of normal conscious functioning, such as memory deficits, loss of sense of self and/or loss of ability to sense or control different parts of the body).[5]

Until the 1980s dissociative disorders were considered rare. Recent research indicates "that dissociative symptoms are as common as anxiety and depression and that individuals with dissociative disorders (particularly dissociative identity disorder and depersonalization disorder) are frequently misdiagnosed for many years, delaying effective treatment. Persons suffering from dissociative identity disorder often seek treatment for a variety of other problems, including depression, mood swings, difficulty concentrating, memory lapses, alcohol or drug abuse, temper outbursts, and even hearing voices."[6]

In this chapter I give my view as a clinician on dissociative disorders and try to illustrate the problems, the goals of treatment, and the ways in which LDN can be a helpful medication to achieve those goals. Working in a department of trauma-related disorders that is part of a hospital treating psychosomatic disorders in an in-patient setting, our therapeutic team gets a close look at the consequences of childhood trauma and the problems our clients confront in everyday life.

I frequently let my clients describe their own experiences via case studies so the reader can get a feeling for dissociative symptoms and the change that LDN can bring, as symptoms are highly individual and difficult for a non-dissociative person to imagine.

Complex Traumatization and Dissociation

Complex trauma occurs when an individual suffers from repetitive, prolonged, and/or cumulative stressors during childhood and/or adolescence. Stressors may include sexual abuse; cruelty; neglect, abandonment, and/or antipathy by primary caregivers; continuing humiliation and excessive demands by caregivers; lack of emotional security; being left alone often; and the early loss of important attachment figures.

These events usually have a deep impact on personality development and lasting consequences in later life. Clients who suffer from complex traumatization often suffer from the following:

- Symptoms of post-traumatic stress disorders, including intrusive memories of traumatic events, nightmares, fragmentation of the memories concerning traumatic events, avoidance of trauma-related stimuli, emotional numbing, and chronic hyperarousal.
- Chronic depression.
- Instability of emotions and difficulties with affective regulation.
- Distortion of self-perception, deep-rooted feelings of helplessness, worthlessness, guilt, and shame (often leads people to isolate themselves from others).
- Attachment disorders involving distrust and a fear of getting close to others, but also dependency (often leads people to remain in destructive relationships).
- Chronic pain, anxiety disorders, eating disorders, and addictive disorders.
- Dissociative disorders.

Very often the individual develops complex post-traumatic stress disorder —a syndrome, first conceptualized in 1992, that will be included in the 11th edition of the International Statistical Classification of Diseases (ICD).[7] Our department mainly treats clients with this syndrome.

Clients with complex post-traumatic stress disorder often complain that they are "triggered" by multiple stimuli that are related to traumatic situations and prompt them to relive those situations. They report feelings of being in the past again. They also describe feeling as helpless as if they were once again in one of the traumatic situations. During these episodes, clients often perceive a regression of age, as though they were a child again and had lost their adult faculties. This can be attributed to the fragmentation of information due to traumatic stress. Often the clients develop amnesia for these situations.

Clients commonly describe their reaction to these episodes as follows: "In these situations, I cannot protect myself, I just freeze and try to bear the situation until it is over." This type of description reflects the way in which the client relives the passive defensive response—the main survival mechanism in a traumatic situation.

Most clients have severe attachment problems, fearing other people and especially new situations. Many withdraw from their social contacts because of the interpersonal stress they cause. A certain word, look, or gesture from another person may activate haunting memories of a former, traumatic situation.

Emotional self-regulation is difficult for these clients; many of them tumble from one emotionally overwhelming state to another and are very anxious about recurring memories.

A usual response to a trauma-related signal is dissociation: to shut down, to distract one's attention from the threatening stimulus and turn inward, to drift away. Clients will describe a sensation of their brain going blank. Triggers for a dissociative reaction are not only external but very often internal, such as emotions. Victims of continuing traumatization learned during their early years that emotions are usually overwhelming (for instance, existential fear, horror, loneliness, sadness, or anger). Due to unstable living conditions and lack of emotional care, they never properly learned to regulate their emotions and were often forced to separate their feelings from consciousness in order to keep functioning in everyday life and to survive. As a result, they fear emotions in their adult lives and try to hold them back, as they are unfamiliar and threatening. These people often describe feeling like robots—numb, depressed, unresponsive to others, and lacking vitality and joy. They describe themselves as disconnected from their inner life, alienated in their own bodies. Their emotions often are either numbed or—when unsuppressed—overwhelming. When emotions arise (such as in a situation that reminds them of a former stress situation), they often lead to a reaction similar to that experienced in the trauma. The person freezes with terror, is not able to act or react appropriately, and feels helpless and "left to the mercy of the perpetrator," as one of my patients described.

A dissociative reaction in a traumatic situation is a protective mechanism. It helps suppress the realization of the unfolding horror, much like anesthesia. When an individual dissociates in a traumatic situation (peritraumatic dissociation), their perception changes; everything seems to be distant and less important. Those affected often describe out-of-body experiences. On the one hand, this is a very helpful mechanism. In the case of complex traumatization, however, the individual gets used to this protective skill and dissociation happens automatically in moments that are only slightly similar to traumatic situations. We might say that the body reacts overprotectively, as the traumatization came to an end years ago. As a result, traumatized people dissociate very often in their everyday life. This is especially true when they encounter challenging situations, as these situations evoke emotional responses, unlike situations that are familiar and safe. To minimize dissociation, they focus on safety and being in control, trying to avoid challenges.

As mentioned before, dissociation can appear in different modes:

- Derealization (the external world seems to be unreal)
- Depersonalization (the perception of their own body is distorted)
- Emotional numbing
- Lack of perception of their own body (somatoform dissociation)
- Amnesia for long periods of the past
- Amnestic episodes in everyday life
- Intrusive memories of traumatic events or emotions and bodily sensations associated with trauma
- Immobilization
- Hearing voices

The Goals of Trauma-Oriented Therapy

A dissociative patient's safety and stability in the present is the first concern of therapy. The next step is to try to work through traumatic events that happened in the past to minimize their consequences in the present. To overcome former traumatization and to cope with everyday life, clients have to learn new strategies to differentiate dangerous situations from harmless ones, to know their own strengths and weaknesses, and to protect themselves. They also need to develop mindfulness and self-empathy. They are encouraged to face new situations in order to understand how they are different from traumatic situations. However, if a client is highly dissociative, it is very difficult for them to focus on the present, especially if the situation is challenging and fear provoking. Improving dissociative symptoms is a laborious and slow-moving process. Dissociation is akin to an automatic machine, because it is a reflex that has been trained for many years. Dissociative behavior is often silent and undramatic, which adds another layer of challenge to therapy.

For example, a therapist may get to a significant point or accomplish an important piece of work in therapy. The work may have been demanding for the patient, but the session seems to be a success. In the next session, when the therapist wants to resume the last one, the client says: "Oh, I can't remember anything of the last session, it must have been too much and I just passed out."

Clients usually report an enormous fear of self-perception—of being aware of what is going on in their inner life—because it could evoke trauma-related feelings. It follows that clients must have a "readiness to realize" if they want to overcome dissociation: On the one hand, dissociation is an impairment in everyday life; on the other hand, it is a protective strategy—an avoidance of realizing what is going on inside. The readiness to realize is a very important topic in therapy with complex traumatized clients. Many of them are only able to manage their life, pretending "everything is okay with me as long as I keep going and functioning, as long as I do not take a close look at the state I am in."

Our experience as therapists is thus: The easier it is for a client to be aware of the present moment—to be there with all the senses—and to stay present when things get rough, the easier it is for them to cope with every-day life and with the traumatic experiences of their past. So, in therapy, the main focus is to motivate clients to keep their awareness on the present and to increase their ability to act and feel as safe as possible in the moment.

Minimizing Dissociative Symptoms: How LDN Can Help

Psychotherapy is the first choice for treating dissociative symptoms, but as described above, it can be difficult for the client to make rapid progress with therapy alone. There is no established pharmacological intervention that directly influences dissociation. Medications used in the treatment of psychiatric diseases can help treat certain dissociative symptoms—anxiety, depression, unstable mood—but these are considered off-label uses.

As a clinician, I use LDN without completely understanding its complex working mechanisms—indeed, these mechanisms are still being explored in the wider medical community. When describing the mechanisms of action in clients with dissociative disorders, I refer to the publications of Dr. Ulrich Lanius, from whom I learned about LDN and who motivated me to try it out as a medication to support treatment of dissociative clients.[8]

WHAT IS THE CONNECTION BETWEEN DISSOCIATION AND LDN?—AN OVERSIMPLIFIED MODEL

Dissociation is at least partially mediated by the release of endogenous opioids.[9] Endogenous opioids are released in situations of inescapable danger, when active, sympathetic defense (fight or flight) is not possible anymore. Opioids activate the parasympathetic defense response, which includes immobilization, pain-reducing analgesia, and the numbing of emotional pain: in the words of Dr. Henry Krystal, "In the state of surrender and catatonoid reaction, all pain is stilled and a soothing numbness ensues."[10] A traumatic event is characterized as an "inescapable shock," with activation of passive (parasympathetic) defense reactions mediated by endogenous opioids. When traumatic stress becomes chronic, a continuously increased release of opioids results, followed by a reduction of opioid receptors. With fewer remaining receptors, even a minor release of opioids leads to a saturation of those receptors, instigating a passive defense response and dissociation.

Furthermore, the endogenous opioid system is involved in affective modulation and the regulation of emotional attachment. The downregulation of opioid receptors causes massive impairment in modulation capacities. As a result, coping with stressors gets less flexible, and already little stressors lead to parasympathetic activation and dissociation. Long-term changes in the activity of endogenous opioids can occur very early as a result of childhood stress.

Active (sympathetic) defense reactions are inhibited by endogenous opioids, so it can be concluded that a blockage of the opioid-mediated defense response supports active defense reactions. Since the 1990s the blockage of opioid receptors with naltrexone/naloxone to diminish dissociation has been the subject of pharmacological research. In earlier studies naltrexone was used in the normal dose from 25 to 100 mg,[11] which partially led to overshooting effects with mobilization of traumatic memories or suicidal tendencies.[12]

Supposedly, treatment with high dose naltrexone leads to an almost complete blockage of opioid receptors, and a resultant blockage of the client's ability to dissociate. This can be massively overburdening for highly dissociative clients due to their lack of alternative coping strategies. LDN has a less extensive impact on a client's ability to dissociate. The option to dissociate when necessary makes LDN more tolerable than the higher dose alternative for clients. Furthermore, LDN seems to reactivate the affect-modulatory competence of the endogenous opioid system—this appears to be a special effect of LDN in the treatment of dissociative symptoms.

PRESCRIBING LDN

In our inpatient treatment facility, we prescribed LDN for the first time in 2009 as a way to support clients with severe dissociative symptoms. Reliability in therapy—especially in case of a crisis—and continuing outpatient treatment after dismissal from the clinic were conditions to start the medication. The clients agreed to observe and document any occurring changes of symptoms.

As LDN is not available in Germany, our hospital pharmacy manufactured the capsules from 50 mg tablets. They informed us that they only could produce 2 mg capsules, as a 1 mg dosage could not be reliably measured. Accordingly, we had to set 2 mg LDN as our starting dose. We currently prescribe doses that range from 2 mg up to 6 mg, sometimes up to 12 mg a day. We start the therapy with 2 mg in the morning and wait about a week to observe the effects. The further dosage is adapted to indivdual symptomatology and the patient's assessment. Sometimes we increase the single dose up to 6 mg. It is often helfpul to give another dose of LDN (from 2 mg to 6 mg) at noon, as the effect decreases in the early afternoon due to the short half-life of LDN. Within a few weeks we adjust the dose to the individual requirements of patients. Sometimes it is helpful for them to take an additional dose as needed—for example, when there is more dissociation due to stressful situations. Sometimes it is also necessary to decrease the dose when patients cannot tolerate the effects at certain times. Usually our patients learn to manange their individual dosage according to their symptoms.

Case Report #1

Our first client was a 47-year-old woman who worked as a professor and had suffered from dissociative symptoms for many years. Memories of the first seven years of her life were shrouded by amnesia; she had only some fragmented traumatic memories of sexual abuse. In the four months prior to her admission to the clinic, her symptoms got worse: Traumatic memories increased, and she was "losing time" often in her everyday life and injuring herself severely. It was becoming difficult for her to focus on complex matters such as her lectures. Her mood was unstable and she experienced depressive episodes. She was admitted to our hospital because she could no longer cope with her job. She found it most embarrassing that she often behaved like a child in challenging situations, especially at work.

She showed an ambivalence concerning her dissociative symptoms: On the one hand, she was worried because her symptoms were causing her to lose control. On the other, she stated: "Dissociation helps me to get away when it is too much; it is a kind of relief." She explained that, when she entered a state of dissociation, she drifted into an imaginary inner room of beautiful, colorful patterns.

After taking her first 2 mg of LDN, she stated: "I cannot just switch off my perception anymore." Before taking the medication, she only perceived her surroundings as a "murmuring" when she dissociated; afterward she could differentiate noises and listen properly to conversations. Her ability to concentrate increased, but she felt more challenged by her surroundings.

Before taking LDN, she explained: "I never get angry, I do not know the feeling at all." With LDN, she experienced anger and reported that angry responses to other people came into her mind, which she found very frightening.

Many traumatized people fear anger, because the emotion is connected with the violence they experienced. Expressing anger may have led to punishment in the past. In the present feelings of anger provoke dissociation, which protects them from traumatic experiences. If it is not possible to perceive their own angry feelings, self-protection and self-care are difficult and can lead to revictimization.

When this client began to experience anger, she had to develop appropriate reactions from this change of perception. She learned to protect herself properly when she reached her limits. She reported feeling capable of acting, and described how she felt "aware of myself and alive."

The automatic dissociation decreased, but she could still willingly dissociate when necessary. She elected to increase her LDN dosage from 2 mg to 4 mg after one week, and then to 6 mg after another week, as she made progress in actively dealing with her surroundings. A few weeks later she described feeling "in contact with my fellow men and my environment." Affects like anger and sadness did not threaten her anymore. She could use them to develop new strategies for self-care. Her concentration and awareness improved day by day.

After 19 months of taking LDN, she described the changes as follows:

*Before taking LDN, I spent much time in states of dissociation—
often without purpose—to be in my own world and to protect*

myself from the demanding environment. Partially I was fascinated by this condition; on the other hand, dissociation impaired me as I could not control it. Since I take LDN, I notice when I begin to dissociate. And then I have the choice to withdraw from the world or to go back into the present. I'm able to stop it, and I'm in control. Overall, dissociation occurs more seldom and has lost a lot of its fascination. I feel much more alive and can stand many challenges. Only in excessively demanding situations, I need to dissociate. But in these situations, it is an ability to cope with overwhelming stress. There is more progress in therapy as I can keep my awareness when things get strenuous, and I can go on working.

This client does not take LDN anymore, as she eventually learned to stop dissociation without the aid of the medication.

Case Report #2

A 38-year-old woman diagnosed with dissociative identity disorder was working through traumatic events in our inpatient setting. Before taking LDN, she stated: "After a session of confrontation I was dissociating the whole night; it was as if I were in the traumatic past again. In the morning I awoke with the feeling of immense horror. I felt very exhausted and weak after confrontation for several days."

After she began taking 2 mg LDN in the mornings, she reported: "On the second day of LDN medication, I could differentiate the emotions that were just 'horror' before. My never-ending ruminations vanished; my thinking was clear and well structured."

Several weeks later, she described:

LDN restructured my emotional life. Before taking it, I felt as if there was a foggy wall surrounding me—partially for my protection. It vanished completely. So I could see and feel the emotions resulting from the trauma-confrontation work. I learned to deal with them. Before taking LDN, I had to mobilize all my strength to struggle against dissociation when emotions occurred. Now when flashbacks occur—which were overwhelming before taking LDN—it is much easier for me to use my stabilization strategies and to cope with them.

CLIENTS' TESTIMONIES

- "It's as if somebody turned on the light in my head."
- "I can feel my body, and I feel the strength of my body. For the first time in my life, I can climb the stairs without being exhausted."
- "I recognized that the carpet has a pattern for the first time. And for the first time, I understood what it means and how it feels to put the feet on the ground for stability."
- "I dare to do new activities: I can be part of a group of people I don't know properly. I don't have to be on the watch all the time."
- "I can concentrate on and understand complicated matters. I always thought that I was stupid because I understood so little and forgot so much."

A Retrospective Study

In 2012 we created a retrospective study that examines the impacts of LDN on the first 15 clients with complex trauma whom we treated with this medication. The treatments date back to 2009.[13] Table 9.1 lists the different dissociative symptoms exhibited by the clients, as well as the number of clients who experienced each symptom.

INITIAL RESPONSES TO LDN

Of the 15 clients in the study, 11 described a positive effect after the first or second day of taking LDN, 2 disliked the effect, and 2 didn't notice any change. Within the four to six weeks after the first application of LDN and the first few months after dismissal, a variety of short-term responses were recorded:

Overstimulation: Three of the clients stopped taking LDN, even though they were part of the group of 11 patients who had noticed a positive effect in the first few days. Their decreased dissociation led to an increased perception of their thoughts, emotions, body sensations, and surroundings, which was too challenging for them. Two of the three patients who stopped the medication reported coming into contact with previously suppressed traumatic memories.

TABLE 9.1. Dissociative Symptoms as Described by Clients

Dissociative Symptoms	Number of Clients Who Experienced Symptom (out of 15 total clients)
Amnesia occurring several times a day.	15
Freezing, or being incapable of acting—triggered by a person with a threatening appearance.	9
Freezing and shutting down—triggered by the client's perception of their own emotions.	9
Temporarily foggy, distant, and distorted perception of the environment.	11
Switching into childlike states of personality. Behaving and experiencing stimuli like a traumatized child.	9
Inability to perceive their own emotions.	14
Inability to perceive their physical body and/or body parts.	10
Difficulty concentrating and focusing.	7
Self-injurious behavior.	6
Intrusive memories/flashbacks.	15

The three clients also reported incurring stress more easily in everyday life. One client showed elevated blood pressure after a few weeks of taking LDN, and another reported diffuse, flu-like pain throughout their body. The reported side effects disappeared after these clients quit the medication.

Progressive development despite initial irritation: The two clients who described a negative effect after the first few days of treatment—namely, increased irritation and anxiousness due to clearer perception—reported an interesting development in the two weeks that followed: They noticed an impulse to be more active in everyday situations and the motivation to engage in new experiences.

One of these clients stopped taking LDN after a few weeks because she found this development to be "too much" at the time of her treatment. The other one "accepted the challenge" and made significant progress concerning self-regulation in the weeks that followed.

No effect: In two clients, the LDN didn't show any effect. We concluded their treatment after they had taken 4 mg for two weeks with no detectable change.

LONG-TERM EFFECTS

This study examined treatment durations that ranged from 8 to 27 months. Seven of the 15 clients answered our 2012 questionnaire, which asked about their continued experience with LDN.

TABLE 9.2. Changes in Dissociative Symptoms with LDN

Symptomatic Change	Number of Patients Who Experienced Change	Number of Patients Who Found the Change Subjectively Helpful	Number of Patients Who Found the Change Subjectively Stressful
"Shutting down" occurred less frequently and was easier to regulate.	8	7	1
Increased ability to perceive and regulate (negative) emotions.	8	6	2
Increased ability to maintain awareness in stressful situations.	8	7	1
Increased clarity of perception of surroundings.	2	2	0
Increased ability to think, focus attention, and understand complex concepts.	2	2	0
Ability to perceive their own body.	1	1	0
Increased ability to control self-injurious behavior, with a resultant decrease in injuries.	2	2	0
Increased clarity of traumatic memories (for some clients, these can be regulated more easily with stabilization techniques).	3	1	2
Decreased intensity of flashbacks.	1	1	0

- Nine of the 15 clients continued taking LDN after discharge from our clinic.
- All nine of the patients who continued on LDN reported that the LDN effect persisted and continued to help with their symptoms.
- One client reduced their dose from 6 mg per day to 4 mg due to recurring diffuse pain. With this reduction in dose, the client's pain vanished while the positive effect was undiminished.
- One client stopped taking LDN, despite a continued positive effect, because of multiple changes in her life and therapy setting. She did not comment on the changes in her dissociative symptoms.

Table 9.2 profiles the long-term changes to dissociative symptoms after treatment with LDN, and table 9.3 depicts the different side effects incurred by clients after varying durations of treatment.

TABLE 9.3. Side Effects of LDN after Varying Durations of Use

	Number of Patients with Side Effects
Immediate side effects (often decreasing over time):	
Headaches	4
Sleepiness	3
Drowsiness	5
Anxiety	1
Feeling of fullness	1
Side effects after several days (often lasting):	
Increased blood pressure	1
Increase of traumatic memories	2
Micturition disturbance	1
Side effects after weeks or months:	
Muscle pain (recurring after quitting and restarting LDN)	2
Gastritis	1
Weight gain (unclear whether an effect of LDN)	1

A 2017 Survey of 50 LDN Clients

In 2017 we did a survey of 50 patients who had been treated with LDN beginning in 2009. The patients were asked whether they still took LDN, why they finished the medication if they did, if and how their dissociative symptoms had changed, if and how the effect of the LDN had changed, and whether there were any side effects. Their responses were as follows:

- Thirty-seven of the 50 clients reported a positive effect and have continued taking LDN after discharge from the clinic.
- Fourteen of the above 37 clients reported that, while LDN's effect was still positive, they modified their dosage protocol. Some of their individual responses are as follows:
  - "When I reduced the dose, dissociative symptoms came back, so I continued the medication."
  - "I adapt the dose of LDN to the particular situation I am in. When I have to be fully focused, I increase the dose."
  - "I take LDN on demand when I think it is necessary to affect."
- Four clients reported that they could do without LDN after various time frames approximating one year. They stated:
  - "The medication gave an impulse; something got in motion and development is going on by itself now."
  - "After stopping LDN, I noticed that I learned to minimize dissociation. I can use my new abilities without LDN now."
- Two clients stopped taking LDN because the medication was too expensive.
- Six clients out of 50 did not notice any effect from taking LDN.

The majority of the 50 clients treated with LDN reported a lasting effect that did not reverse over time. Some clients had the impression that the effect decreased, so they had to temporarily increase their dose. Two clients reported that after a time, they could not notice the effect anymore. The cause of the changing effect over time remains unclear.

Frequently Asked Questions

Is it possible to predict who will benefit from taking LDN?
Our impression is that the extent to which the effect of LDN is helpful for clients seems at least partially dependent on their ability to cope with

CLIENTS' TESTIMONIES AFTER LONG-TERM LDN USE (2–5 YEARS)

- "As I am dissociating less, I have been able to cope with difficult tasks in therapy and my life. I am stabilized in my work life and have fewer sick days."
- "I am feeling alive and in contact with my emotions."
- "I don't feel as isolated as I did before taking LDN. I'm in contact with other people and my environment."
- "I am able to sense my needs and my limits and can protect myself."
- "I have fewer psychic crises."
- "Unfortunately, I cannot dissociate my chronic pain anymore; the perception of my pain also increased."

everyday problems. Clients who see themselves as needing protection and who tend to avoid challenges seem to experience the effect of LDN as a burden. Clients who are "progressive" or "hands-on" often experience short-lived irritation, followed by remarkable progress in therapy and coping. It is still unclear why some clients do not notice any effect at all.

Is LDN to be used as a short-term or long-term medication?
Given our experience, LDN is suitable as both a short- and a long-term medication. Taking the client off LDN for a period of time is useful in verifying whether the LDN effect is still present and medication is helpful. We have evolved three strategies of treatment based on the different ways clients deal with the effects of LDN:

- Permanent medication in cases where LDN is effective over time, with individual adaptions of dose depending on the situation.
- Short-term medication in cases where LDN's effect can no longer be felt, or when the effect is no longer necessary.
- Situational medication during times of need—for instance, when the client is dealing with a difficult topic in therapy or attempting to cope with an especially challenging situation.

Can LDN have an effect on dissociative amnesia?

Our impression is that LDN doesn't mobilize new traumatic material, and dissociative barriers seem to remain unbroken. However, clearer and less fragmented perception and increased personal realization can increase the client's burdensome confrontation with traumatic content in the short run. On the other hand, it often appears that LDN can facilitate the client's development of stabilization techniques and methods of distancing themselves from traumatic memories so that coping with those memories becomes easier.

What differentiates LDN from other medications?

Other medications (such as antidepressants, neuroleptics, and mood stabilizers) generally soften symptoms. As a result clients feel more distant from themselves, sometimes as though they're having an out-of-body experience. With LDN they feel connected to themselves and even gain access to feelings they weren't aware of before. When clients gain access to their emotions and self-empathy, they often describe feeling alive and in touch with their inner life and other people. This is usually noticeable in the relationship between the therapist and the client and, in my experience, is often a very touching moment in therapy. I experience many of these moments when clients describe their feelings of change after a few days of taking LDN. It is as if a connection is restored for these clients who often feel disconnected from themselves.

Conclusion

In our experience LDN can be a very helpful medication in the treatment of complexly traumatized clients with dissociative disorders. Emotional regulation, self-empathy, self-care, and mindfulness are likely to increase under the influence of LDN. Clients we treat with LDN find it easier to stay present, even in difficult situations. As a result, the integration of traumatic memories and emotions is more easily achieved, as clients are able to withstand distressing situations during trauma confrontation, to stay within the "window of tolerance," and to soothe themselves when threatening emotions arise.

Furthermore, compared with drugs previously used in treating dissociation and complex PTSD, there is something new about the effects that occur in patients who are treated with LDN. Not only does the anxious symptomatology decline, but it seems as if a new connection arises between cognitive thinking and emotional perception, which may lead to expanded self-awareness, self-reflection, and self-empathy. After 10 years of prescribing LDN off-label, we conclude that it is a psychotherapeutic drug, as it helps clients gently get in touch with their inner life and past suffering. It can be supportive in psychotherapy, considering psychotherapy's effort to develop strategies of self-care. Indeed, LDN treatment should be accompanied by psychotherapy, as the medication's effects need to be mediated and integrated. The same effect can be interpreted differently by different individuals.

At the moment we can only speculate, given our experiences so far, what the preconditions are for patients to benefit from LDN. An individualized assessment of the client's situation, coping capacity, and motivation to change and develop is required, but a prediction of therapeutic success remains difficult. We hope that future research will further illuminate these prospects.

TEN

Post-Traumatic Stress Disorder

ULRICH LANIUS, PHD,
AND GALYN FORSTER, MS

Post-traumatic stress disorder (PTSD) is a chronic response to traumatic life events that include but are not limited to military combat, natural disaster, motor vehicle accidents, sexual assault, medical trauma, or unexpected loss of a loved one. PTSD symptoms typically include hyperarousal, intrusive thoughts, exaggerated startle response, flashbacks, nightmares, sleep disturbances, emotional numbness, and persistent avoidance of trauma-associated stimuli. Lifetime prevalence rates of PTSD in community samples have been reported to be about 8 percent.[1] Generally, PTSD is associated with a wide range of physical health problems and mental health issues, including difficulties at work and social dysfunction.

In this chapter we discuss the use of naltrexone, particularly LDN, for the treatment of post-traumatic stress disorder. At the time of publication, there have been no randomized controlled trials examining the treatment of PTSD with LDN. However, in our clinical experience based on several hundred cases, LDN provides a promising option as an intervention for intractable PTSD, particularly in individuals who have a history of multiple traumatization and developmental trauma.

PTSD, Complex PTSD, Developmental Trauma, and Dissociation

Complex PTSD (C-PTSD), as compared with simple PTSD, is typically diagnosed when there is a history of childhood trauma that includes chronic abuse, neglect, or other types of adversity while growing up. Central to the development of C-PTSD is a prolonged, repeated experience of interpersonal trauma in a context in which the individual has little or no chance of escape. Individuals with C-PTSD commonly have an increased incidence of comorbid disorders, including but not limited to major depressive disorder, generalized anxiety disorder, substance use disorder, panic disorder, and obsessive-compulsive disorder.[2] C-PTSD has recently been included in the International Classification of Diseases (ICD-11). The *Diagnostic and Statistical Manual of Mental Disorders*, fifth edition (DSM-5), diagnosis that bears the closest resemblance to C-PTSD is PTSD—dissociative subtype.[3]

C-PTSD is also related to the concept of developmental trauma, which occurs when a child is exposed to overwhelming stress and their caregiver does not help reduce this stress, or is the cause of the stress. Some of these children will go on to develop PTSD or other mental health disorders, though many do not. Nevertheless, they are at risk for a host of complex emotional, cognitive, and physical disorders that commonly affect them throughout their lives.[4] Thus individuals with a history of developmental trauma often present with a wide variety of mental and physiological symptoms, including significant dissociative symptoms.[5] They tend to be difficult to treat, and frequently only respond minimally or not at all to standard trauma treatment approaches.[6]

Individuals with C-PTSD have significantly higher levels of dissociative experiences compared to those with simple PTSD.[7] Dissociative symptoms vary by type and severity. They commonly affect the person's sense of identity, memory, and consciousness, as well as self-awareness and awareness of their surroundings. They may include the following:

- Depersonalization: feeling disconnected from oneself.
- Derealization: feeling as though the world is distorted or not real.
- Amnesia: memory problems without a medical explanation.
- Identity confusion: not feeling oneself; behaving in a way that one would normally find offensive or abhorrent.
- Significant memory lapses, such as forgetting important personal information.
- Affect dysregulation: problems with handling intense emotions.
- Sudden and unexpected shifts in mood, such as feeling very sad for no reason.
- Depression and/or anxiety.

- Other cognitive (thought-related) problems such as concentration problems.
- Obsessive symptoms: feeling compelled to behave in a certain way.
- Vulnerability to pain disorders: increased issues with chronic/persistent pain.

In our experience LDN has a beneficial effect on PTSD, particularly when there are significant dissociative symptoms, and it has clear benefits as an adjunctive pharmacological intervention to psychotherapy above and beyond that offered by more traditional pharmacological interventions such as antidepressants.

PTSD and Physical Health

There is a growing body of literature highlighting the increased risk for other chronic physical diseases in persons with PTSD and other psychiatric disorders. In addition to the accepted psycho-social symptoms of PTSD, there is substantial evidence suggesting a complex interplay of multiple biological factors associated with traumatic stress disorders that require us to broaden our conceptualization of what PTSD is. While PTSD is currently diagnosed based solely on psychological and behavioral symptoms, there likely is a link between PTSD and alterations in the immune and inflammatory systems.[8]

For instance, in a large sample of Vietnam veterans with PTSD, Boscarino found an increased incidence of common autoimmune diseases, including rheumatoid arthritis, psoriasis, insulin-dependent diabetes, and thyroid disease. He suggested that chronic PTSD—particularly PTSD with multiple comorbidities or C-PTSD—is associated with all of these conditions. He specifically noted the presence of biological markers consistent with a broad range of inflammatory disorders, including both cardiovascular and autoimmune diseases (for example, clinically higher T-cell counts, hyperreactive immune responses on standardized delayed cutaneous hypersensitivity tests, clinically higher immunoglobulin-M levels, and clinically lower dehydroepiandrosterone levels).[9]

Similarly, a more recent study of 666,269 Iraq and Afghanistan veterans confirmed such an association between PTSD and autoimmune disorders: Veterans with PTSD had twice the risk of being diagnosed with an autoimmune disorder compared with those without any psychiatric disorders, and a greater than 50 percent increased risk compared to veterans with psychiatric disorders other than PTSD. By comparison, the effect size for all other psychiatric disorders was smaller than for PTSD.[10]

Specifically, in a review, Miller et al. suggest:

> *Medical comorbidities are common, including chronic pain, cardiometabolic disease, neurocognitive disorders, and dementia. The hallmark symptoms of post-traumatic stress—recurrent sensory-memory re-experiencing of the trauma(s)—are associated with concomitant activations of threat- and stress-related neurobiological pathways that occur against a tonic backdrop of sleep disturbance and heightened physiological arousal. Emerging evidence suggests that the molecular consequences of this stress-perpetuating syndrome include elevated systemic levels of oxidative stress and inflammation.[11]*

Stress-induced alterations or impairments in opioid system functioning directly affect immunomodulatory functioning through their effects on the hypothalamic-pituitary-adrenal (HPA) axis, thus potentially accounting for compromised immune system functioning not only after exposure to extreme stress, but also due to early childhood trauma. This makes interventions in the opioid system with LDN a logical venue for potential treatment interventions.[12]

Endogenous Opioids, Stress, and Dissociation

Dissociation is at least in part mediated by endorphins and endogenous opioids, which may account for dissociative phenomena such as numbing, confusion, and cognitive impairment, including amnesia.[13] Researchers have known for decades that exposure to overwhelming trauma often results in a sustained period of analgesia. Soldiers wounded in battle frequently require much lower doses of morphine than the doses needed by patients injured in noncombat contexts.[14]

Stress-induced analgesia (SIA) is a well-documented phenomenon in many forms of traumatic stress. The release of endorphins at the time of acute stress has distinct survival benefits. An animal ministering to its wounds to subdue pain during a life-threatening situation would significantly compromise its defensive capabilities. Multiple animal models may be relevant to our understanding of traumatic dissociation. These include models that look at SIA, learned helplessness (LH), and tonic immobility (TI).[15] All of these phenomena are common animal responses to stress that are, at least in part, opioid-mediated. Moreover, these responses are part of a hardwired affective response that occurs not only in animals but also in humans.[16]

Feelings, Emotions, Defensive Responses, and PTSD

Defensive responses are hardwired emotional responses to threat, designed to maximize survival. Fight and flight are the defensive responses that most commonly come to mind when we think of PTSD and threat in general, but there are others. Panksepp identifies the following hardwired mammalian defensive emotions: SEEKING for protection, RAGE (or fight), FEAR (or flight), and PANIC (or immobilization).[17] These defensive responses commonly occur in a hierarchical fashion, and are in part expressed based on individual differences, including genetic predisposition, as well as the nature and context of the threat.

The initial response is the seeking of proximity to others for safety, or, in the case of a child, SEEKING a primary attachment figure for protection—usually Mom or Dad. If such support is unavailable in the face of threat, RAGE is usually mobilized to ward off an attacker. If the attacker is much larger or happens to be the primary attachment figure, RAGE is unlikely to be fully mobilized, and the next defensive response, FEAR, is mobilized. The mounting of such an active defensive response—flight—by a small child is more often than not unsuccessful: There is no escape. This then leads to PANIC and immobilization, with an eventual parasympathetic collapse. This parasympathetic activation of the nervous system coincides with SIA, ultimately leading to TI with concomitant LH.

In the case of a small child trying to escape, immobilization—also referred to as tonic immobility—is a last-resort defensive behavior that is mediated, at least in part, by opioid activation. It is an inborn, hardwired defensive behavior characterized by a temporary state of profound motor inhibition.[18] TI is related to restraint stress, which has similar features. TI is mediated, in part, by endogenous opioids acting upon opioid receptors in the periaqueductal gray (PAG), a structure in the upper midbrain. For instance, when beta-endorphin is injected directly into the PAG, it produces profound catatonia reminiscent of immobilization.[19] Moreover, opioidergic stimulation of the ventrolateral PAG increases immobilization, an effect that can be reversed with the opioid antagonist naloxone.[20] Altered PAG function and connectivity recently has been reported to be associated with PTSD.[21] Indeed, immobilization may be the juncture between traumatic stress and immune system functioning: Farabollini et al. suggest that immobilization as a result of acute restraint induces opioid-mediated immune system effects, particularly in the ventromedial hypothalamus and the PAG.[22]

Attachment, Trauma, and Endogenous Opioids

The endogenous opioid system also plays a major role in human attachment. Brain circuits involved in the maintenance of affiliative behavior are precisely those most richly endowed with opioid receptors.[23] The separation distress response can be inhibited with morphine, abolishing the separation cry in infants as well as the maternal response to it.[24] This suggests that the endogenous opioid system plays an important role in the maintenance of social attachment.[25]

Schore suggests that abuse and/or neglect, including inadequate amounts of sensory input, particularly touch, over the first two years, negatively impacts the major regulatory system in the human brain, the orbital prefrontolimbic system.[26] Animal research suggests that lack of caregiving during the first few weeks of life decreases the number of opioid receptors in the cingulate gyrus.[27] This raises the question of whether neglect and a lack of caregiving in humans has a similar impact on the opioid system, resulting in fewer opioid receptors. This potentially reduces the human capacity to experience pleasure, at the same time as it makes the brain more vulnerable to the effects of opioids due to the reduced number of opioid binding sites, resulting in a predisposition toward dissociation.

In addition, Schore (2001) suggests that hyperarousal and dissociation, resulting from adverse childhood experiences, create the template for later childhood, adolescent, and adult PTSD.[28] Altered opioid functioning in C-PTSD may also contribute to many of the multiple comorbidities associated with traumatic stress syndromes, including major depression and anxiety disorders.[29] Thus, alterations in the opioid system in childhood are likely further compounded by altered opioid receptor binding secondary to adulthood trauma, making LDN a potential candidate of choice for pharmacological intervention for PTSD and, in particular, C-PTSD.[30]

Treating PTSD with LDN: History and Background

Dr. Ulrich Lanius has had copious experience with regular dose naltrexone in PTSD dating back to 1999.[31] Although many clients who had been prescribed regular doses of naltrexone benefited greatly, others experienced negative side effects, with about 30 percent experiencing some gastric distress upon initial dosing.[32]

In 2002 a patient presented with severe developmental trauma and early medical trauma. She had a history of fibromyalgia and significant dissociative symptoms, including profound amnesia. She was prescribed regular dose naltrexone (50 mg per day), which successfully addressed ongoing dissociative symptoms. Unfortunately, it also resulted in the breaking of amnestic barriers with spontaneous recall of previously dissociated mnemonic material; the patient became quite overwhelmed by this.

At the time, having just been introduced to low dose naltrexone through another client who was using LDN to treat multiple sclerosis, Dr. Lanius raised the possibility of an empirical trial of low dose naltrexone. The client was prescribed 3 mg of naltrexone per day (about 0.06 mg of naltrexone per 1 kg of body weight). She benefited not only from a reduction in fibromyalgia symptoms, but also from reduced depersonalization and derealization and less uncontrolled switching of self-states—very similar to the benefits noted with regular doses of naltrexone but without the breaking down of amnestic barriers as experienced with the higher dose. Interestingly enough, the client found that increasing the dose to 3 mg twice a day (BID), and on occasion 3 mg three times a day (TID), actually increased the benefits of naltrexone concerning both dissociative symptoms as well as fibromyalgia symptoms. The lowered dose of naltrexone appeared to offer similar benefits to the regular 50 mg dose.

Naltrexone Dosing

At this time there are no recognized, formally established dosing protocols for treating PTSD with LDN. There is some research with regular and high doses of naltrexone (50 to 400 mg a day), but there are only two studies focused on LDN: a pilot trial focused on depression and a study focused on treating dissociation and complex trauma with LDN.[33]

With regard to naltrexone, a nonlinear dosage effect has been reported.[34] That is, the magnitude of the effect is not necessarily proportional to the dosage. It has been suggested that very low and high dosages are most effective, and intermediate ones less so. Belluzzi and Stein report that high dose naltrexone may activate postsynaptic receptor sites, whereas a low dose may act preferentially on presynaptic receptor sites.[35] Some clients may benefit more from presynaptic blockade of mu, delta, and kappa receptors at high doses of naltrexone, while others may respond better to the more subtle effects of low doses, primarily affecting mu receptors.

Adding another layer of complexity, Collin et al. demonstrated that the kappa/dynorphin opioid system (responsible for mediating dysphoria) exerts a regulating effect on the mu/endorphin system, but not on delta receptors.[36] Though unproven, bidirectional regulation may exist, with the mu system also exerting a regulating effect on the kappa system, so that LDN may moderate dysphoria by indirectly downregulating kappa activity.

In contrast with how LDN is typically used to treat immune system dysfunction, we have found that individuals with C-PTSD generally respond more favorably to multiple doses per day—usually twice a day—which enable them to better manage hypervigilance, anxiety, and dissociative symptoms. In some cases PTSD symptoms respond better to dosing regimens of three times a day or even four times a day (QID). Most individuals with C-PTSD respond well to weight-based dosing; we have found the ideal dosage under normal circumstances to be about 0.06 mg per kg of body weight. For instance, for a person who weighs roughly 180 pounds (81.6 kg), this works out to a dosage of about 5 mg taken twice a day. Interestingly, this is the same dose ratio at which alcohol-addicted rats stop seeking alcohol.

Individuals with C-PTSD and co-occurring autoimmune disorder typically show improved response to twice or sometimes more frequent daily dosing. It is unclear whether this response pattern is unique to PTSD and may be attributable to altered opioid receptor binding in PTSD.[37]

While most individuals with C-PTSD will tolerate LDN at a full weight-based dosage immediately, there are some for whom alternative dosing schedules are preferred. In general, it is wise to start trauma survivors at less than the full weight-based LDN dose. Individuals who have a high stress-induced opioid tone in their system (in our experience, about 30 percent of individuals diagnosed with C-PTSD or a dissociative disorder) will exhibit some symptoms suggestive of opioid withdrawal when administered naltrexone. Such withdrawal symptoms—typically nausea and gastric distress—are usually minimal with LDN, but they can be completely avoided by introducing LDN more slowly.

This also avoids a possible flare of autoimmune symptoms in those who are diagnosed with co-occurring autoimmune disorders. In this case we would commonly introduce LDN at 0.5 mg or 1 mg doses and increase the dosage to the target dose by body weight, advancing at a pace the patient can tolerate. It is common for dosing to be modified multiple times during the first few months, as the patient is adjusting to the medication and general biological function is being restored.

EXQUISITE SENSITIVITY AND LOW DOSE NALTREXONE DOSING

For some exquisitely sensitive individuals, an even lower starting dose may be beneficial. For people who have multiple allergies and/or sensitivities—including allergies to medications and to environmental substances—and for those who appear to have generally hypersensitive nervous systems, we suggest different initial dosing to further minimize side effect potential: for example, starting at 1 mg and increasing to a twice-daily schedule before introducing increments of 1 mg. The dosage is titrated upward until the amount recommended by the application of the formula outlined above is reached. If, for some reason, the patient feels overwhelmed or is experiencing any negative effects, the lower dose can be maintained or further reduced until they adjust to it. For some people, a daily dosage less than that suggested by the formula will be preferable. For individuals who are exquisitely sensitive, even doses of 0.5 mg or 1 mg can be too much. They may require doses as low as 0.01 mg (usually prescribed in liquid formulation), and they may need to titrate up very slowly. This is also the case for some individuals with severe dissociative identity disorder (DID), where sometimes a dosage difference of as little as 2 mg a day can make the difference between accessing and not accessing a suicidal part of the self.

While most individuals with C-PTSD report improved sleep and decreased nightmares on LDN, a subset will respond with more disrupted sleep, especially during the early stages when getting used to LDN. In such cases the last dose should either be given earlier in the day, decreased, or, in some cases, avoided altogether. Sometimes clients who did not benefit from the evening dose early on will respond favorably later on in treatment.

COMPLICATING EFFECTS:
AFFECT PHOBIA AND AFFECT INTOLERANCE

Fear and/or avoidance of emotions, as well as emotional numbness and/ or an inability to feel, are common to PTSD, especially C-PTSD. It has been our experience that an inability, unpreparedness, or unwillingness to access emotional experience will compromise the person's capacity to tolerate normal LDN dosages. This is common in individuals who have adverse attachment histories, have a compartmentalized sense of self, and have learned to avoid feeling emotions at any cost. In some cases, there is a distinct positive-affect phobia: The person has learned that it is not safe to feel good or to be relaxed.[38] Patients in recovery from addictions should be screened for this issue.

Psycho-education is important when working with this population. LDN's reduction of dissociation sets some patients up to initially mistake an increased experience of their own emotions as a bad thing. Without the buffer of dissociation, feeling all affect more distinctly, and particularly experiencing positive affect, can feel overwhelming and may at first be experienced as aversive. In these individuals, especially when they are also exquisitely sensitive to other environmental stimuli, regular LDN dosing (especially early in treatment) may trigger anxiety or overwhelm, and very slow titration of LDN dosage or lower baseline dose is commonly preferred. Often, psychotherapeutic interventions in a safe relationship will allow the person to increase tolerance to their own emotions and to LDN.

In general, when patients treated with LDN report feeling emotional distress or discomfort that goes beyond the initial transient side effects referenced elsewhere (see chapter 1), clinicians should rule out the possibility that the reaction is due to an affect phobia. This concept of shared positive-affect phobia can be challenging for clinicians as well as the general population, since the idea that positive feelings might feel bad defies common logic.

A client raised in a chaotic, neglectful, single-parent home reported that in the first six hours after taking LDN, he experienced all his emotions more intensely, and positive affect was particularly intimidating. Nevertheless, he stated that it was worth it to him because the positive effects outweighed the negative: Neuropathy in his feet was eliminated, mental fog lifted, he could find his thoughts and keep problems in perspective, and he was much more productive at home and work.

Another client reported that, when she started LDN, "It felt exhausting at first to feel things, but now it is a relief to have feelings and be able to cry instead of disconnecting from feelings." She also observed, "Early on, it was important to be in counseling; being stuck in the same old mindset, I would not have known what to do with my newfound clarity."

Naltrexone and Dissociation: The Issue of Drug Absorption

Lanius and Corrigan suggest that dissociative processes in C-PTSD may interfere with the normal absorption of medications or with their metabolism.[39] This may, in part, account for both the lack of effectiveness, as well as the paradoxical effects, of medications in this population. Altered absorption of drugs taken concurrently with LDN is a concern for patients who are on medications that need to be at specific blood levels, or for those on high doses of other medications.

Specific blood levels are an issue for patients who are on warfarin, a blood thinner and anticoagulant. The individual dose is determined by the measurement of the international normalized ratio (INR). Lanius and Corrigan report the case of a client on warfarin for whom the addition of LDN significantly altered the INR ratio, resulting in the need to adjust the warfarin dosage.[40]

Accordingly, adding LDN when someone is already on high doses of other medications may increase the probability of side effects. Lanius and Corrigan describe a patient with a history of pervasive neglect who presented with a developmental disorder, schizophrenia, and C-PTSD. The patient had been prescribed high doses of atypical neuroleptics and had not responded significantly to them. After the addition of LDN, the patient suddenly developed significant side effects to the antipsychotic medication. The neuroleptic side effects abated with a lowering of the antipsychotic dose, and significant improvement in functioning occurred. This response is consistent with the literature that suggests opioid antagonists can increase response to neuroleptic medication.[41]

Lanius and Corrigan further describe several cases where neither LDN alone nor antidepressant alone had significant therapeutic effects. However, the addition of LDN increased the therapeutic effects of other medications. This phenomenon has been described in the literature where response to antidepressants has been augmented by opioid antagonists.[42] Similar effects have been reported in patients with OCD, treatment-refractory depression, eating disorders, and smoking cessation.[43]

These clinical observations of augmented drug effects and increased blood levels of medications suggest that LDN may have an effect on absorption that may be secondary to or concomitant with reducing dissociative symptoms. Given such experience with altered blood levels, as well as the development of side effects to other medications after initiation of LDN, we recommend significant caution and close monitoring in the case of patients who are on high doses of other medications or have been prescribed medications that rely on specific blood levels.

Clinical Effects of LDN: Increased Self-Regulation

Lanius and Corrigan (2014) suggest that opioid antagonists, including LDN, significantly help traumatized patients with C-PTSD to stay within their window of tolerance by reducing dissociative symptoms.[44] LDN appears to decrease hyperarousal, flashbacks, intrusive symptoms, and hypervigilance with a concomitant increase in attentional functioning. Emotional regulation and/or self-regulation, as well as tolerance of emotions and body sensations, commonly improve. Both alexithymia (emotional numbing) and self-harming behavior typically decrease. Eating to soothe emotions is reduced, and appetite and food intake tend to be better regulated in most clients, though eating disorders typically respond much better to higher doses (minimum of 50 to 100 mg per day).

Uncontrolled and unpredictable switching between self-states is reduced, with a simultaneous increase in co-consciousness among parts of the self, and thus an increased continuity in the person's sense of self. With decreased dissociative symptoms, there is commonly not only decreased immobility and helplessness, but also an increase in assertive behavior accompanied by an increased sense of personal agency.

Patients who have been amnestic for significant periods of their life tend to experience a decrease in amnesia. With LDN this usually occurs very gradually. In conjunction with increased affect tolerance, this tends to be unproblematic: Rather than breaking through dissociative barriers, patients are able to choose the issues they want to focus on, and obsessive thinking and ruminating tend to be reduced.

Given that the opioid system plays a crucial role in the modulation of anxiety, one would suspect an increase in anxiety, as has sometimes been reported in the literature.[45] Among our clients, all of whom were in a psychotherapeutic relationship when LDN was initiated, this almost never occurred. However, agitation is often interpreted as anxiety in patients with unresolved affect phobia until they learn to tolerate the experience of feeling emotions. In the absence of a stable interpersonal or therapeutic relationship, LDN has some potential to be aversive, usually at the initiation of treatment. Usually, this can be managed by reducing the dosage, though on very rare occasions patients have responded better to regular doses of naltrexone.

Case Studies

Below is a small sample of case studies of our many patients with C-PTSD, chosen to give an idea of the wide range of clientele and the variety of trauma-related symptoms for which LDN typically provides relief. Dr. Lanius has provided additional case studies and discussion in an earlier publication.[46]

VIETNAM VETERAN WITH MILITARY PTSD: ANGER, DEPRESSION, AND ANXIETY

A male Vietnam veteran with extensive combat experience as well as childhood trauma was diagnosed with C-PTSD. He was a self-described survivor and adrenaline junkie, always on the run, often moving on just when success was within his grasp. He had an explosive temper and significant anger management problems, and he suffered from bouts of depression that included what he described as "a black hole" feeling. He had twice participated in Veterans Administration residential PTSD treatment programs, and reported he had "tried every prescribed and non-prescription drug [he] could find to try to help [himself] feel better." He smoked marijuana daily to help with mood and took zolpidem nightly to improve his sleep.

While in psychotherapeutic treatment, he began taking 2 mg LDN once a day and increased this to twice a day after experiencing minimal side effects. He maintained this dosage (half the standard of 0.06 mg/kg/b/w) and frequency of use for roughly two years. With LDN serving as an adjunctive to eye movement desensitization and reprocessing (EMDR) psychotherapy, over these two years he reduced his marijuana use and eliminated zolpidem as a sleep aid.

He described the effect of LDN as follows:

> *Prior to LDN, I constantly had the feeling of being right on the edge of panic: fear on steroids. When I first began taking naltrexone, I felt a benzedrine/amphetamine-like speediness, but this only*

lasted a few days. Nevertheless, I immediately felt grounded and was able to focus on the "now" of life. "Grounded" is the keyword here for me. Most of my life, I have felt like I was trying to stay afloat in an agitating washing machine. Now I'm able to feel all my emotions and see my thoughts first instead of instantly acting out, like a slave to my own reactions. With LDN, I have that extra second to think before acting or not acting . . . I feel free and alive like I did at 10 before I knew what "scared to death" was.

Due to poor communication, his dose had been left at 2 mg instead of titrating up to his target dose of 4 mg. When he increased the dose to 3.5 mg, he experienced a further reduction in anxiety and episodic depressive symptoms. In his next pool tournament, instead of choking under pressure, as was his habit, he took first place. After increasing the dose to 4 mg, he phoned and exclaimed, "I'm healed! I feel centered and a deep sense of well-being, and I'm not waiting for the other shoe to drop all the time!"

This patient has taken LDN for over eight years without complications.

AFGHANISTAN VETERAN WITH MILITARY PTSD: HYPERVIGILANCE, CONCENTRATION AND SLEEP DIFFICULTIES

A 26-year-old male veteran of three tours of military service in Afghanistan with extensive combat experience met the criteria for PTSD. He also reported a history of severe depression. His bouts of depression typically lasted for two weeks every few months. He was raised in a military family that moved frequently. He reported that he had no close friends growing up. He was sleeping up to 10 hours a night, but his sleep quality was very poor. A sleep study revealed he was waking up roughly 200 times during the night, but interestingly, he did not have sleep apnea. He reported racing thoughts, difficulty completing thoughts, obsessive-compulsive-type thinking, and concentration and memory problems.

Extreme hypervigilance caused him to feel exposed, vulnerable, and highly mistrustful of other people. In restaurants and lecture halls, he always sat with his back to a wall or in a position where he could see his surroundings, but he still had difficulty concentrating. Concentration and focus-related memory problems resulted in academic issues. He reported that when he tried an SSRI antidepressant, it blunted his emotions and motivation, adding to rather than lifting his depression.

Early in his psychotherapy trauma treatment, he began LDN at a full dose of 5.5 mg (0.06 mg/kg/b/w) in the evening. He immediately found it easier to fall asleep (previously he needed to read for an hour or more), and he began sleeping through the night and waking rested.

When he started taking LDN in the morning, he found his hypervigilance in classroom settings diminished, and he was more relaxed around other students. He reported that, when standing in the raucous student section at football games, he was able to enjoy himself instead of feeling angry and agitated at being jostled. No longer having to avoid crowds, he was able to do grocery shopping during the day instead of late at night, and instead of feeling suspicious and angry most of the time, he "felt playful and friendly."

After using LDN for a couple of months, he discontinued the morning dose for a few weeks but noticed that hypervigilance returned, along with greater irritability and greater difficulty concentrating during the day. When he resumed the morning dose, hypervigilance immediately diminished as before.

This patient cut 50 mg pills into doses approximating 5 to 6 mg because he was not able to get the Veterans Administration to pay for compounding. He took LDN for eight months prior to leaving psychotherapeutic treatment.

PTSD WITH OCD SYMPTOMS, SUBSTANCE USE, AND GUT ISSUES

A 190-pound (86.2 kg), 30-year-old male was diagnosed with PTSD. He had childhood trauma, as well as trauma related to a security job that exposed him to ongoing threat. He exhibited extreme hypervigilance, OCD-type symptoms (including trichotillomania), phobia of positive affect, anxiety, panic attacks, and sleep disturbance/deprivation.

He had chronic stomach and digestion issues that had been treated unsuccessfully with conventional medications. Treatment with an sn-1 monolaurin supplement improved a possible candida overgrowth, but gut issues persisted. Three months prior to LDN treatment, he appeared to effectively work through trauma with EMDR therapy. However, his hypervigilance and anxiety remained high, and he continued to ruminate extensively.

With his first LDN treatment of 4.5 mg in the morning, he noticed little change initially but reported the next day that he felt more positive and was slightly less anxious. After adding an afternoon dose, anxiety and reactivity to triggering events were reduced. While anxiety and ruminating occurred, they were less intense and less persistent. Ten hours following a dose, anxiety and depression returned until he took his next LDN dose. A midday dose of 3 mg boosted LDN levels and reduced both anxiety and depressed feelings.

His mental clarity increased. He stopped agonizing over decisions and became more decisive. Reading descriptions of violent crime—part of his graduate program studies—affected him more strongly with LDN, probably due to the disruption of dissociative responses and emotional numbing. He also reported that hypervigilance was reduced so that he no longer felt a need to track what everyone in a restaurant, bar, or classroom was doing. Previously, this had interfered with his ability to socialize comfortably in public settings.

In his words: "Much of my adult life I have observed myself in the third person; with LDN I find myself experiencing life in the first person. Talking with people while on LDN, I was able to be funny, like I was before all the trauma. And after a social outing, it didn't feel necessary to mentally rehash the whole event, as was typical in the past."

LDN appeared to interrupt his moderate smoking habit. He reported: "After smoking half a cigarette, I throw it away because I don't like the taste or smell. Eleven or 12 hours after taking LDN, the old pattern returns, and I smoke the whole cigarette." Alcohol consumption followed a similar pattern. When out with friends, if he had recently taken LDN, he was able to stop after two or three drinks.

It appears that 11 or 12 hours after a dose, the LDN was no longer sufficient to disrupt the dissociative trance that contributed to his smoking and drinking, and old patterns reemerged. But when LDN was at full strength, he was more fully present in the moment rather than in a trance state.

With LDN gut issues quickly began improving, allowing him to eat without bloating and pain. At week 2 he increased his regimen to 4.5 mg at 7 AM, 3 mg at 11 AM and 3 PM, and 4.5 mg before bedtime. Gut issues almost fully resolved two weeks after starting this regimen. After years of gut pain, he began digesting food normally again. He no longer had heartburn "every day, all day" and no longer needed antacids or a proton pump inhibitor (PPI). Thinking it was no longer needed, he stopped taking the sn-1 monolaurin supplement, and a few weeks later, LDN stopped working for him. Resuming the supplement, LDN again quickly and effectively reduced anxiety and supported healthy gut functioning.

The first few nights on LDN, he slept through the night, then resumed a long-standing pattern of waking up at 2:30 AM (in his old neighborhood, bars close at 2 AM). Taking 3 mg at 2:30 AM, he got back to sleep in half an hour. Taking 5 mg LDN at bedtime (about midnight), he started sleeping through the night.

Initially his concentration and reading retention were disrupted. We attribute this difficulty to his having developed a study strategy of constantly checking the internet, organized to accommodate his long-standing hyper-vigilance and his need to scan his environment for threat. This resolved after approximately four weeks; at about the same time, his gut issues were resolving, supporting parasympathetic relaxation, rest, and restoration. LDN appeared to be helping his brain and gut adjust to his safer present-time reality.

LDN reduced a multitude of his PTSD symptoms and increased the speed of trauma resolution. At the time of this writing, he has been taking LDN roughly two to three times daily for 18 months.

PTSD, NEGLECT, KIDNAPPING, AND DOMESTIC VIOLENCE: AUTOIMMUNE DISORDER AND EMOTIONAL EATING

A 48-year-old female survivor of early neglect and abuse, a kidnapping, and long-term domestic violence was diagnosed with PTSD. Even though she was two years out of an abusive relationship when she entered psychother-apy, her ex-partner had an ongoing negative impact on her life. Her symp-toms included extreme hypervigilance, constant anxiety, frequent panic attacks, and restricted social interactions. Her sleep was severely disrupted, in part due to trauma-themed nightmares that made her fearful of sleeping. She was also being treated by a rheumatologist for familial cold-induced autoinflammatory syndrome (FCAS)—a rare genetic syndrome—and irri-table bowel syndrome (IBS).

Her FCAS was being treated prophylactically in the winter months with colchicine to protect against kidney damage and to control flare-ups in reac-tion to being chilled. Flare-ups involved fever, joint inflammation, swelling, and pain. She reported that high-CBD marijuana edibles, used within the first half an hour of symptoms, usually controlled FCAS symptoms and prevented a flare-up. Naproxen was also used for inflammation-related pain.

She initiated LDN with one daily dose of 2.5 mg and quickly increased the frequency of dosing to three times a day. Two and a half months later, without titrating it up, she doubled the dose to 5 mg TID. This worked extremely well for her. Three days after increasing the dose to 5 mg three times a day, her symptoms reduced markedly: in her words, "Immediately, I stopped feeling like a spring too tightly wound. I feel so normal! . . . I didn't realize how badly I was experiencing that anxiety feeling until it went away."

Prior to initiating treatment with Galyn Forster, this client was briefly treated with sertraline but discontinued use because it caused her to become suicidal. She initiated treatment of depression and anxiety with buspirone at the same time she began treatment with LDN. She reported that it worked okay for her, but discontinued it after two months because LDN worked better and without side effects. Prior to starting psychotherapy, she was using the benzodiazepine alprazolam to treat anxiety and panic. She complained that it made her "groggy" and discontinued use after LDN and trauma therapy rendered panic rare and eliminated most intrusive memories.

Amitriptyline was used for a short time to treat insomnia, but she stopped regular use because she was drinking wine while in a sleep state in the middle of the night. LDN significantly reduced insomnia, so she restricted her use of amitriptyline to instances of extreme insomnia, when she had been lying awake for a couple of hours.

Along with reducing anxiety, LDN also eliminated her need to use food to manage emotions, and her IBS symptoms diminished almost as rapidly as her anxiety, to the point of full remission. At this point, treatment with omeprazole was briefly discontinued, but because of a hiatal hernia, she resumed the use of omeprazole to reduce the risk of additional damage to her throat.

In a matter of weeks, she transformed from being a person who frequently left work early—disabled by anxiety and panic—to one who rarely missed work and became a leader and mentor in her department. She stated, "Co-workers have been making comments about how much brighter my personality has been lately. It's nice to not be crippled by anxiety and to be able to laugh and relax." She became a model of courage and creativity, figuring out how to deal more effectively with difficult or angry customers and finding ways to make the workplace enjoyable for her co-workers and customers.

After using LDN for one month, she reported increased mental health and quality-of-life benefits, as well as ongoing remission of IBS. Chronic pain in her left knee went away, insomnia disappeared, and she reported the absence of her normal PMS symptoms of irritability and weepiness.

At two months, she reported a significant reduction in the frequency and intensity of her FCAS flare-ups. When a flare-up occurred, it only lasted a few hours to a day instead of three days or longer, as had been typical in the past. She reduced naproxen use from twice daily to once daily. She reported having an FCAS flare-up with the typical inflammation and joint pain, but, for the first time in 10 years, the flare-up did not include a debilitating fever.

Adding LDN as an adjunctive to psychotherapy accelerated her EMDR therapy since she was better able to stay present during sessions, with only minimal dissociation. She was also able to more quickly resolve traumatic memories.

She has transformed from a victim, literally crippled by anxiety and fear, to an empowered and happy individual living a rich and rewarding life. LDN didn't resolve the trauma by itself, but it played a major role in the process and continues to help manage anxiety and hypervigilance, as well as her autoimmune disorder.

PTSD: EMOTIONAL NEGLECT AND SEXUAL ABUSE

A 30-year-old female survivor of emotional neglect and childhood sexual abuse was diagnosed with PTSD. When LDN was introduced as an adjunctive treatment to psychotherapy, it made EMDR therapy easier to tolerate. She reported that LDN helped her keep things in perspective when she had conflicts with her husband. She became pregnant and stopped LDN after the second trimester because of fears of premature labor. When her delivery date passed, she reinitiated LDN.

The client reported:

> LDN has helped me a lot with PTSD symptoms. I used to have terrible nightmares two to three times a week. After starting LDN, I have only had nightmares maybe once a month, every two months. It has dramatically helped with that sense of "I know I'm triggered, and I understand the fact, but I just can't stop being freaked out." It has helped my relationship with my husband, too. I am better able to talk calmly about emotional issues and feel like we're approaching a problem together instead of feeling hyper-critical and sensitive.

> *I've noticed negative experiences bother me more when I stop*
> *taking LDN, so I feel confident that LDN does have a significant*
> *effect independent of other things. It hasn't had any negative*
> *side effects. I recently was experiencing postpartum depression;*
> *sertraline helped me a long time ago with depression, so I went on*
> *sertraline again, and yuck and ew! It was so gross, so I went off of*
> *it and went back to LDN, which didn't have negative side effects.*
> *When I take LDN, it is subtle, but it leaves me feeling like something*
> *good just happened. At the same time, I will say that I don't really*
> *need it as much as I used to because I've gotten so much better.*

This client used LDN regularly for over 3 years and has continued to use it episodically for 10 years to help deal with more challenging episodes in her life.

Conclusion

Current pharmaceutical and psychological treatments frequently fall short of meeting the treatment needs of many individuals suffering from PTSD, especially those who meet diagnostic criteria for C-PTSD. Multiple factors, including compelling evidence of opioid system involvement in many symptoms common to C-PTSD, suggest that LDN may be a useful tool that can help fill this gap.

C-PTSD is commonly associated with both attachment disruption and chronic traumatization. Research suggests that early attachment disruption likely results in alteration of opioid receptor density that may help set the stage for adult PTSD, which in turn has been associated with changes in opioid receptor binding. Based on this research and our clinical experience, we hypothesize that exposure to stress-driven high levels of endogenous opioids, in combination with decreased opioid receptor density, not only results in significant dissociative symptoms that are the hallmark of C-PTSD but also likely contributes to the autoimmune and inflammatory vulnerabilities that are frequently experienced by individuals who have been exposed to chronic traumatization and/or developmental trauma.

Moreover, endogenous opioid system alterations are likely involved in multiple dissociative and C-PTSD related symptoms, such as depersonalization, derealization, state switching, amnesia, alexithymia, affect dysregulation, and additional phenomena related to dissociation. Opioid activation also plays a key role in the related phenomena of learned help-lessness, stress-induced analgesia, and tonic immobility.[47]

Given the involvement of endogenous opioid activity in the expression of dissociative symptoms, a trial of LDN is a logical choice and a promising treatment strategy for patients with traumatic stress syndromes who often exhibit dissociative symptoms. Adding to its attractiveness is its established track record as a treatment for inflammation and autoimmune issues.

Our clinical experience supports the notion that LDN is a viable intervention in multiply traumatized clients. Not only are classic PTSD symptoms such as hyperarousal, intrusive thoughts, exaggerated startle, flashbacks, nightmares, sleep disturbance, and emotional numbness reduced, but clients tend to experience increased emotional stability, including decreased anger, improved self-regulation, increased awareness, and a greater capacity for mindfulness. Dissociative symptoms like sponta-neous state switching, depersonalization, and derealization are commonly decreased. In addition, LDN seems to moderate depressive symptoms, and it commonly lowers anxiety.

LDN appears to have a regulating influence on the opioid system, directly moderating dissociative symptoms characteristic of C-PTSD. In addition to targeting traditional PTSD symptoms, it also appears to moderate symptoms associated with autoimmune issues and associated systemic inflammation commonly found in this population. In addition, LDN has a proven safety record, is nontoxic, has few side effects, and is inexpensive and readily available. Compared to other pharmaceutical interventions, LDN is notable for its relative absence of negative side effects and its positive impact on quality of life. This combination of effects makes LDN a promising candidate for the treatment of PTSD, especially C-PTSD.

All the patients in the cases described here either met criteria for C-PTSD or had not significantly responded to treatment as usual. Given their success with LDN, it is worthwhile for researchers to investigate the use of LDN in both C-PTSD and simple PTSD, as well as how LDN compares with other interventions. Regardless, while the above-described therapeutic effects appear promising, the use of LDN as a treatment for traumatic stress syndromes must be considered experimental until these effects can be confirmed in placebo-controlled, double-blind trials. Finally, we recommend further research concerning whether the apparent benefits of multiple dosing for clients with autoimmune disorders co-occurring with PTSD and C-PTSD may be attributable to alterations of the opioid system, in addition to the impact LDN has on inflammation and other biological structures related to immune system function.

ELEVEN

Lyme Disease and Other Tick-Borne Illnesses

DARIN INGELS, ND, FAAEM, FMAPS

Lyme disease is one of the fastest-growing infectious diseases in the world, with more than 329,000 new cases each year in the United States and more than 85,000 new cases in Europe.[1] These numbers may seem staggering, but the reality is that the incidence is much higher, as many cases of Lyme disease go misdiagnosed or unreported. The symptoms of Lyme disease can often be vague, and many people go months to years without getting a proper diagnosis or treatment. To compound the problem, there is no real consensus in the medical and scientific community about the best ways to diagnose and treat Lyme disease.

In this chapter I discuss how Lyme disease is transmitted, the complexity of diagnosing the disease, and conventional and alternative methods for treating Lyme. I also look at the relationship between Lyme disease and the immune system, and the corresponding application of LDN in treatment.

History and Transmission

In the late 1970s a group of children living in Lyme, Connecticut, reported mysterious joint pain that was believed to be a form of juvenile rheumatoid arthritis (JRA). JRA is a relatively rare condition, so it was odd that so many children in this small town were experiencing similar symptoms. Public health officials started to look at a possible infectious cause. They sent blood samples to entomologist and microbiologist Dr. Willy Burgdorfer, a government researcher and an expert in insect-transmitted diseases. After several years of research, Dr. Burgdorfer was finally able to identify the causative agent: a newfound bacteria, *Borrelia burgdorferi*, that was named after its discoverer.

While *Borrelia burgdorferi* continues to be the most common cause of Lyme disease in the United States, research has shown there are more than 100 strains of *Borrelia* in North America and more than 300 strains worldwide, although not all strains make people sick. In North America, *B. burgdorferi*, *B. miyamotoi*, and *B. mayonii* are the more widespread strains, while *B. afzelii* and *B. garinii* are most commonly seen in Europe. There is evidence that some of the strains may produce more intense symptoms than others, but more research is needed to verify this observation.[2]

The majority of Lyme disease cases are caused by a tick bite—specifically that of a deer tick (technically known as the *Ixodes* tick). Most public health officials believe the tick needs to be attached to your skin for at least 24 to 48 hours to transmit Lyme disease, but research has shown that Lyme can be transmitted within 16 hours of a tick bite.[3] Many people think they can only be exposed if they are out hiking in the woods or camping, but the reality is that Lyme disease can strike anywhere, as birds have carried ticks to places where they did not exist before. Even those living in urban areas like Los Angeles, Chicago, London, Sydney, and New York City contract Lyme disease. It has been reported in more than 80 countries around the world.[4]

The possibility of Lyme disease transmission from other insects—such as mosquitoes, fleas, and flies—has been speculated, but is not clearly shown in the medical literature. There is now evidence that pregnant mothers can pass Lyme disease to their unborn children, leading to birth defects, stillbirth, or developmental delays.[5] Sexual transmission of Lyme disease has not been well researched, although Dr. Ray Stricker found the Lyme organism in the semen of some men and vaginal secretions of some women with Lyme disease, suggesting that sexual transmission may be possible.[6] However, there are no current studies showing that sexual transmission of Lyme disease occurs, so it remains unclear whether Lyme disease can be spread through sexual contact.

The increased incidence of Lyme disease has been attributed to several factors connected with climate change, including warmer winter temperatures, migration of birds away from their normal habitats, decreased populations of natural predators for ticks, and more people spending time outdoors in warmer weather.[7] The World Health Organization predicts that insect-borne illnesses such as Lyme disease will continue to affect more and more people every year.

The Diagnosis of Lyme Disease

Lyme disease has been hailed as "the Great Mimic," as its symptoms often look like those of numerous other diseases. There are upward of 100 different symptoms associated with Lyme disease, so it's no surprise that this notorious microbial condition can be so difficult to diagnose. Because the symptoms are often mistaken for something else, people can go decades without getting a proper diagnosis or treatment. They might see countless doctors and specialists, get several diagnoses, and find no real answers for why they feel sick. There are upward of 300 different conditions that may be associated with Lyme disease, including the following:

- Multiple sclerosis
- Rheumatoid arthritis
- Lupus
- Polymyalgia rheumatic
- Fibromyalgia
- Chronic fatigue syndrome
- Parkinson's disease
- Amyotrophic lateral sclerosis (ALS or Lou Gehrig's disease)
- Alzheimer's disease
- Mononucleosis (mono)
- Depression
- Meningitis
- Tourette's syndrome
- Irritable bowel syndrome (IBS)
- Migraine headaches
- Restless legs syndrome
- Pediatric autoimmune neuropsychiatric syndrome (PANS)

If you have been given one of these diagnoses and have struggled for months or years trying to find answers, it may be helpful to get tested for Lyme disease and other co-infections to at least rule them out as possibilities. I have seen many people in my practice for whom Lyme was the real cause of their illness, and once we identified it and started appropriate treatment, the symptoms started to improve. Getting the right information is the first step to better health and wellness. Lack of early diagnosis and treatment can lead to chronic inflammation in the joints, nervous system, and gut, as well as an autoimmune syndrome that can attack any organ. Untreated Lyme disease can lead to severe neurological impairment, inflammation in the heart, and, rarely, death.

The diagnosis of Lyme disease has become controversial over the past decade. The Centers for Disease Control and Prevention (CDC) recommends a two-tiered testing system, starting with a Lyme screen test that measures antibodies against the Lyme organism. If that test is positive, then a second, more specific antibody test called a western blot is performed. If the second test is positive, then the CDC considers this a confirmatory test for Lyme exposure. Unfortunately, the initial screening test for Lyme disease is not sensitive, which means it does not pick up many instances of the disease. Research suggests the current Lyme screening test detects less than 46 percent of Lyme disease cases.[8] Other studies have corroborated these findings, suggesting that Lyme blood testing is not reliable in diagnosing Lyme disease.

I was a medical technologist before becoming a naturopathic physician, and I used to run Lyme tests in the laboratory. False positive tests are uncommon, but false negatives are quite common. This means that a negative test does not exclude the possibility of having Lyme disease. Since it is an antibody test, results may vary depending on how well an individual's immune system can make antibodies; whether they take immunosuppressive medications, such as steroids, that could interfere with the tests; the length of time since their tick bite (immunity wanes over time); and whether they have an inherited or acquired immune deficiency or other condition that influences antibody production. These factors are not considered when doctors interpret Lyme test results, so some doctors will ignore patients who have a negative Lyme test, even when they have many of the symptoms.

Furthermore, the many strains of *Borrelia* make Lyme testing additionally problematic, as the standard commercial tests only look for *Borrelia burgdorferi*. Outside North America, this is not even the most common strain, so the test will miss anyone infected with other types of *Borrelia*. There are labs that do offer more comprehensive testing and will test for other strains of *Borrelia*, but this is not the standard of care, and many doctors are unaware of these labs. This adds to the list of reasons why so many people do not get a proper diagnosis in a timely manner.

According to the CDC, Lyme disease is a clinical diagnosis, which means it is based on the presence of signs and symptoms of Lyme disease, particularly for those who live in areas where deer ticks are endemic.[9]

Therefore, Lyme testing is really meant to confirm exposure to the bacteria. It is important to rule out other potential causes of symptoms, including autoimmune diseases such as lupus or rheumatoid arthritis; other tick-borne infections such as bartonellosis, babesiosis, or anaplasmosis; and environmental exposures like mold or mycotoxins, to name a few.

Since Lyme disease gets overlooked so often, how do you know if you have it? Acute Lyme disease can occur within 3 to 30 days of a tick bite, and often feels like a bad case of flu. One of the hallmark signs of Lyme disease is a rash that looks like a bull's-eye or target, technically called an erythema migrans (EM) rash. The CDC claims that up to 80 percent of those with Lyme disease get this classic rash, but other research suggests that less than 50 percent of Lyme-infected people actually develop it.[10] The presence of an EM rash confirms exposure to Lyme disease, but the absence of the rash does not exclude potential exposure to Lyme disease.

Most people with acute Lyme disease feel unwell enough to seek medical help. Some of the signs and symptoms of acute Lyme disease include:

- Fever
- Chills
- Pounding, throbbing headache
- Persistent, debilitating fatigue
- Numbness and tingling
- Joint and/or muscle pain
- Swollen lymph nodes
- Bell's palsy (loss of muscle tone in the face, where one or both sides droop)
- Erythema migrans (EM) rash

If you are fortunate enough to catch Lyme disease early and get treatment right away, your symptoms may subside quickly and you may feel well again. If not, then the picture starts to change. You might end up visiting multiple doctors, trying to find answers for your mysterious symptoms. Many people with Lyme disease are told they have chronic fatigue syndrome, fibromyalgia, restless legs syndrome, multiple sclerosis, depression, neuropathy, or another condition. The suffering continues, and the condition gets worse.

When Lyme disease is not treated early, it can become chronic. Some people go on to develop symptoms that get progressively worse and involve multiple body systems. With so many different presentations of Lyme disease, there is no specific set of symptoms that are consistent from person to person. Some of the most common symptoms of chronic Lyme disease include:

- Wandering joint pain (moves frequently from joint to joint—this is somewhat unique to Lyme disease)
- Brain fog and forgetfulness
- Insomnia
- Chronic swollen glands
- Unexplained fever or night sweats
- Mood swings and irritability
- Depression
- Muscle twitching
- Ringing in ears (tinnitus)
- Heart palpitations or chest pain
- Irritable bowel syndrome
- Thyroid problems (often hypothyroid)
- Changes in handwriting or mixing up words
- Sexual function problems
- Worsening neuropathy with balance, coordination problems
- Chronic headaches or migraines
- New onset of allergies or hypersensitivity to foods, mold, pollen, or chemicals
- Extremely low blood pressure or difficulty maintaining body temperature

As stated above, part of diagnosing Lyme disease is to rule out other conditions that look similar. In 20 years of practice, I have seen countless people who have been diagnosed with other diseases, only to find out later that the symptoms they experienced were due to Lyme. However, the opposite is also true. There is an old saying that goes, "If you only have a hammer, then everything looks like a nail," and this couldn't be more pertinent to the approach taken by some Lyme doctors. It is easy for Lyme doctors to see the whole world through a Lyme lens and forget that there can be other reasons why people feel the way they do.

I once had a young woman come to my office with severe joint pain, headaches, and mood swings. She had seen another practitioner who had diagnosed her with Lyme disease based on her symptoms (she had a negative blood test) and began treating her as such. She had undergone over a year of treatment with no significant improvement in her symptoms. When I met with her, she mentioned that her migraines had started when she was a child, while her other symptoms came on much later in her life. She also complained of chronic gastrointestinal symptoms, which had never been specifically addressed.

After our initial consultation, we decided to see if she had any food allergies or sensitivities. Testing showed she was highly reactive to multiple foods, so we began a regimen of elimination of the problematic foods and sublingual immunotherapy, a technique used to help desensitize people to their allergies (much like allergy shots). After a month of this regimen, her headaches had almost completely gone away, and her joint pain and mood swings were both markedly improved. Over the next few months, all of her symptoms completely resolved, and she felt well again.

Her case is a great example of a set of symptoms that initially looked like Lyme disease, but actually had nothing to do with it. In my experience, when you treat someone for Lyme disease and have tried multiple regimens that have failed, there is likely another culprit that has yet to be identified. Other common conditions that get mistaken for Lyme include infection with another microbe, mold toxicity, small intestinal bacterial overgrowth (SIBO), and mast cell activation syndrome (MCAS), to name a few.

Co-Infections

As if Lyme weren't enough, many ticks that carry Lyme disease also transmit other infectious diseases. Public health departments report that, in parts of the world where deer ticks are endemic, more than 30 percent of the ones that carry Lyme disease also carry multiple other microbes that can make you sick. Some of the more common microbes that cause co-infections with Lyme include:

> **Bartonella:** A bacterium mostly known for causing cat-scratch fever, which can cause joint pain, fatigue, fever, numbness, tingling, and purple discoloration marks (called tracts) that look like stretch marks, but are unrelated to weight changes.
> **Babesia:** A blood parasite that is a cousin of malaria and can cause cyclical fevers, joint or muscle pain, fatigue, night sweats, and the feeling of needing to take a deep breath (called air hunger).

Anaplasma: A bacterium that causes severe headache, fever, chills, nausea, vomiting, muscle pain, diarrhea, loss of appetite, and low white blood cell count; in serious cases it leads to organ failure and bleeding problems.

Ehrlichia: A bacterium that is similar to anaplasma. It also causes severe headache, fever, chills, nausea, vomiting, muscle pain, diarrhea, loss of appetite, mental confusion, low white blood cell count, and sometimes a rash (seen mostly in children). Ehrlichia can cause damage to the brain or nervous system. Like anaplasma, it can also lead to organ failure and bleeding problems.

Rickettsia: A bacterium best-known for causing Rocky Mountain spotted fever, which often starts with a fever and is followed by a splotchy or spotted rash two to four days after the fever begins. It can also cause headaches, fever, chills, nausea, vomiting, muscle pain, and loss of appetite.

Mycoplasma: This is the primary agent for walking pneumonia, which causes a dry, hacking cough that lasts for weeks. The microbe is spread via inhalation of droplets from another infected person who coughs or sneezes on you. However, you can also get mycoplasma through a tick bite and might never develop classic walking pneumonia symptoms. Mycoplasma can cause joint pain, fatigue, headaches, and inflammation in the eyes.

Coxiella: These bacteria cause fever, chills, muscle aches, fatigue, and intestinal problems, but joint pain is rare. They are responsible for the disease called Q fever.

In addition to the microbes above, researchers suspect that a different strain of *Borrelia* might be responsible for an illness known as southern tick associated rash illness (STARI), though this has yet to be proven. STARI presents similarly to Lyme disease, with a smaller bull's-eye rash. It can cause fatigue, headaches, muscle pain, and fever. This illness is not transmitted through deer ticks, but rather through Lone Star ticks found mostly in the southwestern United States.

Many other microbes can be transmitted through tick bites. Every year I attend a conference on tick-borne illnesses, and it seems that each year we learn about new microbes that cause illness following a tick bite. Some of the newer illnesses that look like Lyme disease include Powassan virus,

Colorado tick fever, tularemia, and relapsing tick fever. It is important to be tested for other pathogens if you have Lyme symptoms, as there is a lot of clinical overlap among symptoms caused by different microbes.

Treatment of Lyme Disease

The CDC recommends giving 10 to 21 days of oral antibiotics for early-stage Lyme disease, or 14 to 28 days of intravenous antibiotics if the doctor suspects Lyme has caused meningitis or early neurological symptoms. For adults who find a deer tick on their skin and pull it out, or know their exposure was within the past 72 hours, a single 200 mg dose of doxycycline is recommended. However, there is no evidence that this single-dose approach is effective. There is only one study that has examined it, and the patients were only followed for six weeks. While the study did find that doxycycline suppressed the bull's-eye rash, it did not necessarily prevent more systemic Lyme disease.[11]

As of the writing of this chapter, the Infectious Diseases Society of America (IDSA) is finalizing new guidelines on the treatment of Lyme disease that will be more conservative than before, calling for only 7 to 14 days of antibiotic therapy. Many public health authorities, including the CDC, have used the IDSA guidelines in shaping public policy and the standard of care in Lyme treatment. What this means is that physicians are directed to follow these recommendations for Lyme treatment, which can be problematic for those who complete their treatment and still have symptoms.

Borrelia happens to be an extremely slow-growing organism, and has the ability to evade our immune system, unlike other bacteria in our body. Most bacteria in our body replicate every 10 to 20 minutes, but *Borrelia* replicates every 1 to 16 days. It is also a true shape-shifter, and can morph from a long, coiled bacteria into a small ball (called the round body form). When it does this, it seems to go dormant; the immune system does not recognize it at all.[12] As a result, it is more difficult for antibiotics to do the job that we want them to do.

The conventional approach to Lyme treatment often misses the mark, leaving millions of people worldwide suffering from chronic Lyme disease. Studies show that up to two-thirds of people with Lyme disease will fail to have their symptoms resolved with conventional antibiotic therapy.[13] Once 72 hours have passed after a tick bite, antibiotics are less likely to be successful at eradicating Lyme.[14] Antibiotic therapy may help certain symptoms subside temporarily, but those symptoms often come back later, as the recommended 10 to 21 days may not be adequate to completely halt the organism in its tracks. The International Lyme and Associated Diseases Society (ILADS) has produced a different set of guidelines on Lyme treatment and suggests a much longer course of treatment—six weeks of antibiotics or longer, depending on how people feel after that duration. Since there is no objective test to determine when a patient is better, their symptoms are the best marker of whether or not the treatment has been successful.

Antibiotics can help some people with Lyme disease; once they are treated, they never have symptoms again. But countless others do not respond to short-course antibiotics and continue to have symptoms. While a longer course of antibiotics may be more beneficial, there are also associated risks. Antibiotics not only target the *Borrelia*, but will kill off some of the beneficial bacteria living in your body—especially the gut, where most of these bacteria live. This can lead to the overgrowth of certain bacteria, yeast, and other bugs that harm us in larger quantities. Since each person with Lyme disease can be affected differently, the patient and doctor have to weigh the benefits and risks of longer-term antibiotic regimens.

My passion for treating Lyme stems from my own personal experience with the disease. I contracted Lyme disease in 2002, just a couple of weeks before I was scheduled to open my own clinic. I found the tick bite early (yes, I had the classic bull's-eye rash) and started on antibiotics right away. I was symptom-free after just 4 days of treatment, but finished a 21-day course of antibiotics. However, I was working long hours getting my new business off the ground, and after eight months I started to relapse. I had joint pain, fatigue, numbness, tingling, and headaches again. I started antibiotics again and saw no improvement. I cycled through various antibiotic regimens over almost nine months and continued to worsen, and my gut was a mess.

Fortunately, I knew of a Chinese medicine doctor in New York City who treated Lyme disease, and I had a few patients who had seen him and responded well to his therapies. I saw him, and he started me on a series of Chinese herbal formulas and acupuncture. Within a month I felt 80 percent better. I realized that I was not taking care of myself in the right way—I hadn't been sleeping or eating properly, and my body needed to heal. So I continued with the Chinese herbs, was more diligent with my sleep and diet, and, after almost three years of treatment, was living a symptom-free life.

I used my own personal experience to help shape how I approached Lyme disease with others, and found that the formula works well for most of the Lyme patients I treat. I developed a five-step plan that addresses the whole of the body and does not solely rely on killing Lyme. Like any other infection, why is it that some people get really ill from Lyme and other people are fine? It comes down to the *terrain*. Getting your gut, immune system, hormones, and other essential signaling molecules to work at their highest level is the key to helping your cells and organs repair themselves and heal. The five steps are:

1. **Heal your gut:** Your gut is the cornerstone of good health and accounts for up to 80 percent of your immune function. Making sure you digest and absorb your food, reduce inflammation, and treat underlying infection is essential for restoring your health. Many Lyme patients develop leaky gut, where food substances that should be filtered out pass through the intestinal wall and stimulate inflammation, which may cause gas, bloating, abdominal pain, and changes in bowel habits. Things like digestive enzymes, probiotics, fish oil, and other nutrients can help repair the damage and heal the gut lining.

2. **Diet:** I recommend following an alkaline diet, which means eating foods that help alkalinize your body after you eat them. Most of your cells function best at an alkaline pH, so eating foods to keep that pH in balance helps reduce inflammation and facilitates the repair of the cells. It also allows the enzymes in the cells to do their work, making the cells function more efficiently. An alkaline diet means eating a mostly plant-based diet, limiting animal proteins and fruits to no more than 20 percent of your total intake for the week, and eliminating highly acidic foods such as junk or processed foods, dairy products, and coffee. After having tried numerous other diets, I find this one to be sustainable for people and nutrient-dense.

3. **Treat the active infection:** Although it is not known whether it's possible to completely eradicate *Borrelia* from your body, you can certainly get it under control and live with it without having symptoms. It's kind of like getting chicken pox when you are 5 years old and then getting shingles when you are 55 years old. It's

the same virus that has been dormant for 50 years because your immune system kept it in check. But once your immune system is compromised, the virus becomes opportunistic and starts to create symptoms. Lyme may very well be the same situation. I prefer to use herbs, as they are effective at killing *Borrelia* without damaging your normal gut bugs the way antibiotics do. Herbs also have other health benefits, including helping to reduce inflammation, support the immune system, improve blood flow, and increase energy, to name a few. There are several herbs and herbal protocols used to treat Lyme disease, so I recommend working with a practitioner knowledgeable about herbal medicine to find the right combination for you.

4. **Control your environment:** There are so many things in the environment that harm us and impair our ability to heal, many of which we are completely unaware of. From the chemicals used in and around our homes, to the personal care products we use on our skin, to the products we use to clean our clothes and dishes, these chemicals and toxins can build up in the body to the point where our liver can't keep up and symptoms arise. Swapping out any items that might be harmful with safer, more natural products is a good place to start. One of the biggest environmental factors in illness that I see in my practice is mold. Mold can be found just about anywhere in the world, but water-damaged buildings pose a serious risk to health, and the symptoms of mold exposure look strikingly similar to Lyme disease. If you live in an older home or in a climate that has a lot of humidity and moisture, it would be wise to have your home checked for mold to make sure it is not adversely affecting your health.

5. **Lifestyle management:** Your quality of sleep, how you manage your stress, and how you move your body all play a role in health and healing. Our brain and cells detoxify and repair damaged tissue during deep sleep. Many people with Lyme disease complain that they have restless sleep and wake feeling unrefreshed. Ensuring that you sleep well is essential to recovery. This means following a regular routine of going to bed at the same time each night, avoiding stimulants and electronics before bedtime, and having a dark, quiet environment to get

your proper sleep. Lyme disease can be stressful for you and your loved ones, so having strategies to master your stress helps with the physical and emotional impact of a chronic illness. Meditation, biofeedback, and other techniques can ease the tension you carry during the day. Movement helps increase blood flow, which brings more oxygen and nutrients to your cells. When you're tired and not feeling like doing anything, gentle exercise like stretching, walking, yoga, or swimming can be a nice way to move your body without putting additional stress on it. All of these strategies help improve your physical and mental well-being.

The bottom line is, there is no single treatment for Lyme disease that works for everyone, and you have to find the right treatments that work for you. Having a Lyme-literate practitioner can make this process much easier. For more information on my comprehensive, whole-body approach to Lyme treatment, see *The Lyme Solution: A 5-Part Plan to Fight the Inflammatory Auto-Immune Response and Beat Lyme Disease*.[15]

Lyme and the Immune System

Our immune system is a complicated organization of cells, organs, and chemicals that are all designed to "talk" with one another in ways that we do not fully understand. Each part plays a role in keeping foreign microbes and allergens from harming our body. From the time we are born, our immune system learns to identify what is part of us and what is not. This process is important for helping our bodies fight off infection when needed and then turn that reaction off once the infection has been eradicated.

However, when some people are exposed to a certain microbe or toxin, their immune system can begin to lose tolerance to "self." In the effort to fight an infection, the immune system accidentally attacks healthy tissue, causing inflammation and damage. Normal, healthy cells and organs, including those of the gut, joints, muscles, skin, and brain, all become targets of the immune system. This is the hallmark of autoimmune disease. A growing body of evidence has shown that bacteria and viruses can trigger the immune system to start working against itself.[16]

So how does the immune system get so confused? The answer is what is known as molecular mimicry. This happens when the invading microbe contains proteins that are similar to those found in your own cells. As the immune system gears up to fight the invading microbe, the antibodies produced to target that microbe also target parts of your body that have similar markers. The antibodies no longer discriminate against what is you and what is the microbe, but rather attack both. Many of the symptoms of Lyme disease can be attributed to the immune reaction to Lyme more so than what the *Borrelia* organism does directly to the body.

Many symptoms seen with persistent or chronic Lyme can be attributed to autoimmunity. Research shows there is a specific protein on the outer surface of the *Borrelia* organism called outer surface protein A (ospA), which is structurally similar to a protein in our body called human lymphocyte function associated antigen-1 (hLFA-1).[17] The autoimmune response to this protein is what causes people to develop joint pain and neurological symptoms, even if they have been treated with antibiotics.

Several other proteins also cross-react with the Lyme bacterium, including endothelial cell growth factor (ECGF), apolipoprotein B-100, and annexin A2, which are commonly found in people with other autoimmune diseases such as rheumatoid arthritis and lupus.[18] One study found that antibodies directed at the tail of the Lyme organism (called the flagellum) cross-react with a protein found in the nerves that go to your arms and your legs, causing numbness, tingling, and pain.[19] There is also evidence that Lyme can trigger antibodies that cross-react with the brain, causing various neurological symptoms.[20] With so many different potential immune targets, it's no surprise that Lyme patients end up with long-term autoimmune problems.

Unfortunately, there are no commercial tests for these autoantibodies associated with Lyme. If you developed a fever, swollen glands, and abdominal pain, your doctor would likely run a blood test to look for Epstein-Barr virus, which causes mononucleosis. However, if you have multiple sclerosis or Parkinson's disease, your doctor is less likely to look for an infectious disease that may be causing symptoms. I am always dumbfounded as to why some doctors do not investigate the cause of many chronic diseases. It's no mystery that if you never look for the cause, you won't find it. With so much evidence showing the link between infection and chronic diseases, you would think that the standard of care would be to run a battery of tests to rule out infection, especially as many infections can be determined through a simple blood test. Sadly, this is not the case.

Lyme Disease and Low Dose Naltrexone

I have used low dose naltrexone successfully for many years with my Lyme patients. Although there are currently no studies looking at the effect of LDN on Lyme disease, research has shown how the drug modulates the immune system and helps "turn off" autoimmune reactions. By altering the Th1/Th2 ratio, LDN seems to flip off the switch that activates autoimmunity.

There is evidence that LDN may help protect the brain, in particular, against damage from autoimmunity. In 2011 researchers found that giving LDN to people with multiple sclerosis reduced autoimmune encephalomyelitis, which leads to the breakdown (demyelination) of the protective sheath around the brain and spinal cord.[21] Since there are many overlapping symptoms between multiple sclerosis and Lyme disease, there may be a similar mechanism triggering symptoms for both conditions, suggesting that LDN might have a similar impact on brain health in Lyme patients. However, more research is needed to see if this is true.

Lyme disease often causes muscle pain. One small study found that LDN was effective in reducing muscle pain and inflammation symptoms in fibromyalgia.[22] Other studies have found LDN to help reduce chronic pain and improve quality of life, both of which are important in the treatment of Lyme disease.

Below, I provide the case reports of two patients whom I treated for Lyme disease using a combination of LDN and other therapies.

CASE STUDY #1

Julie was a 47-year-old woman with a 2-year history of joint pain, fatigue, abdominal pain, insomnia, and brain fog. She had been seen by a functional medicine doctor and was found to have elevated inflammatory markers, but her blood tests were negative for various autoimmune diseases (lupus, rheumatoid arthritis, et cetera). Her other stool tests and blood tests showed she had yeast overgrowth, so she was treated with antifungal medication. She had some improvement in her gastrointestinal symptoms and a slight improvement in brain fog.

Diet changes also helped reduce her joint pain and further improved her gastrointestinal symptoms, but after six months her progress plateaued. Her insomnia had not changed significantly. Her doctor tested her for Lyme disease, and her test was positive. She was then referred to my office for evaluation and treatment for Lyme.

Julie was started on an herbal protocol to treat active Lyme, and low dose immunotherapy, a treatment used to modulate the immune system against Lyme. This protocol helped her fatigue and brain fog over the next six weeks. Her joint pain also improved slightly, but she still did not sleep well. I started her on 1 mg of low dose naltrexone at bedtime to help with her pain and sleep. After two weeks there was no improvement, so I had her increase to 2 mg LDN at bedtime. Soon after increasing her dose, she reported better sleep and a slight improvement in her joint pain. She told me she was sleeping deeper and longer than before.

After two more weeks I increased Julie's dose to 3 mg at bedtime. After this increase she reported that she slept consistently through the night, experienced regular bowel movements, and had better energy. She continued to experience an overall improvement in her health after three months, but she still had residual joint pain in her shoulders and hands. I continued to increase her dose up to 3.5 mg at bedtime.

One month later Julie was sleeping well, and her hands were no longer painful. Her grip strength was good, and she was able to perform all activities without limitations. Her digestion continued to be well and she no longer complained of brain fog or abdominal pain. She was even able to go skiing for six to eight hours a day without any joint or muscle pain afterward. Julie has continued with 3.5 mg of naltrexone at bedtime and has been able to reduce other nutritional supplements and herbs. She continues to feel well and live her best life.

CASE STUDY #2

Alex had come to see me after struggling with Lyme disease for many years. He had been through various antibiotic and herbal regimens with only modest improvement in his symptoms. He was dealing with joint pain, fatigue, brain fog, gut problems, and difficulty sleeping. Food intolerance testing found he was sensitive to many foods, so I started him on an elimination diet and immune therapy to help build his immune tolerance to the offending foods. After a few weeks his joint pain had improved and his gut felt better.

I then prescribed 1 mg of LDN and had him increase by 1 mg every two weeks, as tolerated, up to 4 mg. When he got to 2 mg at bedtime, he started to sleep better and felt more rested when he woke. His brain fog had also improved, as his sleep was more consistent. I had him continue up to 4 mg, as he was tolerating it well and had no adverse side effects. His energy slowly improved but was still not as good as expected.

Lyme disease can cause damage to the mitochondria, the parts of your cells that generate energy, so I added nutrients such as CoQ10 and acetyl-L-carnitine to his supplement regimen. Over the next couple of months, Alex's energy was markedly improved. He continued with 4 mg of LDN at bedtime, and I raised his dose to 4.5 mg. Over the next several months, Alex felt well enough to start exercising again and was doing many things he had stopped doing due to his health. His health continued to progress, and LDN was an important part of his road to recovery.

Conclusion

I have now treated hundreds of Lyme patients with low dose naltrexone and have been happy with the benefits; I rarely see side effects. Only a handful of patients have complained of vivid dreams or changes in their sleep patterns. I find many Lyme patients to be overly sensitive to medication, so I start conservatively with low doses, such as 0.5 to 1 mg at bedtime, and increase every two weeks up to 6 mg as tolerated. I have had some Lyme patients respond well at 1 mg, and others who have needed 6 mg to see the difference in their health. My approach is to start small with everything and increase doses slowly. I find this minimizes adverse side effects and allows the body to get used to new medications and supplements.

Given the excellent safety profile of LDN and potential positive benefits, I encourage most of my Lyme patients to try it. For the handful of people who do not tolerate it at bedtime, I recommend taking it during the day, and that often works better. As part of a comprehensive treatment approach to Lyme disease, LDN can be an important medication to provide you with symptomatic relief and alter your immune system so it functions more healthily.

Epilogue

JILL COTTEL, MD

It seems hard to believe that it has already been four years since the first edition of *The LDN Book* was published. So much has happened since then. More studies on LDN have been published in mainstream medical journals than ever before. More and more doctors are becoming familiar with low dose naltrexone, and many have begun prescribing it in their practices. Much of this is due to the efforts of the LDN Research Trust led by Linda Elsegood, who has been unfailing in her quest to bring awareness of low dose naltrexone to prescribers and patients alike. It is no stretch at all to say that the work done by Linda has literally saved lives.

When I wrote the introduction to the first book, I had about 100 patients taking LDN. Up to that point, I had been keeping a spreadsheet with records of every patient taking it. Over the next few years, the number of patients kept increasing. Soon I had over 300 patients taking LDN, and about that time, I stopped keeping track of the number. Eventually it felt like I had more patients in my practice taking LDN than not, although I am sure that was not the case.

My work with the LDN Research Trust and with low dose naltrexone has been an amazing journey. As a general internist and primary care doctor, I previously had a fairly mundane schedule consisting of patients with high blood pressure, diabetes, and high cholesterol. The day would be sprinkled with coughs and colds and the occasional sprained ankle. Whenever there were patients with something interesting, they were sent out to various specialists pretty rapidly. Due to this, there were tons of medical illnesses that I had only ever read about but had never seen personally.

Because of my experience with low dose naltrexone, I have now had the opportunity to see some of the most interesting cases of my entire career. Some of these cases have been very unusual and some rare. Doctors call these rare illnesses zebras—a term that has been historically attributed to the late professor of medicine Dr. Theodore Woodward. Per the website Quote Investigator, the saying goes something like this: "When you hear hoofbeats, don't expect to see a zebra." The term *zebra* in medicine is now commonly used to describe a rare disease or condition, especially when its occurrence is a surprise.

For several years now I have been honored to be a speaker at the LDN Research Trust conferences. In 2017 I gave a presentation titled "Treating Zebras in Primary Care."

Because of how many unusual patients I have seen, I was able to do the entire talk on the zebra patients alone. It is well known that LDN is used for multiple sclerosis, fibromyalgia, and Crohn's disease, and those are the illnesses for which we have the most published data. We also have published case reports and case series of its use for many other illnesses, including inflammatory skin disorders, sarcoidosis, mast cell activation syndrome, ulcerative colitis, and chronic regional pain syndrome.

In addition to seeing patients with all those illnesses, my zebra patients have included those with middle ear myoclonus, eosinophilic esophagitis, ankylosing spondylitis, myasthenia gravis, Ehlers-Danlos syndrome, and pemphigus vulgaris. It has been fascinating to see these cases, but the more meaningful part of my work has been meeting all the remarkable patients who tell me their stories.

I have noticed that there seems to be something different about the patients who come to me seeking treatment with low dose naltrexone. I now expect these patients to have a higher health literacy, be more internet-savvy, and be more connected with their health community.

However, what really comes through in my conversations with patients is that they are fighters. They are not passive about their care or resigned to their fate. They have a determinedness, and are persistent in their search for help. They refuse to settle for the idea of "learning to live with it," which so often seems to be the answer of Western medicine to an illness for which there is no obvious treatment. This resolute attitude is helpful, and I think it has been one of the main factors in how well my patients have fared.

I may have been destined to work with these types of patients because my life has since led me on a completely new journey. Two years ago I moved across the country from one coast to the other, giving up my private solo practice to work in a free and charitable clinic of which I am now medical director. The patients I work with now, while in many ways very different from those of my previous practice, have something in common with those doggedly determined LDN patients of mine. They are also survivors, coming from difficult backgrounds and situations, struggling to make ends meet, often while trying to also deal with health problems.

One of my main concerns when I began work in the new clinic was how to practice medicine without being able to prescribe low dose naltrexone. We are blessed to have our own pharmacy at the clinic, and we are able to provide most medications to patients either free or at a nominal charge. However, LDN is not something that is readily obtainable as it needs to be compounded and individualized. In addition, even though LDN is not expensive compared with most other treatments, our patients do not have the resources to be able to afford it on an ongoing basis.

To my delight and surprise, CareFirst Specialty Pharmacy in New Jersey stepped up and offered to make a very generous donation to the clinic. Because of their support, we are now able to prescribe LDN to some of our patients. This has been life changing for many of them, so much so that some of the patients have chosen to pay for the prescription out of pocket on their own after they have left the clinic and gone on to obtain private insurance.

There are many challenges in working with the underserved. Patients often seek care later in the course of their illness. There is often a lack of consistency with their previous health care services. They may struggle with a language barrier or have literacy and educational issues. Others may have a low health literacy, which makes simple things like reading a prescription bottle or following the instructions of their provider difficult.

Our patients also have limited financial resources. They struggle with basic needs such as food, clothing, transportation, and housing. Having warm winter clothes, wearing proper footwear, and being able to get to doctor appointments are things they do not take for granted. Stress management and self-care time is nearly nonexistent. Food insecurity leads to problems with nutrition. Patients eat whatever is most easily available, often food that is both nutrient-depleted and high in sugar, salt, and fat, which is more inflammatory. Getting patients onto a gluten-free diet is near impossible.

Having said all of this, my initial thought was that LDN was not going to be quite as effective in the free clinic as it was in my previous practice. Many of those patients were already doing well from an integrative medicine standpoint. Their diets were clean, high in nutrients, low-inflammation, and usually gluten-free. Their vitamin levels and hormones had already been optimized. Most had good stress management programs, and the opportunity for regular exercise. All these things are important when treating a patient for any disease state.

With all this in mind, I began to treat a small number of patients with LDN for chronic pain. When I discovered that the patients were responding, I was thrilled. The first 20 patients to be treated were reported in a case series presentation, which was recorded for the most recent LDN conference. Of the 20 patients, the majority were women, and greater than half were over 50 years of age. About half of the patients had myofascial pain, and the other half had either inflammatory or neurogenic pain.

Only 3 of the 20 patients discontinued the medication for side effects, which included the typical complaints of digestive symptoms, headache, and anxiety. Three other patients discontinued early (less than three months) due to a perceived lack of benefit. Of the 14 who continued treatment past three months, 11 of them experienced at least some improvement in their symptoms. Their diagnoses included fibromyalgia or myofascial pain syndrome, chronic regional pain syndrome, localized neuralgia, and chronic pain syndrome not otherwise specified. Most of these patients had already tried all the standard therapies for their medical problems without any success, so to find something that helped at all was greeted with much appreciation.

The experience that I have had so far in treating the free clinic patients with LDN speaks to the effectiveness of the treatment. Studies are often done in pristine environments, with a lot of time and attention spent with patient guidance and education. Many times the patient groups have already been screened for the ones most likely to respond. High rates of response might be reported in the study, but then out in the community, practitioners do not see the same results in their practices. However, I can now say that I have seen LDN work for patients who are in the least ideal circumstances.

If you are a practitioner who is considering treating patients with low dose naltrexone, you should be encouraged by these words. If LDN can work in our less-than-ideal real-world free clinic, then it is certainly worth a try in a typical practice. Even if only half your patients respond, your practice is still better off than before. And even if some only have modest responses, those patients are still better off than before, especially if they are in chronic pain.

If you are a patient who is considering treatment with low dose naltrexone, you should be encouraged as well. The majority of prescribers would tell you that there is nothing to lose, myself included. LDN is safe, well tolerated, well studied, and used widely throughout the world.

If you are a practitioner like myself who already prescribes LDN, Linda and I want to express our gratitude. The more of us that are out there, the more the knowledge of LDN will spread. Our goal is to see awareness of low dose naltrexone continue to grow among practitioners and patients—and along with that, increased prescribing of LDN for patients who need it.

Together we can make a change, and our patients and their lives will be better for it.

ACKNOWLEDGMENTS

I want to thank Chelsea Green Publishing for the opportunity to compile *The LDN Book, Volume 2*. Thanks to the staff, who did an excellent job of editing and proofreading; to all the contributors for their dedication and hard work, without which there would be no second book; and last but not least, to Paula Johnson for her work on the endnotes—a long, tedious task!

Dosing Protocols

Sarah J. Zielsdorf, MD, MS

with contribution from Mark Mandel, PharmD

Low dose naltrexone is an inexpensive prescription medication that is used to treat a variety of conditions.* Because it is administered in such low doses, it must be compounded. Patients should be sure to have their prescription compounded by a reputable pharmacy to guarantee that quality and safety checks have been carried out.

My own personal journey with LDN began in 2014 as I was suffering from a severe Hashimoto's autoimmune thyroid flare when I was three months postpartum with my daughter. LDN gave me my life back within a month, and I was able to complete my residency. I have now had the honor of treating thousands of chronically ill patients as an attending internist and diagnostician. My autoimmune symptoms are controlled on 4.5 mg of LDN. I've taken time off of it and chose to restart it.

When I was 29 years old, I was unable to get out of my car after driving only six miles to work, paralyzed by stabbing back and body pain. With the aid of LDN, I no longer have daily chronic pain, and my overall attitude is much more positive. I've become a fiercely passionate advocate for LDN. There really is something to say for its correction of that low endorphin state.

During my first LDN conference in 2017, the consensus among researchers and clinicians, including myself, was that there were only a few therapeutic dosing regimens, namely taking 1.5 to 4.5 mg compounded naltrexone nightly (or in the morning if it caused insomnia or severe nightmares).

---

* A list of conditions can be found on the LDN Research Trust website: www.ldn researchtrust.org/conditions.

In only two years, as I learned at the 2019 conference, our regimens have seemingly exploded with creativity and variability. With the customization of treatment regimens and customized dosing forms, our medical and research advisers to the LDN Research Trust and LDN clinicians have been able to share insights, thus expanding the medical knowledge and treatment paradigms for patient care. We are reaching more patients using social media, patients are inquiring about LDN use with their clinicians, and more collaborative research is being undertaken. In short, we've come a long way since Dr. Ian Zagon hypothesized that endogenous opioids acted as growth factors in the 1970s, and Dr. Bernard Bihari tested using LDN to enhance the immune response for infection (AIDS), autoimmunity, and cancer in the early 1980s.

Compounded Forms of Naltrexone

Naltrexone can be compounded into a number of different forms, including capsules, tablets, gummy bears, sublingual drops, liquids, eye drops, troches, topical lotions, and transdermal creams.

> **Oral-liquid LDN** allows for titration of dosing from 0.1 mg to 16 mg and anything in between.
>
> **LDN sublingual drops** are best for patients with swallowing difficulties, or those who do not experience any benefits from ingested, oral-liquid formulations, as sublingual LDN drops are absorbed directly through the oral mucosa. This allows for faster absorption and can reduce gastrointestinal side effects.
>
> **LDN capsules** can be made from 0.1 mg to whatever dose the prescribers would prefer. Fillers can vary from pharmacy to pharmacy but

TABLE A.1. Dose Definitions

Naltrexone Strength	Dose
Full dose naltrexone	50–100 mg
Low dose naltrexone	0.5–16 mg*
Very low dose naltrexone (VLDN)	50–500 mcg
Ultra low dose naltrexone (ULDN)	1–20 mcg

* Traditionally, the upper limit of what was defined as LDN was 4.5 mg, but this definition has been slightly broadened.

generally include sucrose, Avicel, or a probiotic depending on a patient's individual sensitivities.

LDN tablets can be compounded and scored so doses can be easily titrated.

LDN topical lotions and creams are normally used for children and skin conditions such as psoriasis.

LDN troches can be made into any dosage and can be split into four. They dissolve under the tongue in one to two minutes. The benefits are comparable to those of sublingual drops.

Dosing Guide

As the chapters in this book make clear, dosing protocols can and do vary widely depending on the condition or patient type.

Autoimmune diseases: The rule of thumb for autoimmune diseases is "Go low, go slow." Start slow and build up slowly: 1 mg daily for 14 days, increasing by 0.5 to 1 mg every two weeks until at 4.5 mg or highest tolerated dose at or above 3 mg.

Cancer: 1.5 mg daily for seven days, increasing by 1.5 mg weekly until at 4.5 mg. Once in remission, dose of 4.5 mg for seven days; start alternating three days on, three days off if indicated.

Chronic pain: Start slow and build up slowly: 1 mg daily for 14 days, increasing by 0.5 to 1 mg every two weeks until at 4.5 mg or highest tolerated dose at or above 3 mg.

Fertility/pregnancy: Start slow and build up slowly: 1 mg daily for 14 days, increasing by 0.5 to 1 mg every two weeks until at 4.5 mg or highest tolerated dose at or above 3 mg.

Anxiety / depression / post-traumatic stress disorder / traumatic brain injury: Start slow and build up slowly: 1 mg daily for 14 days, increasing by 0.5 to 1 mg every two weeks until at 4.5 mg or highest tolerated dose at or above 3 mg. Though LDN is generally used once per day, it can be used up to four times a day for mental health conditions.

Chronic fatigue syndrome / myalgic encephalomyelitis: Twice-daily dosing could be prescribed (between 1.5 and 4.5 mg per dose).

Allergies: Some clinicians dose up to three times per day in higher
doses for allergy patients (up to 8 mg per dose).

Behavioral health issues: Up to four times a day could be prescribed
in low doses.

Children: Children under 40 kg: 0.1 mg per kg, starting at 0.1 mg
and increasing over a period of four weeks to calculated dose.
Creams have little published evidence of efficacy, but are available
for topical administration. Children > 40 kg: Treat as adults. In
children take special care that the status as an unlicensed medicine
is well known by family members.

Pets: Doses of up to 15 mg daily have been used in dogs for cancer and
chronic pain conditions. Give at the same time every day; day or
night is irrelevant.

Opioid addiction: In doses of 1 mcg (ultra low dose naltrexone /
ULDN), it can be used alongside opioids; over time, titrate the
opioid down and the ULDN up until the patient is on LDN. This
should always be under medical supervision. See below for opioid
weaning considerations.

Dosing Time

Normally, LDN is taken or administered in the evening, although many
people prefer to take it in the morning to avoid sleep disturbance. Of note,
some patients see the greatest benefit by skipping one night per week, which
may help with receptor sensitivity. It used to be recommended to use on/off
cycling by taking LDN for three days and then skipping days to maximize
effect, but as of the last LDN conference, many LDN prescribers believe that
the time period between daily doses reflects the rebound effect of opioid/
enkephalin production, and thus that receptors are reset.

Drug Compatibility

If taking any of the treatments below, please discuss your individual case
with your clinician before initiating LDN.

Biologics: Compatible with LDN as long as being monitored and
stable before LDN initiation. Includes daclizumab (Zinbryta),

QUALITY ASSURANCE OF COMPOUNDED LDN
by Mark Mandel, PharmD

Accredited compounding pharmacies are required to have very stringent quality control of the medications that they compound. They use pure raw ingredients (active pharmaceutical ingredients / APIs) with known and documented potency of each batch of raw chemical (Certificate of Assay). Batches are relatively small and can be easily monitored. As a result of the overwatch function of accreditation boards, and their very stringent rules, patients should be receiving consistent compounded products that are uniform in content and potency.

Warnings

The chemical naltrexone is a water-soluble drug and is available commercially as a 50 mg generic tablet. It might seem a simple process to take a tablet, drop it into about 11 ml of water, and get about 4.5 mg per ml. However, this method isn't recommended. It isn't accurate for a variety of reasons, including the variability of dose found in commercial generic tablets, and can easily become contaminated.

Purchasing naltrexone or LDN without a prescription online is illegal and extremely dangerous as you have no way of knowing what is purchased. Counterfeit drugs look exactly the same as the real thing. However, they won't have gone through the same stringent quality checks as pharmaceutical-grade drugs. At best, they could be harmless with no active ingredients, or they could contain harmful components that could be lethal or anything in between. Prescription drugs shipped to other countries that are purchased without a prescription are often confiscated at customs. So a good deal on the surface might be anything but. Remember, always, that the most expensive medication or treatment is the one that fails to work!

dimethyl fumarate (Tecfidera), fingolimod (Gilenya), interferon beta-1a (Avonex, Rebif), mitoxantrone (Novantrone), natalizumab (Tysabri), ocrelizumab (Ocrevus), peginterferon beta-1a (Plegridy), teriflunomide (Aubagio), glatiramer acetate (Copaxone, Glatopa), interferon beta-1b (Betaseron, Extavia).

Antibiotics: Tetracyclines and aminoglycosides compatible with caveats.

Steroids: Prednisone/methylpred compatible as long as daily dose is < 20 mg equivalent prednisolone and not being used for organ replacement anti-rejection therapy. Dexamethasone is compatible at any dose as long as it is being monitored by oncology.

Short-acting painkillers (such as co-codamol/tramadol): Leave a four- to six-hour gap before taking LDN.

Ketamine: Use LDN with caution while using ketamine.

Alcohol and tramadol: Naltrexone is often used to help with alcohol cravings. With regard to low dose naltrexone, individuals have different responses to LDN and concomitant alcohol use. Many are fine consuming a few drinks and have no reactions to their LDN medication. However, in practice I have had some patients develop severe headaches or decreased alcohol tolerance when using LDN. Therefore, I recommend making sure you tolerate LDN without alcohol use prior to trialing small amounts of alcohol within six hours of taking LDN. Anecdotally, some patients with alcohol-LDN interactions have been able to tolerate alcohol if taking their LDN in the morning, and moderate alcohol use so that it is only in the evening. Because tramadol is a synthetic analog of codeine, and acts on the central nervous system (CNS) via selective interaction with the mu-opioid receptor, there is concern for use with LDN. However, tramadol's analgesic effect is only partially inhibited by naltrexone. Researchers therefore believe that tramadol works on other aspects of the CNS.[1] Therefore, it is recommended that tramadol be separated from LDN and alcohol by six hours.

Opioids: Concomitant opioid administration increases the risk of induced withdrawal. Cautionary use with short-acting opioids. Contraindicated in sustained release opioids or high doses (SR morphines or analogs: MST, oxycodone, dipipanone, and fentanyl). If on a sustained release opioid regimen, switch to alternative pain control and leave a four- to six-hour gap between opioid and LDN.

Not compatible: Patients on active clinical trials or taking anti-rejection drugs, anti–tumor necrosis factor, programmed death ligand-1 (PD-1) inhibitors (checkpoint inhibitors including Opdivo and Keytruda, and all in class), anti-cancer vaccines—CAR-T and equivalent plus all in class.

Unless described or cautioned above, all other prescription medications are compatible.

Patient Special Considerations

Over the past five years working with thousands of chronically ill and incredibly complex patients, I have observed that specific conditions require nuanced prescribing of LDN. Patients with the following conditions may have different dosing needs that require careful consideration.

Hashimoto's thyroiditis patients may require closer titration and testing of T3/T4 levels every four to eight weeks during initiation phase. In general, newer thyroid patients start at 0.5 mg, often in liquid form, to titrate in smaller increments, even by 0.1 mg weekly. Long-standing thyroid patients may be able to tolerate regular dosing increments from 0.5 to 1.5 mg and increasing by 0.5 to 1.5 mg every two weeks to a maximum dose of 4.5 mg nightly.

Chronic fatigue syndrome / myalgic encephalomyelitis patients often experience flu-like symptoms and may need slower titration. If exacerbation of symptoms occurs, decrease the dose until able to tolerate titrate accordingly.

Multiple sclerosis patients often experience worsening of symptoms in the first eight weeks. This is normal and is often a sign of good long-term response.

Lyme patients on multiple antibiotics and disease-modifying anti-rheumatic drug agents should seek careful advice from and work with experienced providers and pharmacists before initiating LDN.[2]

Sensitive patients who are unable to tolerate regular drug dosages may need to start with very low dose naltrexone (VLDN), which is often titrated up until on LDN.

Thyroid medication dependent patients may need to reduce their dose once LDN starts taking effect.

Malabsorption cases may require higher doses and/or liquid form.

Opioid weaning considerations: The recommended dose of ULDN is 1 μg twice daily. A randomized, controlled, blinded trial of 719 patients with chronic low back pain were treated concomitantly with 80 mg per day or less of oxycodone and 2 or 4 μg naltrexone daily. The final analysis of 360 patients concluded that 2 μg naltrexone daily showed the fewest opioid-related adverse effects, including constipation, somnolence, and pruritus, in addition to the fewest withdrawal symptoms following active treatment and weaning.[3]

The general recommendation for opioid weaning is to taper by 10 percent monthly if a patient has been taking opioid medications longer than a year. A more aggressive weaning may be considered for a relatively opioid-naive patient (use no longer than weeks to months), such as decreasing by 10 percent weekly. With the use of ULDN, weaning may be done quicker, even for a long-term opioid medication user. This is a general approach and must be individualized to each patient. This must be done with a multidisciplinary approach utilizing primary care, pain management, and other specialists to determine the appropriate treatment plan and closely monitor for adverse effects and the need for greater support. Using these micro doses, alongside opioids titrating one up and one down, the goal is success weaning off the opioid medication; many patients subsequently titrate up to LDN dosing.

ULDN is also utilized for the enhancement of opioid analgesia, especially for chronic pain patients. One group that especially benefits from this combination is the fibromyalgia community. Dr. Ginevra Liptan, a fibromyalgia specialist and internist, puts it best: "The key is finding the dosage sweet spot where LDN is able to calm the glial cells, but not knock the opiates off their receptors." One concern is that opioid-induced tolerance may be secondary to increased irritation of glial cells in the central nervous system. By reducing glial cell sensitivity, opioid effectiveness can be restored and enhanced.[4] ULDN may, in fact, act as a reset button for the opioid response pathway, much like rebooting a frozen computer.[5]

NOTES

Chapter 1: The History and Pharmacology of LDN

1. M. P. Stapleton, "Sir James Black and Propranolol. The Role of the Basic Sciences in the History of Cardiovascular Pharmacology," *Texas Heart Institute Journal* 24, no. 4 (1997): 336–42.
2. M. D. Kertai et al., "A Combination of Statins and Beta-Blockers Is Independently Associated with a Reduction in the Incidence of Perioperative Mortality and Nonfatal Myocardial Infarction in Patients Undergoing Abdominal Aortic Aneurysm Surgery," *European Journal of Vascular and Endovascular Surgery* 28, no. 4 (October 2004): 343–52.
3. M. J. Brownstein, "A Brief History of Opiates, Opioid Peptides, and Opioid Receptors," *Proceedings of the National Academy of Sciences USA* 90, no. 12 (June 1993): 5391–93.
4. O. Schmiedeberg, *Über die Pharmaka in der Ilias und Odysse* (Strassburg: Karl J. Trübner, 1918), 1–29; L. Lewin, *Phantastica* (New York: Dutton, 1931).
5. Reginald L. Campbell and R. Everett Langford, "Brief History of Substance Abuse," in *Substance Abuse in the Workplace* (Boca Raton, FL: Lewis Publishers, 1995).
6. Brownstein, "A Brief History of Opiates."
7. Campbell and Langford, "Brief History of Substance Abuse."
8. J. M. Scott, *The White Poppy: A History of Opium* (New York: Funk & Wagnalls, 1969).
9. India: S. C. Dwarakanath, "Use of Opium and Cannabis in the Traditional Systems of Medicine in India," *Bulletin on Narcotics* 17, no. 1 (1965): 15–19; China: J. Fort, "Giver of Delight or Liberator of Sin: Drug Use and 'Addiction' in Asia," *Bulletin on Narcotics* 17, no. 3 (1965): 1–11.
10. Campbell and Langford, "Brief History of Substance Abuse."
11. Brownstein, "A Brief History of Opiates."
12. Hearne and Van Hout, "'Vintage Meds': A Netnographic Study of User Decision-Making, Home Preparation and Consumptive Patterns of Laudanum," *Substance Use & Misuse* 50, no. 5 (April 2015): 598–608.
13. Hearne and Van Hout, "'Vintage Meds.'"
14. P. Prioreschi, "Medieval Anesthesia—The *Spongia Somnifera*," *Medical Hypotheses* 61, no. 2 (August 2003): 213–19; G. Keil, "*Spongia Somnifera*. Medieval Milestones on the Way to General and Local Anesthesia," *Anaesthesist* 38, no. 12 (December 1989): 643–48.

15. F.W.A. Sertürner, "Darstellung der Reinen Mohnsäure (Opiumsäure), Nebst Einer Chemischen Untersuchung des Opium," *J. Pharm. f. Artze. Apoth Chem.* 14 (1806): 47–93.

16. F.W.A. Sertürner, *Gilbert's Annalen der Physik* 25 (1817): 56–89.

17. D. Noble, "Claude Bernard, the First Systems Biologist, and the Future of Physiology," *Experimental Physiology* 93, no. 1 (January 1993): 16–26.

18. Noble, "Claude Bernard."

19. J. Sawynok, "The Therapeutic Use of Heroin: A Review of Pharmacological Literature," *Canadian Journal of Physiology and Pharmacology* 64, no. 1 (January 1986): 1–6.

20. M. C. Michel, "An Anthology from Naunyn-Schmiedeberg's Archives of Pharmacology," *Naunyn-Schmiedeberg's Archives of Pharmacology* 373, no. 2 (May 2006): 139.

21. C. C. Scott and K. K. Chen, "The Action of 1,1-diphenyl-1-(dimethylaminoiso-propyl)-butanone-2, a Potent Analgesic Agent," *Journal of Pharmacology and Experimental Therapeutics* 87, no. 1 (May 1946): 63–71.

22. S. Hosztafi, T. Friedmann, and Z. Furst, "Structure-Activity Relationship of Synthetic and Semisynthetic Opioid Agonists and Antagonists," *Acta Pharmaceutica Hungarica* 63, no. 6 (November 1993): 335–49.

23. Sankyo Co., *New morphinone and codeinone derivatives and process for preparing the same, GB Patent 939287 A*, filed March 9, 1962, and issued October 9, 1963; M. J. Lewenstein, *Morphine derivative, US Patent 3254088*, filed March 14, 1961, and issued May 31, 1966.

24. "Essential Medicines," World Health Organization, http://www.who.int/medicines/services/essmedicines_def/en.

25. Endo Lab, *14-hidroxydihydronormorphinone derivatives*, filed December 6, 1966, and issued July 25, 1967.

26. C. B. Pert and S. H. Snyder, "Opiate Receptor: Demonstration in Nervous Tissue," *Science* 179, no. 4077 (March 1973): 1011–14.

27. M. R. Hutchinson et al., "Evidence That Opioids May Have Toll-Like Receptor 4 and MD-2 Effects," *Brain, Behavior, and Immunity* 4, no. 1 (January 2010): 83–95.

28. M. Galanter and H. D. Kleber, *The American Psychiatric Publishing Textbook of Substance Abuse Treatment*, 4th ed. (Washington, DC: American Psychiatric Publishing, April 2008).

29. K. Miotto et al., "Naltrexone and Dysphoria: Fact or Myth?," *American Journal on Addictions* 11, no. 2 (Spring 2002): 151–60; E. R. Zaaijer et al., "Effect of Extended-Release Naltrexone on Striatal Dopamine Transporter Availability, Depression and Anhedonia in Heroin-Dependent Patients," *Psychopharmacology* 232, no. 14 (July 2015): 2597–607; "Naltrexone Hydrochloride 50 mg Film-Coated Tablets," medicines.org.uk, last updated March 5, 2014, https://www.medicines.org.uk/emc/medicine/25878.

30. J. E. Blalock and E. M. Smith, "A Complete Regulatory Loop between the Immune and Neuroendocrine Systems," *Federation Proceedings* 44, no. 1 (January 1985): 108–11.

31. Blalock and Smith, "A Complete Regulatory Loop."

32. Blalock and Smith, "A Complete Regulatory Loop."
33. B. Bihari, "Low Dose Naltrexone in the Treatment of HIV Infection," lowdose naltrexone.org, last modified September 1996, http://www.lowdosenaltrexone .org/ldn_hiv_1996.htm.
34. Bihari, "Low Dose Naltrexone."
35. I. S. Zagon and P. J. McLaughlin, "Opioid Antagonist-Induced Modulation of Cerebral and Hippocampal Development: Histological and Morphometric Studies," *Brain Research* 393, no. 2 (August 1986): 233–46; I. S. Zagon and P. J. McLaughlin, "Opioid Antagonist (Naltrexone) Modulation of Cerebellar Development: Histological and Morphometric Studies," *Journal of Neuroscience* 6, no. 5 (May 1986): 1424–32.
36. R. N. Donahue et al., "The Opioid Growth Factor (OGF) and Low Dose Naltrexone (LDN) Suppress Human Ovarian Cancer Progression in Mice," *Gynecologic Oncology* 122, no. 2 (August 2011): 382–88.
37. S. Gupta et al., eds., "Mechanisms of Lymphocyte Activation and Immune Regulation X: Innate Immunity," *Advances in Experimental Medicine and Biology*, Vol. 560 (New York: Springer, 2005), 41–45.
38. Gupta et al., "Mechanisms of Lymphocyte Activation."
39. C. Giuliani, "NF-kB Transcription Factor: Role in the Pathogenesis of Inflammatory, Autoimmune, and Neoplastic Diseases and Therapy Implications," *Clinical Therapeutics* 152, no. 4 (July–August 2001): 249–53; B. O'Sullivan et al., "NF-kappa B as a Therapeutic Target in Autoimmune Disease," *Expert Opinion on Therapeutic Topics* 11, no. 2 (February 2007): 111–22.
40. C. S. Mitsiades, "Activation of NF-kappa B and Upregulation of Intracellular Anti-Apoptotic Proteins via the IGF-1/Akt Signalling in Human Multiple Myeloma Cells: Therapeutic Implications," *Oncogene* 21, no. 37 (August 2002): 5673–83.
41. M. R. Hutchinson et al., "Non-Stereoselective Reversal of Neuropathic Pain by Naloxone and Naltrexone: Involvement of Toll-Like Receptor 4 (TLR4)," *European Journal of Neuroscience* 28, no. 1 (July 2008): 20–29.
42. Hutchinson et al., "Non-Stereoselective Reversal of Neuropathic Pain;" Rachel Cant, Angus G. Dalgleish, and Rachel L. Allen, "Naltrexone Inhibits IL-6 and TNFα Production in Human Immune Cell Subsets following Stimulation with Ligands for Intracellular Toll-Like Receptors," *Frontiers in Immunology* 8 (July 2017): 809, https://doi.org/10.3389/fimmu.2017.00809.
43. Hutchinson et al., "Non-Stereoselective Reversal of Neuropathic Pain."
44. Cant, Dalgleish, and Allen, "Naltrexone Inhibits IL-6 and TNFα Production in Human Immune Cell Subsets following Stimulation with Ligands for Intracellular Toll-Like Receptors."
45. A. Marshak-Rothstein, "Toll-Like Receptors in Systemic Autoimmune Disease," *Nature Reviews Immunology* 6, no. 11 (November 2006): 823–35; V. D. Pradhan et al., "Toll-Like Receptors in Autoimmunity with Special Reference to Systemic Lupus Erythematosus," *Indian Journal of Human Genetics* 18, no. 2 (May–August 2012): 155–60; D. Singh and S. Naik, "The Role of Toll-Like Receptors in Autoimmune Diseases," *Journal of Indian Rheumatology Association* 13 (2005): 162–65.
46. L.A.J. O'Neill, "Toll-Like Receptors in Cancer," *Oncogene* 27 (2008): 158–60.

Chapter 2: Chronic Pain

1. S. E. Mills et al., "Chronic Pain: A Review of Its Epidemiology and Associated Factors in Population-Based Studies," *British Journal of Anaesthesia* 123, no. 2 (2019): e273–e283.
2. T. P. Jackson et al., "The Global Burden of Chronic Pain," *ASA Monitor* 78, no. 6 (2014): 24–27.
3. J. Barcellos de Souza et al., "Prevalence of Chronic Pain, Treatments, Perception, and Interference on Life Activities: Brazilian Population-Based Survey," *Pain Research and Management* 2017 (2017): Article ID 4643830.
4. Jackson et al., "The Global Burden of Chronic Pain."
5. Barcellos de Souza et al., "Prevalence of Chronic Pain."
6. Barcellos de Souza et al., "Prevalence of Chronic Pain."
7. E. Wambre and D. Dong, "Oral Tolerance Development and Maintenance," *Immunology and Allergy Clinics of North America* 38, no. 1 (2018): 27–37.
8. Wambre and Dong, "Oral Tolerance Development and Maintenance."
9. S. Akbari and A. A. Rasouli-Ghahroudi, "Vitamin K and Bone Metabolism: A Review of the Latest Evidence in Preclinical Studies," *Hindawi BioMed Research International* (2018): Article ID 4629383.
10. V. Nurminen et al., "Primary Vitamin D Target Genes of Human Monocytes," *Frontiers in Physiology* 10 (2019): Article 194.
11. M.A.M. Rogers and D. Aronoff, "The Influence of Non-Steroidal Anti-Inflammatory Drugs on the Gut Microbiome," *Clinical Microbiology and Infection: The Official Publication of the European Society of Clinical Microbiology and Infectious Diseases* 22, no. 2 (2016): 178.e1–178.e9.
12. L. P. James et al., "Acetaminophen-Induced Hepatotoxicity," *Drug Metabolisn and Disposition* 31 (2003): 1499–506.
13. D. Hota et al., "Off-Label, Low-Dose Naltrexone for Refractory Painful Diabetic Neuropathy," *Pain Medicine* 17, no. 4 (April 2016): 790–91.
14. D. Trofimovitch and S. J. Baumrucker, "Pharmacology Update: Low-Dose Naltrexone as a Possible Nonopioid Modality for Some Chronic, Nonmalignant Pain Syndromes," *American Journal of Hospice and Palliative Care* 36, no. 10 (October 2019): 907–12.
15. Hota et al., "Off-Label, Low-Dose Naltrexone."
16. F. Birklein and V. Dimova, "Complex Regional Pain Syndrome-Up-to-Date," *Pain Reports* 2, no. 6 (November 2017): e624.
17. G. M. Alexander et al., "Changes in Cerebrospinal Fluid Levels of Pro-Inflammatory Cytokines in CRPS," *Pain* 116, no. 3 (August 2005): 213–19; L. Parkitny et al., "Inflammation in Complex Regional Pain Syndrome: A Systematic Review and Meta-Analysis," *Neurology* 80, no. 1 (January 2013): 106–17.
18. L. Del Valle et al., "Spinal Cord Histopathological Alterations in a Patient with Longstanding Complex Regional Pain Syndrome," *Brain, Behavior and Immunity* 23, no. 1 (January 2009): 85–91; P. Chopra and M. S. Cooper, "Treatment of Complex Regional Pain Syndrome (CRPS) Using Low Dose Naltrexone (LDN)," *Journal of Neuroimmune Pharmacology* 8, no. 3 (June 2013): 470–76.

19. Chopra and Cooper, "Treatment of Complex Regional Pain Syndrome."

20. L. R. Webster, "Oxytrex: An Oxycodone and Ultra-Low-Dose Naltrexone Formulation," *Expert Opinion on Investigational Drugs* 16, no. 8 (August 2007): 1277–83; Y.H.J. Kim and K. West, "Treating Chronic Pain with Low Dose Naltrexone and Ultralow Dose Naltrexone: A Review Paper," *Journal of Pain Management and Therapy* 3, no. 1 (February 2019): 1–5.

21. V. L. Chindalore et al., "Adding Ultralow-Dose Naltrexone to Oxycodone Enhances and Prolongs Analgesia: A Randomized, Controlled Trial of Oxytrex," *Journal of Pain* 6, no. 6 (June 2005): 392–99.

22. K. Toljan and B. Vrooman, "Low-Dose Naltrexone (LDN)—Review of Therapeutic Utilization," *Medical Sciences (Basel, Switzerland)* 6, no. 4 (September 2018): 82.

23. Z. Li et al., "Low-Dose Naltrexone (LDN): A Promising Treatment in Immune-Related Diseases and Cancer Therapy," *International Immunopharmacology* 61 (August 2018): 178–84.

24. D. Segal et al., "Low Dose Naltrexone for Induction of Remission in Crohn's Disease," *Cochrane Database of Systematic Reviews* 2 (February 2014): CD010410; J. P. Smith et al., "Low-Dose Naltrexone Therapy Improves Active Crohn's Disease," *American Journal of Gastroenterology* 102, no. 4 (April 2007): 820–28.

25. G. Raknes et al., "The Effect of Low-Dose Naltrexone on Medication in Inflammatory Bowel Disease: A Quasi Experimental Before-and-After Prescription Database Study," *Journal of Crohn's and Colitis* 12, no. 6 (May 2018): 677–86.

26. M. Lie et al., "Low Dose Naltrexone for Induction of Remission in Inflammatory Bowel Disease Patients," *Journal of Translational Medicine* 16, no. 1 (March 2018): 55.

27. C. E. Parker et al., "Low Dose Naltrexone for Induction of Remission in Crohn's Disease," *Cochrane Database of Systematic Reviews* 4 (April 2018): CD010410.

28. G. Raknes and L. Småbrekke, "Low Dose Naltrexone: Effects on Medication in Rheumatoid and Seropositive Arthritis. A Nationwide Register-Based Controlled Quasi-Experimental Before-After Study," *PLoS One* 14, no. 2 (February 2019): e0212460.

29. S. J. Peterson et al., "An Online Survey of Hypothyroid Patients Demonstrates Prominent Dissatisfaction," *Thyroid* 28, no. 6 (2018): 707–21.

30. S. J. Zielsdorf, "Just Try LDN: 3 Years of Insight from Over 1,000 Patients' Use of Low Dose Naltrexone." Research presented at the LDN AIIC 2019 Conference, Portland, OR, June 7–9, 2019.

31. A. Alonso and M. A. Hernan, "Temporal Trends in the Incidence of Multiple Sclerosis: A Systematic Review," *Neurology* 71, no. 2 (July 2008): 129–35.

32. M. T. Wallin et al., "The Prevalence of MS in the United States: A Population-Based Estimate Using Health Claims Data," *Neurology* 92, no. 10 (July 2019): e1029–e1040.

33. Michael D. Ludwig, Ian S. Zagon, and Patricia J. McLaughlin, "Featured Article: Serum [Met5]-Enkephalin Levels Are Reduced in Multiple Sclerosis and Restored by Low-Dose Naltrexone," *Experimental Biology and Medicine (Maywood)* 242, no. 15 (September 2017): 1524–33.

34. K. A. Rahn et al., "Prevention and Diminished Expression of Experimental Autoimmune Encephalomyelitis by Low Dose Naltrexone (LDN) or Opioid

Growth Factor (OGF) for an Extended Period: Therapeutic Implications for Multiple Sclerosis," *Brain Research* 1381 (March 2011): 243–53.

35. Ludwig, Zagon, and McLaughlin, "Featured Article: Serum [Met(5)]-Enkephalin Levels Are Reduced."

36. M. D. Ludwig et al., "Featured Article: Modulation of the OGF–OGFr Pathway Alters Cytokine Profiles in Experimental Autoimmune Encephalomyelitis and Multiple Sclerosis," *Experimental Biology and Medicine (Maywood)* 243, no. 4 (February 2018): 361–69.

37. M. Gironi et al., "A Pilot Trial of Low-Dose Naltrexone in Primary Progressive Multiple Sclerosis," *Multiple Sclerosis Journal* 14, no. 8 (September 2008): 1076–83.

38. B. A. Cree et al., "Pilot Trial of Low-Dose Naltrexone and Quality of Life in Multiple Sclerosis," *Annals of Neurology* 68, no. 2 (August 2010): 145–50; A. P. Turel et al., "Low Dose Naltrexone for Treatment of Multiple Sclerosis: A Retrospective Chart Review of Safety and Tolerability," *Journal of Clinical Psychopharmacology* 35, no. 5 (October 2015): 609–11.

39. N. Sharafaddinzadeh et al., "The Effect of Low-Dose Naltrexone on Quality of Life of Patients with Multiple Sclerosis: A Randomized Placebo-Controlled Trial," *Multiple Sclerosis Journal* 16, no. 8 (August 2010): 964–69.

40. G. Raknes and L. Småbrekke, "Low Dose Naltrexone in Multiple Sclerosis: Effects on Medication Use. A Quasi-Experimental Study," *PLoS One* 12, no. 11 (November 2017): e0187423.

41. B. Ghai et al., "Off-Label, Low-Dose Naltrexone for Refractory Chronic Low Back Pain," *Pain Medicine* 15, no. 5 (May 2014): 883–84.

42. L. R. Webster et al., "Oxytrex Minimizes Physical Dependence While Providing Effective Analgesia: A Randomized Controlled Trial in Low Back Pain," *Journal of Pain* 7, no. 12 (December 2006): 937–46.

43. Toljan and Vrooman, "Low-Dose Naltrexone (LDN)—Review of Therapeutic Utilization."

44. D. J. Clauw, "Fibromyalgia: A Clinical Review," *Journal of the American Medical Association* 311, no. 15 (April 2014): 1547–55; L. M. Arnold et al., "AAPT Diagnostic Criteria for Fibromyalgia," *Journal of Pain* 20, no. 6 (June 2019): 611–28.

45. Clauw, "Fibromyalgia: A Clinical Review."

46. Arnold et al., "AAPT Diagnostic Criteria for Fibromyalgia."

47. J. Younger et al., "The Use of Low-Dose Naltrexone (LDN) as a Novel Anti-Inflammatory Treatment for Chronic Pain," *Clinical Rheumatology* 33, no. 4 (April 2014): 451–59.

48. J. Younger and S. Mackey, "Fibromyalgia Symptoms Are Reduced by Low-Dose Naltrexone: A Pilot Study," *Pain Medicine* 10, no. 4 (May–June 2009): 663–72.

49. L. Parkitny and J. Younger, "Reduced Pro-Inflammatory Cytokines after Eight Weeks of Low-Dose Naltrexone for Fibromyalgia," *Biomedicines* 5, no. 2 (April 2017): 16.

50. Younger and Mackey, "Fibromyalgia Symptoms Are Reduced by Low-Dose Naltrexone"; J. Younger et al., "Low-Dose Naltrexone for the Treatment of

Fibromyalgia: Findings of a Small, Randomized, Double-Blind, Placebo-Controlled, Counterbalanced, Crossover Trial Assessing Daily Pain Levels," *Arthritis & Rheumatology* 65, no. 2 (February 2013): 529–38.

51. S. Metyas et al., "Low Dose Naltrexone in the Treatment of Fibromyalgia," *Current Rheumatology Reviews* 14, no. 2 (2018): 177–80.

52. Toljan and Vrooman, "Low-Dose Naltrexone (LDN)—Review of Therapeutic Utilization."

53. A. Coutinho Jr. et al., "MR Imaging in Deep Pelvic Endometriosis: A Pictorial Essay," *RadioGraphics* 2, no. 31 (March 2011).

54. J. Mercier and K. Miller, "Mercier Therapy Helps Infertile Women Achieve Pregnancy," *Midwifery Today* 105 (2013): 40, 68.

55. C. H. Choi et al., "A Rare Case of Post-Hysterectomy Vault Site Iatrogenic Endometriosis," *Obstetrics and Gynecology Science* 54, no. 5 (2015): 319–22.

56. O. Laghzaoui and M. Laghzaoui, "Nasal Endometriosis: Apropos of 1 Case," *Journal de Gynécologie Obstétrique et Biologie de la Reproduction (Paris)* 30, no. 8 (2001): 786–88.

57. Timothy A. Deimling, Milton S. Hershey Medical Center, "Low-Dose Naltrexone in Combination with Standard Treatment in Women with Endometriosis," Clinical Trials.gov. Identifier: NCT03970330, https://clinicaltrials.gov/ct2/show/NCT03970330.

58. F. Malfait et al., "The 2017 International Classification of the Ehlers-Danlos Syndromes," *American Journal of Medical Genetics: Seminars in Medical Genetics* 175, no. 1 (March 2017): 8–26.

59. Z. Zhou et al., "Management of Chronic Pain in Ehlers-Danlos Syndrome: Two Case Reports and a Review of Literature," *Medicine (Baltimore)* 97, no. 45 (November 2018): e13115.

60. D. K. Patten et al., "The Safety and Efficacy of Low-Dose Naltrexone in the Management of Chronic Pain and Inflammation in Multiple Sclerosis, Fibromyalgia, Crohn's Disease, and Other Chronic Pain Disorders," *Pharmacotherapy* 38, no. 3 (March 2018): 382–89.

61. G. Raknes and L. Småbrekke, "A Sudden and Unprecedented Increase in Low Dose Naltrexone (LDN) Prescribing in Norway. Patient and Prescriber Characteristics, and Dispense Patterns. A Drug Utilization Cohort Study," *Pharmacoepidemiology and Drug Safety* 26, no. 2 (February 2017): 136–42.

62. Patten et al., "The Safety and Efficacy of Low-Dose Naltrexone."

Chapter 3: Gut Health

1. Jill P. Smith and Leonard B. Weinstock, "Inflammatory Bowel Disease," in *The LDN Book: How a Little-Known Generic Drug—Low Dose Naltrexone—Could Revolutionize Treatment for Autoimmune Diseases, Cancer, Autism, Depression, and More*, ed. Linda Elsegood (White River Junction, VT: Chelsea Green, 2016), pp. 55–68.

2. Yi-Zhen Zhang and Yong-Yu Li, "Inflammatory Bowel Disease: Pathogenesis," *World Journal of Gastroenterology* 20, no. 1 (2014): 91–99, https://www.ncbi.nlm.nih.gov/pmc/articles/PMC3886036/pdf/WJG-20-91.pdf.

3. Laurent Peyrin-Biroulet et al., "The Natural History of Adult Crohn's Disease in Population-Based Cohorts," *American Journal of Gastroenterology* 105, no. 2 (February 2010): 289–97, https://doi.org/10.1038/ajg.2009.579.

4. Peyrin-Biroulet et al., "The Natural History of Adult Crohn's Disease."

5. Claire E. Parker et al., "Low Dose Naltrexone for Induction of Remission in Crohn's Disease," *Cochrane Database of Systematic Reviews* 4 (April 2018): CD010410, https://doi.org/10.1002/14651858.CD010410.pub3.

6. Dina Ibrahim Tawfik et al., "Evaluation of Therapeutic Effect of Low Dose Naltrexone in Experimentally-Induced Crohn's Disease in Rats," *Neuropeptides* 59 (October 2016): 39–45, https://doi.org/10.1016/j.npep.2016.06.003.

7. Tawfik et al., "Evaluation of Therapeutic Effect."

8. Gwenny Fuhler et al., "Low Dose Naltrexone Reduces In Vitro Endoplasmic Reticulum Stress and Stimulates Wound Healing in Intestinal Epithelial Cells" (poster presentation), European Crohn's and Colitis Organisation, 2016.

9. K. Shard, "Norwegian LDN Documentary," https://www.youtube.com/watch?v =rBd2gv8UGU0&feature=youtu.be&fbclid=IwAR2TqrplHgQ6eWSYmcBsYJ db336aES0rXcTswaySchativVljxb8eXufGaw.

10. Guttorm Raknes et al., "The Effect of Low Dose Naltrexone on Medication in Inflammatory Bowel Disease: A Quasi Experimental Before-and-After Prescription Database Study," *Journal of Crohn's and Colitis* 12, no. 6 (June 2018): 677–86, https://doi.org/10.1093/ecco-jcc/jjy008.

11. Mitchell R.K.L. Lie et al., "Low Dose Naltrexone for Induction of Remission in Inflammatory Bowel Disease Patients," *Journal of Translational Medicine* 16 (March 2018): Article 55, https://doi.org/10.1186/s12967-018-1427-5.

12. Jill P. Smith et al., "Therapy with the Opioid Antagonist Naltrexone Promotes Mucosal Healing in Active Crohn's Disease: A Randomized Placebo-Controlled Trial," *Digestive Diseases and Sciences* 56, no. 7 (July 2011): 2088–97.

13. Leonard B. Weinstock, "Naltrexone Therapy for Crohn's Disease and Ulcerative Colitis," *Journal of Clinical Gastroenterology* 48, no. 8 (September 2014): 742, https://doi.org/10.1097/MCG.0000000000000093.

14. Hans Törnblom et al., "Gastrointestinal Motility and Neurogastroenterology," *Scandinavian Journal of Gastroenterology* 50, no. 6, (March 2015): 685–97, https://doi.org/10.3109/00365521.2015.1027265.

15. Michael Gershon, "Review Article: Serotonin Receptors and Transporters— Roles in Normal and Abnormal Gastrointestinal Motility," *Alimentary Pharmacology and Therapeutics* 20, no. 7 (November 2004): 3–14, https://doi .org/10.1111/j.1365-2036.2004.02180.x.

16. Michael Camilleri, "New Treatment Options for Chronic Constipation: Mechanisms, Efficacy and Safety," *Canadian Journal of Gastroenterology* 25, Supplement B (October 2011): 29B–35B.

17. J. Grider and G. M. Makhlouf, "Role of Opioid Neurons in the Regulation of Intestinal Peristalsis," *American Journal of Physiology* 253 (August 1987): G226–31, https://doi.org/10.1152/ajpgi.1987.253.2.G226.

18. J. Grider et al., "Interplay of Somatostatin, Opioid, and GABA Neurons in the Regulation of the Peristaltic Reflex," *American Journal of Physiology* 267 (October 1994): G696–701, https://doi.org/10.1152/ajpgi.1994.267.4.G696.

19. Raymond Jian et al., "Influence of Metenkephalin Analogue on Motor Activity of the Gastrointestinal Tract," *Gastroenterology* 93 (1987): 114–20.

20. Peter Holzer, "Opioid Receptors in the Gastrointestinal Tract," *Regulatory Peptide* 155 (June 2009): 11–17.

21. Aitak Farzi et al., "Toll-Like Receptor 4 Contributes to the Inhibitory Effect of Morphine on Colonic Motility in Vitro and in Vivo," *Scientific Reports* 5, no. 9499 (March 2015), https://doi.org/10.1038/srep09499.

22. M. Jiménez et al., "Opioid-Induction of Migrating Motor Activity in Chickens," *Life Sciences* 50, no. 7 (1992): 465–72, https://doi.org/10.1016/0024-3205(92)90385-3.

23. Jennifer Ploesser et al., "Low Dose Naltrexone: Side Effects and Efficacy in Gastrointestinal Disorders," *International Journal of Pharmaceutical Compounding* 14, no. 2 (March–April 2010): 171–73.

24. Beth Livengood, "Gastroparesis—Case Study," https://www.ldnresearchtrust.org /video-categories/gastroparesis.

25. Henry Parkman, "Naloxegol for Opioid-Related Gastroparesis," ClinicalTrials.gov. Identifier: NCT03036891, https://clinicaltrials.gov/ct2/show/NCT03036891.

26. George F. Longstreth et al., "Functional Bowel Disorders," *Gastroenterology* 130, no 5 (April 2006): 1480–91; A.P.S. Hungin et al., "Irritable Bowel Syndrome in the United States: Prevalence, Symptom Patterns and Impact," *Alimentary Pharmacology and Therapeutics* 21, no. 11 (June 2005): 1365–75; Yuri A. Saito et al., "The Epidemiology of Irritable Bowel Syndrome in North America: A Systematic Review," *American Journal of Gastroenterology* 97, no. 8 (August 2002): 1910–15.

27. Longstreth et al., "Functional Bowel Disorders"; Hungin et al., "Irritable Bowel Syndrome in the United States."

28. Hungin et al., "Irritable Bowel Syndrome in the United States"; Saito et al., "The Epidemiology of Irritable Bowel Syndrome in North America."

29. Hungin et al., "Irritable Bowel Syndrome in the United States"; Saito et al., "The Epidemiology of Irritable Bowel Syndrome in North America"; Bradley C. Martin et al., "Utilization Patterns and Net Direct Medical Cost to Medicaid of Irritable Bowel Syndrome," *Current Medical Research and Opinion* 19, no. 8 (October 2003): 771–80, https://doi.org/10.1185/030079903125002540.

30. Hungin et al., "Irritable Bowel Syndrome in the United States"; Longstreth et al., "Functional Bowel Disorders."

31. Brooks D. Cash and William D. Chey, "Diagnosis of Irritable Bowel Syndrome," *Gastroenterology Clinics of North America* 34, no. 2 (2005): 205–20; Brooks D. Cash et al., "The Utility of Diagnostic Tests in Irritable Bowel Syndrome Patients: A Systematic Review," *American Journal of Gastroenterology* 97, no. 11 (November 2002): 2812–19.

32. W. Grant Thompson, "The Road to Rome," *Gastroenterology* 130, no. 5 (April 2006): 1552–56, https://doi.org/10.1053/j.gastro.2006.03.011.

33. Mark Pimentel et al., "Lower Frequency of MMC Is Found in IBS Subjects with Abnormal Lactulose Breath Test, Suggesting Bacterial Overgrowth," *Digestive Diseases and Sciences* 47, no. 12 (December 2002): 2639–43.

34. Mark Pimentel et al., "Autoimmunity Links Vinculin to the Pathophysiology of Chronic Functional Bowel Changes Following *Campylobacter Jejuni* Infection in a Rat Model," *Digestive Diseases and Sciences* 60, no. 5 (May 2015): 1195–1205.

35. Walter Morales et al., "Second-Generation Biomarker Testing for Irritable Bowel Syndrome Using Plasma Anti-Cdtb and Anti-Vinculin Levels," *Digestive Diseases and Sciences* 64, no. 11 (May 2019): 3115–21, https://doi.org/10.1007/s10620-019-05684-6.

36. Ali Rezaie et al., "Hydrogen and Methane-Based Breath Testing in Gastrointestinal Disorders: The North American Consensus," *American Journal of Gastroenterology* 112, no. 5 (May 2017): 775–84, https://doi.org/10.1038/ajg.2017.46.

37. Mark Pimentel et al., "Eradication of Small Intestinal Bacterial Overgrowth Reduces Symptoms of Irritable Bowel Syndrome," *American Journal of Gastroenterology* 95, no. 12 (December 2000): 3503–06.

38. Cash and Chey, "Diagnosis of Irritable Bowel Syndrome."

39. Cash and Chey, "Diagnosis of Irritable Bowel Syndrome."

40. Mark Pimentel et al., "Effects of Rifaximin Treatment and Retreatment in Non-Constipated IBS Subjects," *Digestive Diseases and Sciences* 56, no. 7 (July 2011): 2067–72, https://doi.org/10.1007/s10620-011-1728-5; Mark Pimentel et al., "Rifaximin Therapy for Patients with Irritable Bowel Syndrome without Constipation," *New England Journal of Medicine* 364 (January 2011): 22–32, https://doi.org/10.1056/NEJMoa1004409; Jun Li et al., "Rifaximin for Irritable Bowel Syndrome: A Meta-Analysis of Randomized Placebo-Controlled Trials," *Medicine (Baltimore)* 95, no. 4 (January 2016): e2534, https://doi.org/10.1097/MD.0000000000002534.

41. Ali Rezaie et al., "Lactulose Breath Testing as a Predictor of Response to Rifaximin in Patients with Irritable Bowel Syndrome with Diarrhea," *American Journal of Gastroenterology* 114, no. 12 (December 2019): 1886–93, https://doi.org/10.14309/ajg.0000000000000444.

42. Anthony Lembo et al., "Repeat Treatment with Rifaximin Is Safe and Effective in Patients with Diarrhea-Predominant Irritable Bowel Syndrome," *Gastroenterology* 151, no. 6 (December 2016): 1113–21, https://doi.org/10.1053/j.gastro.2016.08.003.

43. Mark Pimentel et al., "Low-Dose Nocturnal Tegaserod or Erythromycin Delays Symptom Recurrence after Treatment of Irritable Bowel Syndrome Based on Presumed Bacterial Overgrowth," *Gastroenterology & Hepatology (New York)* 5, no. 6 (June 2009): 435–42; Leonard B. Weinstock, "Long-Term Outcome of Rifaximin Therapy in Non-Constipation Irritable Bowel Syndrome," *Digestive Diseases and Sciences* 56, no. 11 (November 2011): 3389–90, https://doi.org/10.1007/s10620-011-1889-2.

44. Revital Kariv et al., "Low-Dose Naltrexone for the Treatment of Irritable Bowel Syndrome: A Pilot Study," *Digestive Diseases and Sciences* 51, no. 12 (December 2006): 2128–33.

45. Ploesser et al., "Low Dose Naltrexone."

46. Lawrence B. Afrin et al., "Characterization of Mast Cell Activation Syndrome," *American Journal of the Medical Sciences* 353, no. 3 (March 2017): 207–15, https://doi.org/10.1016/j.amjms.2016.12.013.

47. Gerhart J. Molderings et al., "Familial Occurrence of Systemic Mast Cell Activation Disease," *PLOS One* 8, no. 9 (September 30, 2013): e76241, https://doi.org/10.1371/journal.pone.0076241.

48. Cash and Chey, "Diagnosis of Irritable Bowel Syndrome."

49. Mark Pimentel et al., "Normalization of Lactulose Breath Testing Correlates with Symptom Improvement in Irritable Bowel Syndrome: A Double-Blind, Randomized, Placebo-Controlled Study," *American Journal of Gastroenterology* 98, no. 2 (February 2003): 412–19.

50. Lawrence B. Afrin and Gerhard J. Molderings, "A Concise, Practical Guide to Diagnostic Assessment for Mast Cell Activation Disease," *World Journal of Hematology* 3, no. 1 (February 6, 2014): 1–17.

51. Leonard B. Weinstock et al., "The Significance of Mast Cell Activation in the Era of Precision Medicine," *American Journal of Gastroenterology* 113, no. 11 (November 2018): 1725–26, https://doi.org/10.1038/s41395-018-0257-7.

52. Giovanni Barbara et al., "Activated Mast Cells in Proximity to Colonic Nerves Correlate with Abdominal Pain in Irritable Bowel Syndrome," *Gastroenterology* 126, no. 3 (March 2004): 693–702, https://doi.org/10.1053/j.gastro.2003.11.055; Giovanni Barbara et al., "Mast Cell-Dependent Excitation of Visceral-Nociceptive Sensory Neurons in Irritable Bowel Syndrome," *Gastroenterology* 132, no. 1 (January 2007): 26–37, https://doi.org/10.1053/j.gastro.2006.11.039; Stefan Wirz and Gerhard J. Molderings, "A Practical Guide for Treatment of Pain in Patients with Systemic Mast Cell Activation Disease," *Pain Physician* 20, no. 6 (September 2017): E849–E861.

53. Rezaie et al., "Lactulose Breath Testing as a Predictor of Response to Rifaximin."

54. Gabrio Bassotti et al., "Increase of Colonic Mast Cells in Obstructed Defecation and Their Relationship with Enteric Glia," *Digestive Diseases and Sciences* 57, no. 1 (January 2012): 65–71, https://doi.org/10.1007/s10620-011-1848-y.

55. Cash and Chey, "Diagnosis of Irritable Bowel Syndrome"; Mark J. Hamilton, "Nonclonal Mast Cell Activation Syndrome: A Growing Body of Evidence," *Immunology and Allergy Clinics of North America* 38, no. 3 (August 2018): 469–81; Fred H. Hsieh, "Gastrointestinal Involvement in Mast Cell Activation Disorders," *Immunology and Allergy Clinics of North America* 38, no. 3 (August 2018): 429–41.

56. Anupam Aich et al., "Mast Cell-Mediated Mechanisms of Nociception," *International Journal of Molecular Sciences* 16, no. 12 (December 2015) 29069–92, https://doi.org/10.3390/ijms161226151.

57. Harissios Vliagoftis et al., "Mast Cells at Mucosal Frontiers," *Current Molecular Medicine* 5, no. 6 (October 2005): 573–89, https://doi.org/10.2174/1566524054863915.

58. Leonard B. Weinstock et al., "Mast Cell Deposition and Activation May Be a New Explanation for Epiploic Appendagitis," *British Medical Journal Case Report* 2018, bcr-2018-224689, http://doi.org/10.1136/bcr-2018-224689.

59. T. Frieling, "Evidence for Mast Cell Activation in Patients with Therapy-Resistant Irritable Bowel Syndrome," *Zeitschrift für Gastroenterologie* 49, no. 2 (February 2011): 191–94, http://doi.org/10.1055/s-0029-1245707; Lei Zhang et al., "Mast Cells and Irritable Bowel Syndrome: From the Bench to the Bedside," *Neurogastroenterology and Motility* 22, no. 2 (April 2016): 181–92, http://doi.org/10.5056/jnm15137; Beatriz Lobo et al., "Downregulation of Mucosal Mast Cell Activation and Immune Response in Diarrhoea-Irritable Bowel Syndrome by Oral Disodium Cromoglycate: A Pilot Study," *United European Gastroenterology Journal* 5, no. 6 (October 2017): 887–97, http://doi.org/10.1177/2050640617691690; Tamira K. Klooker et al., "The Mast Cell Stabiliser Ketotifen Decreases Visceral Hypersensitivity and Improves Intestinal Symptoms in Patients with Irritable Bowel Syndrome," *Gut* 59, no. 9 (September 2010): 1213–21, http://doi.org/10.1136/gut.2010.213108.

60. Leonard B. Weinstock et al., "Small Intestinal Bacterial Overgrowth Is Common in Mast Cell Activation Syndrome," *American Journal of Gastroenterology* 114, no. 2019 ACG Annual Meeting Abstracts (October 2019).

61. Anneleen B. Beckers et al., "Gastrointestinal Disorders in Joint Hypermobility Syndrome/Ehlers-Danlos Syndrome Hypermobility Type: A Review for the Gastroenterologist," *Neurogastroenterology & Motility* 29, no. 8 (August 2017): e13013, https://doi.org/10.1111/nmo.13013; John K. DiBaise, "Postural Tachycardia Syndrome (POTS) and the GI Tract: A Primer for the Gastroenterologist," *American Journal of Gastroenterology* 113, no. 10 (October 2018): 1458–67, https://doi.org/10.1038/s41395-018-0215-4.

62. Suranjith L. Seneviratne et al., "Mast Cell Disorders in Ehlers-Danlos Syndrome," *American Journal of Medical Genetics Part C: Seminars in Medical Genetics* 175, no. 1 (March 2017): 226–36, https://doi.org/10.1002/ajmg.c.31555; Emily M. Garland, "Postural Tachycardia Syndrome: Beyond Orthostatic Intolerance," *Current Neurology and Neuroscience Reports* 15, no. 60 (July 2015), https://doi.org/10.1007/s11910-015-0583-8; Taylor A. Doherty et al., "Postural Orthostatic Tachycardia Syndrome and the Potential Role of Mast Cell Activation," *Autonomic Neuroscience* 215 (December 2018): 83–88, https://doi.org/10.1016/j.autneu.2018.05.001.

63. Pimentel et al., "Normalization of Lactulose Breath Testing Correlates with Symptom Improvement"; Susan V. Jennings et al., "The Mastocytosis Society Survey on Mast Cell Disorders: Patient Experiences and Perceptions," *Journal of Allergy and Clinical Immunology* 2, no. 1 (January–February 2014): 70–76, https://doi.org/10.1016/j.jaip.2013.09.004; Jill Schofield and Lawrence B. Afrin, "Recognition and Management of Medication Excipient Reactivity in Patients with Mast Cell Activation Syndrome," *American Journal of the Medical Sciences* 357, no. 6 (June 2019): 507–11, https://doi.org/10.1016/j.amjms.2019.03.005; Lawrence B. Afrin et al., "Mast Cell Activation Disease and Microbiotic Interactions," *Clinical Therapeutics* 37, no. 5 (February 2015): 941–53, http://doi.org/10.1016/j.clinthera.2015.02.008; Aarane M. Ratnaseelan et al., "Effects of Mycotoxins on Neuropsychiatric Symptoms and Immune Processes," *Clinical Therapeutics* 40, no. 6 (June 2018): 903–17, https://doi.org/10.1016/j.clinthera.2018.05.004.

64. Leonard B. Weinstock et al., "Successful Treatment of Postural Orthostatic Tachycardia and Mast Cell Activation Syndromes Using Naltrexone, Immunoglobulin and Antibiotic Treatment," *British Medical Journal Case Reports* 2018 (January 2018): bcr-2017-221405, https://doi.org/10.1136/bcr-2017-221405.

65. K. Iida et al., "Analysis of T Cell Subsets and Beta Chemokines in Patients with Pulmonary Sarcoidosis," *Thorax* 52, no. 5 (May 1997): 431–37, https://doi.org/10.1136/thx.52.5.431.

66. Robert P. Baughman and Jan C. Grutters, "New Treatment Strategies for Pulmonary Sarcoidosis: Antimetabolites, Biological Drugs, and Other Treatment Approaches," *Lancet Respiratory Medicine* 3, no. 10 (October 2015): 813–22, https://doi.org/10.1016/S2213-2600(15)00199-X.

67. Miguel Giovinale et al., "Atypical Sarcoidosis: Case Reports and Review of the Literature," *European Review for Medical and Pharmacological Sciences* 13, no. 1 (March 2009): 37–44.

68. Leonard B. Weinstock et al., "Low-Dose Naltrexone for the Treatment of Sarcoidosis," *Sarcoidosis Vasculitis and Diffuse Lung Disease* 34, no. 2 (August 2017): 184–97, https://doi.org/10.36141/svdld.v34i2.5303.

69. Gaelle Guettrot-Imberta et al., "Mesenteric Panniculitis," *La Revue de Médecine Interne* 33, no. 11 (November 2012): 621–27, https://doi.org/10.1016/j.revmed.2012.04.011.

70. Mahmoud R. Hussein and Saad R. Abdelwahed, "Mesenteric Panniculitis: An Update," *Expert Review of Gastroenterology & Hepatology* 9, no. 1 (January 2015): 67–78, https://doi.org/10.1586/17474124.2014.939632.

71. Mamoon H. Al-Omari et al., "Mesenteric Panniculitis: Comparison of Computed Tomography Findings in Patients with and without Malignancy," *Clinical and Experimental Gastroenterology* 2019, no. 12 (August 2018): 1–8, https://doi.org/10.2147/CEG.S182513.

72. Eli D. Ehrenpreis et al., "Clinical Significance of Mesenteric Panniculitis-Like Abnormalities on Abdominal Computerized Tomography in Patients with Malignant Neoplasms," *World Journal of Gastroenterology* 22, no. 48 (December 2016): 10601–08, https://doi.org/10.3748/wjg.v22.i48.10601.

73. Nienke van Putte-Katier et al., "Mesenteric Panniculitis: Prevalence, Clinicoradiological Presentation and 5-Year Follow-Up," *British Institute of Radiology* 87, no. 1044 (December 2014): 20140451, https://doi.org/10.1259/bjr.20140451.

74. Michael S. Green et al., "Sclerosing Mesenteritis: A Comprehensive Clinical Review," *Annals of Translational Medicine* 6, no. 17 (September 2018): 336, https://doi.org/10.21037/atm.2018.07.01.

75. Roberto Mazure et al., "Successful Treatment of Retractile Mesenteritis with Oral Progesterone," *Gastroenterology* 114, no. 6 (June 1998): 1313–17, https://doi.org/10.1016/S0016-5085(98)70438-X.

76. Prabin Sharma et al., "Sclerosing Mesenteritis: A Systematic Review of 192 Cases," *Journal of Clinical Gastroenterology* 10, no. 2 (April 2017): 103–11, https://doi.org/10.1007/s12328-017-0716-5.

77. Grigory Roginsky et al., "Initial Findings of an Open-Label Trial of Low-Dose Naltrexone for Symptomatic Mesenteric Panniculitis," *Journal of Clinical Gastroenterology* 49, no. 9 (October 2015): 794–95, https://doi.org/10.1097/MCG.0000000000000398.

78. Angus G. Dalgleish and Wai M. Liu, "Cancer," in Elsegood, *The LDN Book*; S. Zagon and Patricia J. McLaughlin, "Opioid Growth Factor (OGF) Inhibits Anchorage-Independent Growth in Human Cancer Cells," *International Journal of Oncology* 24, no. 6 (July 2004): 1443–48.

79. Wai M. Liu et al., "Naltrexone at Low Doses Upregulates a Unique Gene Expression Not Seen with Normal Doses: Implications for Its Use in Cancer Therapy," *International Journal of Oncology* 49, no. 2 (June 2016): 793–802, https://doi.org/10.3892/ijo.2016.3567.

80. Renee N. Donahue et al., "Low-Dose Naltrexone Targets the Opioid Growth Factor–Opioid Growth Factor Receptor Pathway to Inhibit Cell Proliferation: Mechanistic Evidence from a Tissue Culture Model," *Experimental Biology and Medicine (Maywood)* 236, no. 9 (September 2011): 1036–50, https://doi.org/10.1258/ebm.2011.011121.

81. Staci D. Hytrek et al., "Inhibition of Human Colon Cancer by Intermittent Opioid Receptor Blockade with Naltrexone," *Cancer Letters* 101, no. 2 (March 1996): 159–64, https://doi.org/10.1016/0304-3835(96)04119-5.

82. Qiush Wang et al., "Methionine Enkephalin (MENK) Improves Lymphocyte Subpopulations in Human Peripheral Blood of 50 Cancer Patients by Inhibiting Regulatory T Cells (Tregs)," *Human Vaccines & Immunotherapeutics* 10, no. 7 (April 2014): 1836–40, https://doi.org/10.4161/hv.28804.

83. Diego M. Avella et al., "The Opioid Growth Factor–Opioid Growth Factor Receptor Axis Regulates Cell Proliferation of Human Hepatocellular Cancer," *American Journal of Physiology—Regulatory, Integrative and Comparative Physiology* 298, no. 2 (February 2010): 459–66, https://doi.org/10.1152/ajpregu.00646.2009.

84. Xiaonon Wang et al., "The Novel Mechanism of Anticancer Effect on Gastric Cancer through Inducing G0/G1 Cell Cycle Arrest and Caspase-Dependent Apoptosis in Vitro and in Vivo by Methionine Enkephalin," *Cancer Management and Research* 2018, no. 10 (October 18, 2018): 4773–87, https://doi.org/10.2147/CMAR.S178343.

85. Burton M. Berkson et al., "The Long-Term Survival of a Patient with Pancreatic Cancer with Metastases to the Liver after Treatment with the Intravenous Alpha-Lipoic Acid/Low-Dose Naltrexone Protocol," *Integrative Cancer Therapies* 5, no. 1 (March 1, 2006): 83–89, https://doi.org/10.1177/1534735405285901.

86. Burton M. Berkson et al., "Revisiting the ALA/N (Alpha-Lipoic Acid/Low-Dose Naltrexone) Protocol for People with Metastatic and Non-Metastatic Pancreatic Cancer: A Report of 3 New Cases," *Integrative Cancer Therapies* 8, no. 4 (December 2009): 416–22, https://doi.org/10.1177/1534735409352082.

87. Jill P. Smith et al., "Opioid Growth Factor Improves Clinical Benefit and Survival in Patients with Advanced Pancreatic Cancer," *Open Access Journal of Clinical Trials* 2010, no. 2 (March 2010): 37–48, https://doi.org/10.2147/OAJCT.S8270.

88. Laurent Schwartz et al., "Metabolic Treatment of Cancer: Intermediate Results of a Prospective Case Series," *Anticancer Research* 34, no. 2 (February 2014): 973–80.

89. Moshe Rogosnitzky et al., "Opioid Growth Factor (OGF) for Hepatoblastoma: A Novel Non-Toxic Treatment," *Investigational New Drugs* 31, no. 4 (August 2013): 1066–70, https://doi.org/10.1007/s10637-012-9918-3.

90. Ruizhe Wang et al., "Interaction of Opioid Growth Factor (OGF) and Opioid Antagonist and Their Significance in Cancer Therapy," *International Immunopharmacology* 75 (October 2019): 105785, https://doi.org/10.1016/j.intimp.2019.105785.

Chapter 4: Dermatologic Conditions

1. I. S. Zagon et al., "The Biology of the Opioid Growth Factor Receptor," *Brain Research Reviews* 38 (2002): 351–76.

2. P. L. Bigliardi et al., "Opioids and the Skin, Where Do We Stand?," *Experimental Dermatology* 18, no. 5 (May 2009): 424–30.

3. P. L. Bigliardi et al., "Specific Stimulation of Migration of Human Keratinocytes by Mu Opiate Receptor Agonists," *Journal of Receptors and Signal Transduction* 22 (2012): 191–99.

4. M. Bigliardi-Qi et al., "Beta-Endorphin Stimulates Cytokeratin 16 Expression and Downregulates Mu Opiate Receptor Expression in Human Epidermis," *Journal of Investigative Dermatology* 114 (2000): 527–32; M. Bigliardi-Qi et al., "Characterization of Mu Opiate Receptor in Chronic and Acute Wounds and the Effect of Beta-Endorphin on Transforming Growth Factor Beta Type II Receptor and Cytokeratin 16 Expression," *Journal of Investigative Dermatology* 120 (2003): 145–52.

5. Bigliardi et al., "Specific Stimulation of Migration of Human Keratinocytes."

6. P. L. Bigliardi et al., "Activation of the Delta Opioid Receptor Promotes Cutaneous Wound Healing by Affecting Keratinocyte Intercellular Adhesion and Migration," *British Journal of Pharmacology* 172 (2015): 501–14.

7. P. L. Bigliardi et al., "Opioids and Skin Homeostasis, Regeneration and Ageing—What's the Evidence?," *Experimental Dermatology* 6, no. 25 (2016): 586–91.

8. P. L. Bigliardi and M. Bigliardi-Qi, "Peripheral Opioids," in E. A. Carstens and T. Akiyama, *Itch: Mechanisms and Treatment* (Boca Raton, FL: CRC Press, 2014); S. Kauser et al., "Regulation of Human Epidermal Melanocyte Biology by Beta-Endorphin," *Journal of Investigative Dermatology* 120 (2003): 173–80.

9. F. Yuan, H. Xiaozhou, Y. Yilin, et al., "Current Research on Opioid Receptor Function," *Current Drug Targets* 13, no. 2 (February 2012): 230–46.

10. Z. Dembic, "The Function of Toll-Like Receptors," *Madame Curie Bioscience Database*, Landes Bioscience (2000–13).

11. D. K. Patten et al., "The Safety and Efficacy of Low Dose Naltrexone in the Management of Chronic Pain and Inflammation in Multiple Sclerosis, Fibromyalgia, Crohn's Disease and Other Chronic Pain Disorders," *Pharmacotherapy* 38 (2018): 382–89.

12. A. J. Bower et al., "Longitudinal in Vivo Tracking of Adverse Effects Following Topical Steroid Treatment," *Experimental Dermatology* 25, no. 5 (May 2016): 362–67.

13. A. D. Papoiu and G. Yosipovitch, "Topical Capsaicin—the Fire of a 'Hot' Medicine Is Reignited," *Expert Opinion on Pharmacotherapy* 11, no. 8 (2010): 1359.

14. J. Rivard and H. W. Lim, "Ultraviolet Phototherapy for Pruritus," *Dermatologic Therapy* 18, no. 4 (2005): 344.

15. M. Metz and S. Stander, "Chronic Pruritis—Pathogenesis, Clinical Aspects and Treatment," *Journal of the European Academy of Dermatology and Venereology* 24, no. 11 (2010): 1249.

16. M. O'Donoghue and M. D. Tharp, "Antihistamines and Their Role as Antipruritics," *Dermatologic Therapy* 18, no. 4 (2005): 333.

17. T. A. Kouwenhoven et al., "Use of Oral Antidepressants in Patients with Chronic Pruritus: A Systematic Review," *Journal of the American Academy of Dermatology* 77, no. 6 (October 2017): 1068.

18. B. M. Matsuda et al., "Gabapentin and Pregabalin for the Treatment of Chronic Pruritus," *Journal of the American Academy of Dermatology* 75, no. 3 (May 2016): 619.

19. D. Sharma and S. G. Kwatra, "Thalidomide for the Treatment of Chronic Refractory Pruritus," *Journal of the American Academy of Dermatology* 74, no. 2 (2016): 363.

20. L. P. Bigliardi-Qi et al., "Mu Opiate Receptor System in Skin and Relationship to Itch," *Journal of the American Academy of Dermatology* 50, no. 3 (March 2004): 29.

21. J. Lee et al., "Clinical Efficacy and Safety of Naltrexone Combination Therapy in Older Patients with Severe Pruritus," *Annals of Dermatology* 28 (2016): 159–63; W. Siemens et al., "Pharmacological Interventions for Pruritus in Adult Palliative Care Patients," *Cochrane Database Systematic Review* 11 (November 2016).

22. N. Q. Phan, "Antipruritic Treatment with Systemic Mu Opioid Receptor Antagonists: A Review," *Journal of the American Academy of Dermatology* 63, no. 4 (October 2010): 680–88.

23. P. L. Bigliardi, "Treatment of Pruritis with Topically Applied Opiate Receptor Antagonist," *Journal of the American Academy of Dermatology* 56, no. 6 (June 2007): 979–88.

24. Kent Holtorf, "Thyroid Disorders," in *The LDN Book: How a Little-Known Generic Drug—Low Dose Naltrexone—Could Revolutionize Treatment for Autoimmune Diseases, Cancer, Autism, Depression, and More*, ed. Linda Elsegood (White River Junction, VT: Chelsea Green, 2016).

25. T. Frech et al., "Low Dose Naltrexone for Pruritus in Systemic Sclerosis," *International Journal of Rheumatology* (September 12, 2011).

26. T. Tran et al., "Successful Treatment of Dermatomyositis with Low Dose Naltrexone," *Dermatologic Therapy* 31, no. 6 (September 2018): e12720.

27. Z. Xu, L. Zhang, et al., "A Case of Hailey-Hailey Disease in an Infant with a New ATP2C1 Gene Mutation," *Pediatric Dermatology* 28, no. 2 (2011): 165.

28. S. M. Burge, "Hailey-Hailey Disease: The Clinical Features, Response to Treatment and Prognosis," *British Journal of Dermatology* 126, no. 3 (1992): 275.

29. A. Borghi et al., "Efficacy of Magnesium Chloride in the Treatment of Hailey-Hailey Disease: From Serendipity to Evidence of Its Effect on Intracellular Ca(2+) Homeostasis," *International Journal of Dermatology* 54, no. 5 (2015): 543–48.

30. B. Farahnik et al., "Interventional Treatments for Hailey-Hailey Disease," *Journal of the American Academy of Dermatology* 76, no. 3 (2017): 551.

31. L. N. Albers et al., "Treatment of Hailey-Hailey Disease with Low Dose Naltrexone," *JAMA Dermatology* 153, no. 10 (October 2017): 1018–20.

32. O. Ibrahim et al., "Low Dose Naltrexone Treatment of Familial Benign Pemphigus (Hailey-Hailey Disease)," *JAMA Dermatology* 153, no. 10 (2017): 1015.

33. Albers et al., "Treatment of Hailey-Hailey Disease with Low Dose Naltrexone."

34. S. Cao et al., "Variable Response to Naltrexone in Patients with Hailey-Hailey Disease," *JAMA Dermatology* 154, no. 3 (2018): 362.

35. C. Riquelme-McLoughlin et al., "Low Dose Naltrexone Therapy in Benign Chronic Pemphigus (Hailey-Hailey Disease): A Case Series," *Journal of the American Academy of Dermatology* 81, no. 2 (August 2019): 644–46.

36. M. McBride, "Recalcitrant Hailey-Hailey Disease Treated with Low Dose Naltrexone," *Journal of the American Academy of Dermatology* 81, no. 4 (October 2019): AB264.

37. A. Alajmi et al., "Hailey-Hailey Disease Treated Successfully with Naltrexone and Magnesium," *JAAD Case Report* 5, no. 9 (August 2019): 760–62.

38. S. Sonthalia et al., "Low Dose Naltrexone Induced Remission in Hailey-Hailey Disease Maintained in Remission with Topical Combination of Ketamine and Diphenhydramine," *Indian Dermatology Online Journal* 10, no. 5 (August 2019): 567–70.

39. D. A. Mehregan et al., "Lichen Planopilaris: Clinical and Pathological Study of Forty-Five Patients," *Journal of the American Academy of Dermatology* 27, no. 6, part 1 (December 1992): 935–42.

40. S. Vano-Galvan, "Frontal Fibrosing Alopecia: A Multicenter Review of 355 Patients," *Journal of the American Academy of Dermatology* 70, no. 4 (April 2014): 670–78.

41. A. Tosti et al., "Frontal Fibrosing Alopecia in Post-Menopausal Women," *Journal of the American Academy of Dermatology* 52, no. 1 (January 2005): 55–60.

42. N. Atanaskova Mesinkovska et al., "Association of Lichen Planopilaris with Thyroid Disease: A Retrospective Case Control Study," *Journal of the American Academy of Dermatology* 70, no. 5 (2014): 889.

43. E. Racz et al., "Treatment of Frontal Fibrosing Alopecia and Lichen Planopilaris: A Systematic Review," *Journal of the European Academy of Dermatology and Venereology* 27, no. 12 (March 2013): 1461; C. Chieregato et al., "Lichen Planopilaris: Report of 30 Cases and Review of the Literature," *International Journal of Dermatology* 42, no. 5 (2003): 342.

44. E. K. Ross et al., "Update on Primary Cicatricial Alopecias," *Journal of the American Academy of Dermatology* 53, no. 1 (2005): 1.

45. Mehregan et al., "Lichen Planopilaris."

46. C. Chiang et al., "Hydroxychloroquine and Lichen Planopilaris: Efficacy and Introduction of Lichen Planopilaris Activity Index Scoring System," *Journal of the American Academy of Dermatology* 62, no. 3 (March 2010): 387–92; E. Racz et al., "Treatment of Frontal Fibrosing Alopecia and Lichen Planopilaris: A Systematic Review," *Journal of the European Academy of Dermatology and Venereology* 27, no. 12 (March 2013): 1461.

47. L. C. Strazzulla et al., "Novel Treatment Using Low Dose Naltrexone for Lichen
Planopilaris," *Journal of Drugs in Dermatology* 16, no. 11 (November 2017):
1140–42.
48. National Psoriasis Foundation, "Psoriasis Cause and Triggers," https://www
.psoriasis.org/about-psoriasis/causes (October 2018).
49. J. L. Lopez-Estebaranz et al., "Effect of a Family History of Psoriasis and Age on
Comorbidities and Quality of Life in Patients with Moderate to Severe Psoriasis:
Results from the ARIZONA Study," *Journal of Dermatology* 43, no. 4 (2016): 395.
50. F. Elsholz et al., "Calcium—A Central Regulator of Keratinocyte Differentiation in
Health and Disease," *European Journal of Dermatology* 24, no. 6 (2014): 650–61.
51. E. G. Harper et al., "Th17 Cytokines Stimulate CCL20 Expression in
Keratinocytes in Vitro and in Vivo: Implications for Psoriasis Pathogenesis,"
Journal of Investigative Dermatology 129, no. 9 (2009): 2175; N. J. Wilson
et al., "Development, Cytokine Profile and Function of Human Interleukin
17-Producing Helper T Cells," *Nature Immunology* 8, no. 9 (2007): 950.
52. D. D. Gladman et al., "Psoriatic Arthritis (PSA)—An Analysis of 220 Patients,"
Quarterly Journal of Medicine 62, no. 238 (1987): 127.
53. A. M. Jensen et al., "Calcipotriol Inhibits the Proliferation of Hyperproliferative
CD29 Positive Keratinocytes in Psoriatic Epidermis in the Absence of an Effect
on the Function and Number of Antigen-Presenting Cells," *British Journal of
Dermatology* 139, no. 6 (1998): 984.
54. C. A. Elmets et al., "Joint American Academy of Dermatology–National Psoriasis
Foundation Guidelines of Care for the Management and Treatment of Psoriasis
with Phototherapy," *Journal of the American Academy of Dermatology* 81, no. 3
(2019): 775.
55. R. M. Pujol et al., "Mental Health Self-Assessment in Patients with Moderate to
Severe Psoriasis: An Observational Multicenter Study of 1164 Patients in Spain
(the VACAP Study)," *Actas Dermo-Sifiliográficas* 104, no. 10 (2013): 897–903.
56. A. C. Bridgmen, "Treatment of Psoriasis Vulgaris Using Low Dose Naltrexone,"
Journal of the American Academy of Dermatology 4, no. 8 (September 2018):
827–29.
57. G. Muller et al., "Compound Low Dose Naltrexone for the Treatment of Guttate
Psoriasis: A Case Report," *International Journal of Pharmaceutical Compounding*
22 (2018): 270–78.
58. M.E.P. Beltran, "Low Dose Naltrexone: An Alternative Treatment for Erythrodermic
Psoriasis," *Cureus Journal of Medical Science* 11, no. 1 (January 2019): 3943.
59. P. J. McLaughlin, J. A. Immonen, and I. S. Zagon, "Naltrexone Accelerates Full-
Thickness Wound Closure in Type 1 Diabetic Rats by Stimulating Angiogenesis,"
Experimental Biology and Medicine 238, no. 7 (July 2013): 733–43.

Chapter 5: Parkinson's Disease

1. Martin Parent and André Parent, "Substantia Nigra and Parkinson's Disease: A
Brief History of Their Long and Intimate Relationship," *Canadian Journal of
Neurological Sciences* 37, no. 3 (May 2010): 313–19, https://doi

.org/10.1017167100010209; M. Gourie-Devi, M. G. Ramu, and B. S. Venkataram, "Treatment of Parkinson's Disease in 'Ayurveda' (Ancient Indian System of Medicine): Discussion Paper," *Journal of the Royal Society of Medicine* 84, no. 8 (August 1991): 491–92.

2. Patricia Inacio, "Toxoplasma Brain Parasite Modulates Parkinson's Signaling Pathways," *Parkinson's News Today*, September 20, 2017, https://parkinsons newstoday.com/2017/09/20/toxoplasma-brain-parasite-modulates-signaling -pathways-common-parkinsons-disease; C. Warren Olanow and Patrik Brundin, "Parkinson's Disease and Alpha Synuclein: Is Parkinson's Disease a Prion-Like Disorder?" *Movement Disorders* 28, no. 1 (February 2013): 31–40, https://doi .org/10.1002/mds.25373; Patrik Brundin and Ronald Melki, "Prying into the Prion Hypothesis for Parkinson's Disease," *Journal of Neuroscience* 37, no. 41 (October 2017): 9808–18, http://doi.org/10.1523/JNEUROSCI.1788-16.2017; Leonid Breydo, Jessica W. Wu, and Vladimir N. Uversky, "α-Synuclein Misfolding and Parkinson's Disease," *Biochimica Et Biophysica Acta (BBA)* 1822, no. 2 (2012): 261–85, https://doi.org/10.1016/j.bbadis.2011.10.002.

3. Maria G. Cersosimo and Eduardo E. Benarroch, "Pathological Correlates of Gastrointestinal Dysfunction in Parkinson's Disease," *Neurobiology of Disease* 46, no. 3 (2012): 559–64, https://doi.org/10.1016/j.nbd.2011.10.014.

4. Christine Klein and Ana Westenberger, "Genetics of Parkinson's Disease," *Cold Spring Harbor Perspectives in Medicine* 2, no. 1 (January 2012): a008888, https:// doi.org/10.1101/cshperspect.a008888; Anna Oczkowska et al., "Mutations in PRKN and SNCA Genes Important for the Progress of Parkinson's Disease," *Current Genomics* 14, no. 8 (December 2013): 502–17, https://doi.org/10.2174/138 92029146661312102058339; D. B. Calne et al., "Positron Emission Tomography after MPTP: Observations Relating to the Cause of Parkinson's Disease," *Nature* 317 (September 1985): 246–48, https://doi.org/10.1038/317246a0; K. J. Billingsley et al., "Genetic Risk Factors in Parkinson's Disease," *Cell and Tissue Research* 373, no. 1 (2018): 9–20, https://doi.org/10.1007/s00441-018-2817-y; Petar Podlesniy et al., "Accumulation of Mitochondrial 7S DNA in Idiopathic and LRRK2 Associated Parkinson's Disease," *EBioMedicine* 48 (October 2019): 554–67, https://doi.org/10 .1016/j.ebiom.2019.09.015.

5. Hiroyoshi Ariga et al., "Neuroprotective Function of DJ-1 in Parkinson's Disease," *Oxidative Medicine and Cellular Longevity* 2013 (May 2013): 683920, https://doi .org/10.1155/2013/683920.

6. Ana Pena, "LRRK2 Worthy Target of Research into Parkinson's Therapies, Study Suggests," *Parkinson's News Today*, May 3, 2018, https://parkinsonsnewstoday.com /2018/05/03/parkinsons-lrrk2-mutation-potential-therapy-target-study-suggests.

7. David Sulzer et al., "Erratum: T Cells from Patients with Parkinson's Disease Recognize α-Synuclein Peptides," *Nature* 549, no. 7671 (2017): 292, https:// doi.org/10.1038/nature23896; Stephen Mullin and Anthony H. V. Schapira, "Pathogenic Mechanisms of Neurodegeneration in Parkinson's Disease," *Neurologic Clinics* 33, no. 1 (2015): 1–17, https://doi.org/10.1016/j.ncl.2014 .09.010; Asa Abeliovich and Aaron D. Gitler, "Defects in Trafficking Bridge

Parkinson's Disease Pathology and Genetics," *Nature* 539, no. 7628 (2016): 207–16, https://doi.org/10.1038/nature20414; "Parkinson's Disease Linked to High Iron Intake," American Academy of Neurology, June 2003, https://www .aan.com/PressRoom/Home/PressRelease/30; Marcio S. Medeiros et al., "Iron and Oxidative Stress in Parkinson's Disease: An Observational Study of Injury Biomarkers," *PLoS One* 11, no. 1 (November 2016): e0146129, https://doi.org /10.1371/journal.pone.0146129; Mike A. Nalls et al., "NeuroX, a Fast and Efficient Genotyping Platform for Investigation of Neurodegenerative Diseases," *Neurobiology of Aging* 36, no. 3 (2015): 1605.e7–1605.e12, https://doi .org/10.1016/j.neurobiolaging.2014.07.028; Vera Dias, Eunsung Junn, and M. Maral Mouradian, "The Role of Oxidative Stress in Parkinson's Disease," *Journal of Parkinson's Disease* 3, no. 4 (2013): 461–91, https://doi.org/10.3233/jpd -130230; Henry Jay Forman, Hongqiao Zhang, and Alessandra Rinna, "Glutathione: Overview of Its Protective Roles, Measurement, and Biosynthesis," *Molecular Aspects of Medicine* 30, no. 1–2 (2009): 1–12, https://doi.org/10.1016/j .mam.2008.08.006; Malú G. Tansey and Marina Romero-Ramos, "Immune System Responses in Parkinson's Disease: Early and Dynamic," *European Journal of Neuroscience* 49, no. 3 (October 2018): 364–83, https://doi.org/10.1111/ejn.14290.

8. Gloria E. Meredith and David J. Rademacher, "MPTP Mouse Models of Parkinson's Disease: An Update," *Journal of Parkinson's Disease* 1, no. 1 (2011): 19–33, https:// doi.org/10.3233/JPD-2011-11023; J. William Langston, "The MPTP Story," *Journal of Parkinson's Disease* 7, supplement 1 (2017): S11–S19, https://doi.org /10.3233/JPD-179006; J. W. Langston, "Chronic Parkinsonism in Humans Due to a Product of Meperidine-Analog Synthesis," *Science* 219, no. 4587 (February 1983): 979–80, https://doi.org/10.1126/science.6823561; Serge Przedborski et al., "MPTP as a Mitochondrial Neurotoxic Model of Parkinson's Disease," *Journal of Bioenergetics and Biomembranes* 36, no. 4 (August 2004): 375–79, https:// doi.org/10.1023/B:JOBB.0000041771.66775.d5; N. Schmidt and B. Ferger, "Neurochemical Findings in the MPTP Model of Parkinson's Disease," *Journal of Neural Transmission* 108 (2001): 1263–82, https://doi.org/10.1007 /s007020100004.

9. Angela Spivey, "Rotenone and Paraquat Linked to Parkinson's Disease: Human Exposure Study Supports Years of Animal Studies," *Environmental Health Perspectives* 119, no. 6 (2011): A259, https://doi.org/10.1289/ehp.119-a259a; Elisa Caggiu et al., "Inflammation, Infectious Triggers, and Parkinson's Disease," *Frontiers in Neurology* 10 (2019), https://doi.org/10.3389/fneur.2019.00122; Robert D. Abbott et al., "Midlife Milk Consumption and Substantia Nigra Neuron Density at Death," *Neurology* 86, no. 6 (September 2015): 512–19, https://doi.org /10.1212/wnl.0000000000002254.

10. Michael A. Collins and Edward J. Neafsey, "Potential Neurotoxic 'Agents Provocateurs' in Parkinson's Disease," *Neurotoxicology and Teratology* 24, no. 5 (September–October 2002): 571–77, https://doi.org/10.1016/S0892-0362(02) 00210-6; Edward A. Lock, Jing Zhang, and Harvey Checkoway, "Solvents and Parkinson's Disease: A Systematic Review of Toxicological and Epidemiological

Evidence," *Toxicology and Applied Pharmacology* 266, no. 3 (2013): 345–55, https://doi.org/10.1016/j.taap.2012.11.016.

11. Seung-Jae Lee et al., "Protein Aggregate Spreading in Neurodegenerative Diseases: Problems and Perspectives," *Neuroscience Research* 70, no. 4 (2011): 339–48, https://doi.org/10.1016/j.neures.2011.05.008; Michelle Smeyne and Richard Jay Smeyne, "Glutathione Metabolism and Parkinson's Disease," *Free Radical Biology and Medicine* 62 (September 2013): 13–25, https://doi.org/10.1016/j.freerad biomed.2013.05.001.

12. Smeyne and Smeyne, "Glutathione Metabolism and Parkinson's Disease."

13. Shankar J. Chinta et al., "Inducible Alterations of Glutathione Levels in Adult Dopaminergic Midbrain Neurons Result in Nigrostriatal Degeneration," *Journal of Neuroscience* 27, no. 51 (December 2007): 13997–14006, https://doi.org /10.1523/JNEUROSCI.3885-07.2007.

14. Carolina Cebrián et al., "MHC-I Expression Renders Catecholaminergic Neurons Susceptible to T-Cell-Mediated Degeneration," *Nature Communications* 5, (April 2014): 3633, https://doi.org/10.1038/ncomms4633.

15. David Sulzer et al., "T Cells from Patients with Parkinson's Disease Recognize α-Synuclein Peptides," *Nature* 546, (June 2017): 656–66, https://doi.org/10.1038 /nature22815.

16. Kemal Ugur Tufekci et al., "Inflammation in Parkinson's Disease," *Advances in Protein Chemistry and Structural Biology* 88 (2012): 69–132, https://doi.org/10.1016 /b978-0-12-398314-5.00004-0; Li Qian, Patrick M. Flood, and Jau-Shyong Hong, "Neuroinflammation Is a Key Player in Parkinson's Disease and a Prime Target for Therapy," *Journal of Neural Transmission* 117, no. 8 (2010): 971–79, https://doi .org/10.1007/s00702-010-0428-1; Zhichun Chen, Shengdi Chen, and Jun Liu, "The Role of T Cells in the Pathogenesis of Parkinson's Disease," *Progress in Neurobiology* 169 (2018): 1–23, https://doi.org/10.1016/j.pneurobio.2018.08.002; Sulzer et al., "Erratum: T Cells from Patients with Parkinson's Disease," 292.

17. "Aggressive Immune Cells Aggravate Parkinson's Disease," *ScienceDaily*, July 19, 2018, www.sciencedaily.com/releases/2018/07/180719094349.htm.

18. Richard Gordon et al., "Protein Kinase Cδ Upregulation in Microglia Drives Neuroinflammatory Responses and Dopaminergic Neurodegeneration in Experimental Models of Parkinson's Disease," *Neurobiology of Disease* 93 (2016): 96–114, https://doi.org/10.1016/j.nbd.2016.04.008.

19. Carolina Cebrián, John D. Loike, and David Sulzer, "Neuroinflammation in Parkinson's Disease Animal Models: A Cell Stress Response or a Step in Neurodegeneration?," *Behavioral Neurobiology of Huntington's Disease and Parkinson's Disease* 22 (2014): 237–70, https://doi.org/10.1007/7854_2014_356; Fabio Blandini, "Neural and Immune Mechanisms in the Pathogenesis of Parkinson's Disease," *Journal of Neuroimmune Pharmacology* 8, no. 1 (March 2013): 189–201, https://doi.org/10.1007/s11481-013-9435-y; Sara A. Ferreira and Marina Romero-Ramos, "Microglia Response during Parkinson's Disease: Alpha-Synuclein Intervention," *Frontiers in Cellular Neuroscience* 12, no. 247 (June 2018), https://doi.org/10.3389/fncel.2018.00247.

20. Tansey and Romero-Ramos, "Immune System Responses in Parkinson's Disease"; Susanne Fonseca Santos et al., "The Gut and Parkinson's Disease—A Bidirectional Pathway," *Frontiers in Neurology* 10 (April 2019), https://doi.org/10.3389/fneur .2019.00574; Małgorzata Kujawska and Jadwiga Jodynis-Liebert, "What Is the Evidence That Parkinson's Disease Is a Prion Disorder, Which Originates in the Gut?" *International Journal of Molecular Sciences* 19, no. 11 (December 2018): 3573, https://doi.org/10.3390/ijms19113573; Rodger A. Liddle, "Parkinson's Disease from the Gut," *Brain Research* 1693 (2018): 201–06, https://doi.org /10.1016/j.brainres.2018.01.010; Olanow and Brundin, "Parkinson's Disease and Alpha Synuclein"; Shakshi Sharma, Anupam Awasthi, and Shamsher Singh, "Altered Gut Microbiota and Intestinal Permeability in Parkinson's Disease: Pathological Highlight to Management," *Neuroscience Letters* 712 (November 2019): 134516, https://doi.org/10.1016/j.neulet.2019.134516.

21. Javier Campos-Acuña, Daniela Elgueta, and Rodrigo Pacheco, "T-Cell-Driven Inflammation as a Mediator of the Gut-Brain Axis Involved in Parkinson's Disease," *Frontiers in Immunology* 10 (2019), https://doi.org/10.3389/fimmu .2019.00239.

22. Fredric P. Manfredsson et al., "Induction of Alpha-Synuclein Pathology in the Enteric Nervous System of the Rat and Non-Human Primate Results in Gastrointestinal Dysmotility and Transient CNS Pathology," *Neurobiology of Disease* 112 (April 2018): 106–18, https://doi.org/10.1016/j.nbd.2018.01.008.

23. Chen, Chen, and Liu, "The Role of T Cells in the Pathogenesis of Parkinson's Disease."

24. Valentina Caputi and Maria Giron, "Microbiome-Gut-Brain Axis and Toll-Like Receptors in Parkinson's Disease," *International Journal of Molecular Sciences* 19, no. 6 (June 2018): 1689, https://doi.org/10.3390/ijms19061689; Denise Barbut, Ethan Stolzenberg, and Michael Zasloff, "Gastrointestinal Immunity and Alpha-Synuclein," *Journal of Parkinson's Disease* 9, no. s2 (2019): S313–S322, https://doi .org/10.3233/jpd-191702.

25. Laurie K. Mischley et al., "A Randomized, Double-Blind Phase I/IIa Study of Intranasal Glutathione in Parkinson's Disease," *Movement Disorders* 30, no. 12 (2015): 1696–701, https://doi.org/10.1002/mds.26351.

26. Montserrat Marí et al., "Mitochondrial Glutathione, a Key Survival Antioxidant," *Antioxidants & Redox Signaling* 11, no. 11 (2009): 2685–700, https://doi.org /10.1089/ars.2009.2695.

27. Vicent Ribas, Carmen García-Ruiz, and Jose C. Fernandez-Checa, "Glutathione and Mitochondria," *Frontiers in Pharmacology* 5 (January 2014), https://doi.org /10.3389/fphar.2014.00151.

28. R.K.B. Pearce et al., "Alterations in the Distribution of Glutathione in the Substantia Nigra in Parkinson's Disease," *Journal of Neural Transmission* 104, no. 6–7 (1997): 661–77, https://doi.org/10.1007/bf01291884; Forman, Zhang, and Rinna, "Glutathione: Overview of Its Protective Roles"; I. P. Hargreaves et al., "Glutathione Deficiency in Patients with Mitochondrial Disease: Implications for Pathogenesis and Treatment," *Journal of Inherited Metabolic Disease* 28, no. 1 (2005): 81–88, https://doi.org/10.1007/s10545-005-4160-1; Katalin Sas et al.,

"Mitochondria, Metabolic Disturbances, Oxidative Stress and the Kynurenine System, with Focus on Neurodegenerative Disorders," *Journal of the Neurological Sciences* 257, no. 1–2 (2007): 221–39, https://doi.org/10.1016/j.jns.2007.01.033.

29. Paul Held, "An Introduction to Reactive Oxygen Species: Measurement of ROS in Cells," *Bio Tek Instruments*, January 26, 2015, https://www.biotek.com/assets/tech_resources/ROS%20White%20Paper_2015.pdf.

30. O. W. Griffith and A. Meister, "Origin and Turnover of Mitochondrial Glutathione," *Proceedings of the National Academy of Sciences* 82, no. 14 (January 1985): 4668–72, https://doi.org/10.1073/pnas.82.14.4668.

31. Mario Rango and Nereo Bresolin, "Brain Mitochondria, Aging, and Parkinson's Disease," *Genes* 9, no. 5 (November 2018): 250, https://doi.org/10.3390/genes 9050250.

32. Hansruedi Büeler, "Impaired Mitochondrial Dynamics and Function in the Pathogenesis of Parkinson's Disease," *Experimental Neurology* 218, no. 2 (2009): 235–46, https://doi.org/10.1016/j.expneurol.2009.03.006; Vera Dias, Eunsung Junn, and M. Maral Mouradian, "The Role of Oxidative Stress in Parkinson's Disease," *Journal of Parkinson's Disease* 3, no. 4 (2013): 461–91, https://doi.org /10.3233/jpd-130230.

33. Sinee Weschawalit et al., "Glutathione and Its Antiaging and Antimelanogenic Effects," *Clinical, Cosmetic and Investigational Dermatology* 2017, no. 10 (April 2017): 147–53, https://doi.org/10.2147/ccid.s128339; Smeyne and Smeyne, "Glutathione Metabolism and Parkinson's Disease"; Igor Rebrin and Rajindar S. Sohal, "Pro-Oxidant Shift in Glutathione Redox State during Aging," *Advanced Drug Delivery Reviews* 60, no. 13–14 (2008): 1545–52, https://doi.org/10.1016/j .addr.2008.06.001; Dikran Toroser and Rajindar S. Sohal, "Age-Associated Perturbations in Glutathione Synthesis in Mouse Liver," *Biochemical Journal* 405, no. 3 (2007): 583–89, https://doi.org/10.1042/bj20061868; Honglei Liu et al., "Glutathione Metabolism during Aging and in Alzheimer Disease," *Annals of t he New York Academy of Sciences* 1019, no. 1 (2004): 346–49, https://doi .org/10.1196/annals.1297.059; J. Viña et al., "Effect of Aging on Glutathione Metabolism. Protection by Antioxidants," *Free Radicals and Aging* 62 (1992): 136–44, https://doi.org/10.1007/978-3-0348-7460-1_14; Tadayasu Furukawa, Simin Nikbin Meydani, and Jeffrey B. Blumberg, "Reversal of Age-Associated Decline in Immune Responsiveness by Dietary Glutathione Supplementation in Mice," *Mechanisms of Ageing and Development* 38, no. 2 (1987): 107–17, https:// doi.org/10.1016/0047-6374(87)90071-6.

34. Sara Sepe et al., "Inefficient DNA Repair Is an Aging-Related Modifier of Parkinson's Disease," *Cell Reports* 15, no. 9 (2016): 1866–75, https://doi.org/10.1016/j.celrep .2016.04.071; Chiara Milanese et al., "Activation of the DNA Damage Response in Vivo in Synucleinopathy Models of Parkinson's Disease," *Cell Death & Disease* 9, no. 8 (2018): 818, https://doi.org/10.1038/s41419-018-0848-7.

35. D. J. Kurz, "Chronic Oxidative Stress Compromises Telomere Integrity and Accelerates the Onset of Senescence in Human Endothelial Cells," *Journal of Cell Science* 117, no. 11 (January 2004): 2417–26, https://doi.org/10.1242/jcs.01097;

Consuelo Borrás et al., "Glutathione Regulates Telomerase Activity in 3T3 Fibroblasts," *Journal of Biological Chemistry* 279, no. 33 (July 2004): 34332–35, https://doi.org/10.1074/jbc.m402425200.

36. Dean P. Jones et al., "Redox Analysis of Human Plasma Allows Separation of Pro-Oxidant Events of Aging from Decline in Antioxidant Defenses," *Free Radical Biology and Medicine* 33, no. 9 (2002): 1290–300, https://doi.org/10.1016/s0891-5849(02)01040-7; Marí et al., "Mitochondrial Glutathione."

37. Bernard Schmitt et al., "Effects of N-Acetylcysteine, Oral Glutathione (GSH) and a Novel Sublingual Form of GSH on Oxidative Stress Markers: A Comparative Crossover Study," *Redox Biology* 6 (December 2015): 198–205, https://doi.org /10.1016/j.redox.2015.07.012; Furukawa, Meydani, and Blumberg, "Reversal of Age-Associated Decline in Immune Responsiveness."

38. Robert A. Hauser et al., "Randomized, Double-Blind, Pilot Evaluation of Intravenous Glutathione in Parkinson's Disease," *Movement Disorders* 24, no. 7 (2009): 979–83, https://doi.org/10.1002/mds.22401.

39. M. Otto, T. Magerus, and J. O. Langland, "The Use of Intravenous Glutathione for Symptom Management of Parkinson's Disease: A Case Report," *Alternative Therapies in Health and Medicine* 4 (July 2018): 56–60.

40. Gianpietro Sechi et al., "Reduced Intravenous Glutathione in the Treatment of Early Parkinson's Disease," *Progress in Neuro-Psychopharmacology and Biological Psychiatry* 20, no. 7 (1996): 1159–70, https://doi.org/10.1016/s0278-5846(96) 00103-0.

41. Ines Elbini Dhouib et al., "A Minireview on N-Acetylcysteine: An Old Drug with New Approaches," *Life Sciences* 151 (April 2016): 359–63, https://doi.org/10.1016 /j.lfs.2016.03.003; Edward A. Lock, Jing Zhang, and Harvey Checkoway, "Solvents and Parkinson Disease: A Systematic Review of Toxicological and Epidemiological Evidence," *Toxicology and Applied Pharmacology* 266, no. 3 (2013): 345–55, https:// doi.org/10.1016/j.taap.2012.11.016.

42. A. Sharma et al., "Attenuation of 1-methyl-4-phenyl-1, 2,3,6-tetrahydropyridine Induced Nigrostriatal Toxicity in Mice by N-acetyl cysteine," *Cellular and Molecular Biology* 53, no. 1 (April 2007): 48–55; Negin Nouraei et al., "Investigation of the Therapeutic Potential of N-Acetyl Cysteine and the Tools Used to Define Nigrostriatal Degeneration in Vivo," *Toxicology and Applied Pharmacology* 296 (April 2016): 19–30, https://doi.org/10.1016/j.taap.2016.02.010; Arman Rahimmi et al., "N-Acetylcysteine Prevents Rotenone-Induced Parkinson's Disease in Rat: An Investigation into the Interaction of Parkin and Drp1 Proteins," *Brain Research Bulletin* 113 (April 2015): 34–40, https://doi.org /10.1016/j.brainresbull.2015.02.007.

43. Mary J. Holmay et al., "N-Acetylcysteine Boosts Brain and Blood Glutathione in Gaucher and Parkinson's Diseases," *Clinical Neuropharmacology* 36, no. 4 (2013): 103–06, https://doi.org/10.1097/wnf.0b013e31829ae713; Hunter G. Moss et al., "N-Acetylcysteine Rapidly Replenishes Central Nervous System Glutathione Measured via Magnetic Resonance Spectroscopy in Human Neonates with Hypoxic-Ischemic Encephalopathy," *Journal of Cerebral Blood Flow &*

Metabolism 38, no. 6 (2018): 950–58, https://doi.org/10.1177/0271678x18765828; Jie Zhou et al., "Intravenous Administration of Stable-Labeled N-Acetylcysteine Demonstrates an Indirect Mechanism for Boosting Glutathione and Improving Redox Status," *Journal of Pharmaceutical Sciences* 104, no. 8 (2015): 2619–26, https://doi.org/10.1002/jps.24482.

44. Ajay S. Unnithan et al., "Rescue from a Two Hit, High-Throughput Model of Neurodegeneration with N-Acetyl Cysteine," *Neurochemistry International* 61, no. 3 (2012): 356–68, https://doi.org/10.1016/j.neuint.2012.06.001.

45. M. M. Banaclocha, "Therapeutic Potential of N-Acetylcysteine in Age-Related Mitochondrial Neurodegenerative Diseases," *Medical Hypotheses* 56, no. 4 (2001): 472–77, https://doi.org/10.1054/mehy.2000.1194.

46. Joanne Clark et al., "Oral N-Acetyl-Cysteine Attenuates Loss of Dopaminergic Terminals in α-Synuclein Overexpressing Mice," *PLoS One* 5, no. 8 (2010): e12333, https://doi.org/10.1371/journal.pone.0012333.

47. Daniel A. Monti et al., "N-Acetyl Cysteine Is Associated with Dopaminergic Improvement in Parkinson's Disease," *Clinical Pharmacology & Therapeutics* 106, no. 4 (2019): 884–90, https://doi.org/10.1002/cpt.1548.

48. Todd B. Sherer et al., "Mechanism of Toxicity in Rotenone Models of Parkinson's Disease," *Journal of Neuroscience* 23, no. 34 (2003): 10756–64, https://doi.org/10.1523/jneurosci.23-34-10756.2003.

49. Barry Halliwell and John M. C. Gutteridge, *Free Radicals in Biology and Medicine* (Oxford, U.K.: Clarendon Press, 1989); Volodymyr I. Lushchak, "Glutathione Homeostasis and Function: Potential Targets for Medical Interventions," *Journal of Amino Acids* 2012 (February 2012): 736837, https://doi.org/10.1155/2012/736837; Young-Sam Keum, "Regulation of Nrf2-Mediated Phase II Detoxification and Anti-Oxidant Genes," *Biomolecules and Therapeutics* 20, no. 2 (March 2012): 144–51, https://doi.org/10.4062/biomolther.2012.20.2.144; Young-Joon Surh, Joydeb Kumar Kundu, and Hye-Kyung Na, "Nrf2 as a Master Redox Switch in Turning on the Cellular Signaling Involved in the Induction of Cytoprotective Genes by Some Chemopreventive Phytochemicals," *Planta Medica* 74, no. 13 (2008): 1526–39, https://doi.org/10.1055/s-0028-1088302.

50. Yasushi Honda et al., "Efficacy of Glutathione for the Treatment of Nonalcoholic Fatty Liver Disease: An Open-Label, Single-Arm, Multicenter, Pilot Study," *BMC Gastroenterology* 17 (August 2017): 96, https://doi.org/10.1186/s12876-017-0652-3.

51. Rudie Kortekaas et al., "Blood-Brain Barrier Dysfunction in Parkinsonian Midbrain in Vivo," *Annals of Neurology* 57, no. 2 (2005): 176–79, https://doi.org/10.1002/ana.20369; Annika Sommer et al., "Th17 Lymphocytes Induce Neuronal Cell Death in a Human IPSC-Based Model of Parkinson's Disease," *Cell Stem Cell* 24, no. 6 (2019): 1006, https://doi.org/10.1016/j.stem.2019.04.019; Shaji Theodore et al., "Targeted Overexpression of Human α-Synuclein Triggers Microglial Activation and an Adaptive Immune Response in a Mouse Model of Parkinson's Disease," *Journal of Neuropathology & Experimental Neurology* 67, no. 12 (2008): 1149–58, https://doi.org/10.1097/nen.0b013e31818e5e99.

52. Dilini Rathnayake, Thashi Chang, and Preethi Udagama, "Selected Serum Cytokines and Nitric Oxide as Potential Multi-Marker Biosignature Panels for Parkinson Disease of Varying Durations: A Case-Control Study," *BMC Neurology* 19, no. 1 (April 2019): 56, https://doi.org/10.1186/s12883-019-1286-6; B. Adams et al., "Parkinson's Disease: A Systemic Inflammatory Disease Accompanied by Bacterial Inflammagens," *Frontiers in Aging Neuroscience* 11 (August 2019): 210, https://doi.org/10.3389/fnagi.2019.00210; Donghui Li et al., "Association of Parkinson's Disease–Related Pain with Plasma Interleukin-1, Interleukin-6, Interleukin-10, and Tumour Necrosis Factor-α," *Neuroscience Letters* 683 (September 2018): 181–84, https://doi.org/10.1016/j.neulet.2018.07.027; Xiao-Yan Qin et al., "Aberrations in Peripheral Inflammatory Cytokine Levels in Parkinson Disease: A Systematic Review and Meta-Analysis," *JAMA Neurology* 73, no. 11 (November 2016): 1316–24, https://doi.org/10.1001/jamaneurol.2016.2742; M. Menza et al., "The Role of Inflammatory Cytokines in Cognition and Other Non-Motor Symptoms of Parkinson's Disease," *Psychosomatics* 51, no. 6 (October 2010): 474–79, https://doi.org/10.1176/appi.psy.51.6.474; Ryul Kim et al., "Peripheral Blood Inflammatory Markers in Early Parkinson's Disease," *Journal of Clinical Neuroscience* 58, (December 2018): 30–33, https://doi.org/10.1016/j .jocn.2018.10.079. E-published October 24, 2018.

53. Doris Blum-Degen et al., "Interleukin-1 beta and Interleukin-6 Are Elevated in the Cerebrospinal Fluid of Alzheimer's and de Novo Parkinson's Disease Patients," *Neuroscience Letters* 202, no. 1–2 (1995): 17–20, https://doi.org/10.1016/0304 -3940(95)12192-7; Richard Gordon et al., "Protein Kinase Cδ Upregulation in Microglia Drives Neuroinflammatory Responses and Dopaminergic Neurodegeneration in Experimental Models of Parkinson's Disease," *Neurobiology of Disease* 93 (September 2016): 96–114, https://doi.org/10.1016/j .nbd.2016.04.008; T. Nagatsu and M. Sawada, "Biochemistry of Postmortem Brains in Parkinson's Disease: Historical Overview and Future Prospects," *Neuropsychiatric Disorders: An Integrative Approach* 72 (2007): 113–20, https:// doi.org/10.1007/978-3-211-73574-9_14.

54. Stefan Liebner et al., "Functional Morphology of the Blood-Brain Barrier in Health and Disease," *Acta Neuropathologica* 135 (2018): 311–36, https://doi.org/10.1007 /s00401-018-1815-1; Javier Campos-Acuña, Daniela Elgueta, and Rodrigo Pacheco, "T-Cell-Driven Inflammation as a Mediator of the Gut-Brain Axis Involved in Parkinson's Disease," *Frontiers in Immunology* 10 (February 2019): 239, https://doi.org/10.3389/fimmu.2019.00239.

55. Yuhua Chen et al., "Clinical Characteristics and Peripheral T Cell Subsets in Parkinson's Disease Patients with Constipation," *International Journal of Clinical and Experimental Pathology* 8, no. 3 (2015): 2495–504.

56. Michelle Block, Luigi Zecca, and Jau-Shyong Hong, "Microglia-Mediated Neurotoxicity: Uncovering the Molecular Mechanisms," *Nature Reviews Neuroscience* 8 (2007): 57–69, https://doi.org/10.1038/nrn2038; Bianca Marchetti et al., "Glucocorticoid Receptor–Nitric Oxide Crosstalk and Vulnerability to Experimental Parkinsonism: Pivotal Role for Glia-Neuron Interactions," *Brain*

Research Reviews 48, no. 2 (April 2005): 302–21, https://doi.org/10.1016/j.brain resrev.2004.12.030.

57. L. J. Lawson et al., "Heterogeneity in the Distribution and Morphology of Microglia in the Normal Adult Mouse Brain," *Neuroscience* 39, no. 1 (1990): 151–70, https://doi.org/10.1016/0306-4522(90)90229-w; Doris Blum-Degena et al., "Interleukin-1β and Interleukin-6 Are Elevated in the Cerebrospinal Fluid of Alzheimer's and De Novo Parkinson's Disease Patients," *Neuroscience Letters* 202, no. 1–2 (1995): 17–20, https://doi.org/10.1016/0304-3940(95)12192-7; M. Mogi et al., "Brain β2-Microglobulin Levels Are Elevated in the Striatum in Parkinson's Disease," *Journal of Neural Transmission—Parkinson's Disease and Dementia Section* 9, no. 1 (1995): 87–92, https://doi.org/10.1007/bf02252965; Dariusz Koziorowski et al., "Inflammatory Cytokines and NT-ProCNP in Parkinson's Disease Patients," *Cytokine* 60, no. 3 (2012): 762–66, https://doi.org/10.1016/j.cyto .2012.07.030; Thorsten Schulte et al., "Polymorphisms in the Interleukin-1 Alpha and Beta Genes and the Risk for Parkinson's Disease," *Neuroscience Letters* 326, no. 1 (2002): 70–72, https://doi.org/10.1016/s0304-3940(02)00301-4.

58. Iwona Kurkowska-Jastrzebska et al., "Dexamethasone Protects against Dopaminergic Neurons Damage in a Mouse Model of Parkinson's Disease," *International Immunopharmacology* 4, no. 10–11 (October 2004): 1307–18, https://doi.org/10.1016/j.intimp.2004.05.006; Vincenzo Di Matteo et al., "Aspirin Protects Striatal Dopaminergic Neurons from Neurotoxin-Induced Degeneration: An in Vivo Microdialysis Study," *Brain Research* 1095, no. 1 (2006): 167–77, https://doi.org/10.1016/j.brainres.2006.04.013; Bin Liu, Lina Du, and Jau-Shyong Hong, "Naloxone Protects Rat Dopaminergic Neurons against Inflammatory Damage through Inhibition of Microglia Activation and Superoxide Generation," *Journal of Pharmacology and Experimental Therapeutics* 293, no. 2 (May 2000): 607–17; Ashley S. Harms et al., "Delayed Dominant-Negative TNF Gene Therapy Halts Progressive Loss of Nigral Dopaminergic Neurons in a Rat Model of Parkinson's Disease," *Molecular Therapy* 19, no. 1 (2011): 46–52, https:// doi.org/10.1038/mt.2010.217; Neha Sharma and Bimla Nehru, "Apocyanin, a Microglial NADPH Oxidase Inhibitor Prevents Dopaminergic Neuronal Degeneration in Lipopolysaccharide-Induced Parkinson's Disease Model," *Molecular Neurobiology* 53 (2016): 3326–37, https://doi.org/10.1007/s12035 -015-9267-2; Sushruta Koppula et al., "Reactive Oxygen Species and Inhibitors of Inflammatory Enzymes, NADPH Oxidase, and iNOS in Experimental Models of Parkinson's Disease," *Mediators of Inflammation* 2012 (April 2012): 823902, https://doi.org/10.1155/2012/823902; Richard Gordon et al., "Protein Kinase Cδ Upregulation in Microglia Drives Neuroinflammatory Responses and Dopaminergic Neurodegeneration in Experimental Models of Parkinson's Disease," *Neurobiology of Disease* 93 (September 2016): 96–114, https://doi.org /10.1016/j.nbd.2016.04.008.

59. Shu G. Chen et al., "Exposure to the Functional Bacterial Amyloid Protein Curli Enhances Alpha-Synuclein Aggregation in Aged Fischer 344 Rats and Caenorhabditis Elegans," *Scientific Reports* 6, no. 1 (June 2016): 34477,

https://doi.org/10.1038/srep34477; Timothy R. Sampson et al., "Gut Microbiota Regulate Motor Deficits and Neuroinflammation in a Model of Parkinson's Disease," *Cell* 167, no. 6 (2016): 1469–80, https://doi.org/10.1016/j.cell.2016.11 .018; Heiko Braak et al., "Gastric α-Synuclein Immunoreactive Inclusions in Meissners and Auerbachs Plexuses in Cases Staged for Parkinson's Disease–Related Brain Pathology," *Neuroscience Letters* 396, no. 1 (2006): 67–72, https:// doi.org/10.1016/j.neulet.2005.11.012; Kathleen M. Shannon et al., "Alpha-Synuclein in Colonic Submucosa in Early Untreated Parkinson's Disease," *Movement Disorders* 27, no. 6 (2011): 709–15, https://doi.org/10.1002/mds.23838; Heiko Braak et al., "Idiopathic Parkinson's Disease: Possible Routes by Which Vulnerable Neuronal Types May Be Subject to Neuroinvasion by an Unknown Pathogen," *Journal of Neural Transmission* 110 (2003): 517–36, https://doi.org/10 .1007/s00702-002-0808-2.

60. Francisco Pan-Montojo et al., "Environmental Toxins Trigger PD-Like Progression via Increased Alpha-Synuclein Release from Enteric Neurons in Mice," *Scientific Reports* 2, no. 1 (2012): 898, https://doi.org/10.1038/srep00898.

61. Theodore et al., "Targeted Overexpression of Human α-Synuclein"; Anke Perren et al., "FK506 Reduces Neuroinflammation and Dopaminergic Neurodegeneration in an α-Synuclein-Based Rat Model for Parkinson's Disease," *Neurobiology of Aging* 36, no. 3 (2015): 1559–68, https://doi.org/10.1016/j.neurobiolaging .2015.01.014.

62. Perren et al., "FK506 Reduces Neuroinflammation."

63. Kazuhiro Imamura et al., "Distribution of Major Histocompatibility Complex Class II–Positive Microglia and Cytokine Profile of Parkinson's Disease Brains," *Acta Neuropathologica* 106, no. 6 (January 2003): 518–26, https://doi.org/10.1007 /s00401-003-0766-2; Patrick L. McGeer et al., "Rate of Cell Death in Parkinsonism Indicates Active Neuropathological Process," *Annals of Neurology* 24, no. 4 (1988): 574–76, https://doi.org/10.1002/ana.410240415.

64. Yasuomi Ouchi et al., "Neuroinflammation in the Living Brain of Parkinson's Disease," *Parkinsonism & Related Disorders* 15, supplement 2 (December 2009): S25, https://doi.org/10.1016/s1353-8020(09)70109-9; Denise K. Patten, Bob G. Schultz, and Daniel J. Berlau, "The Safety and Efficacy of Low-Dose Naltrexone in the Management of Chronic Pain and Inflammation in Multiple Sclerosis, Fibromyalgia, Crohn's Disease, and Other Chronic Pain Disorders," *Pharmacotherapy* 38, no. 3 (2018): 382–89, https://doi.org/10.1002/phar.2086; Alexander Gerhard et al., "In Vivo Imaging of Microglial Activation with [11C] (R)-PK11195 PET in Idiopathic Parkinson's Disease," *Neurobiology of Disease* 21, no. 2 (2006): 404–12, https://doi.org/10.1016/j.nbd.2005.08.002; Yasuomi Ouchi et al., "Microglial Activation and Dopamine Terminal Loss in Early Parkinson's Disease," *Annals of Neurology* 57, no. 2 (2005): 168–75, https://doi.org/10.1002 /ana.20338.

65. A. Roy et al., "Attenuation of Microglial RANTES by NEMO-Binding Domain Peptide Inhibits the Infiltration of CD8 T Cells in the Nigra of Hemiparkinsonian Monkey," *Neuroscience* 302 (August 2015): 36–46, https://doi.org/10.1016/j.neuro

science.2015.03.011; Goutam Chandra et al., "Neutralization of RANTES and Eotaxin Prevents the Loss of Dopaminergic Neurons in a Mouse Model of Parkinson's Disease," *Journal of Biological Chemistry* 291, no. 29 (December 2016): 15267–81, https://doi.org/10.1074/jbc.m116.714824.

66. Mona Sadeghian et al., "Neuroprotection by Safinamide in the 6-Hydroxydopamine Model of Parkinson's Disease," *Neuropathology and Applied Neurobiology* 42, no. 5 (2015): 423–35, https://doi.org/10.1111/nan.12263; Shi Zhang et al., "CD200 -CD200R Dysfunction Exacerbates Microglial Activation and Dopaminergic Neurodegeneration in a Rat Model of Parkinson's Disease," *Journal of Neuroinflammation* 8, no. 1 (2011): 154, https://doi.org/10.1186/1742-2094-8-154.

67. Julie Rowin et al., "Granulocyte Macrophage Colony-Stimulating Factor Treatment of a Patient in Myasthenic Crisis: Effects on Regulatory T Cells," *Muscle & Nerve* 46, no. 3 (2012): 449–53, https://doi.org/10.1002/mus.23488; D. Games et al., "Reducing C-Terminal-Truncated Alpha-Synuclein by Immunotherapy Attenuates Neurodegeneration and Propagation in Parkinson's Disease–Like Models," *Journal of Neuroscience* 34, no. 28 (September 2014): 9441–54, https://doi.org/10.1523/jneurosci.5314-13.2014.

68. K. Noon et al., "A Novel Glial Cell Inhibitor, Low Dose Naltrexone, Reduces Pain and Depression, and Improves Function in Chronic Pain: A CHOIR Study," *Journal of Pain* 17, no. 4 (2016): S79, https://doi.org/10.1016/j.jpain.2016.01.395.

69. Jarred Younger et al., "Low-Dose Naltrexone for the Treatment of Fibromyalgia: Findings of a Small, Randomized, Double-Blind, Placebo-Controlled, Counterbalanced, Crossover Trial Assessing Daily Pain Levels," *Arthritis & Rheumatism* 65, no. 2 (2013): 529–38, https://doi.org/10.1002/art.37734; Bruce A. C. Cree, Elena Kornyeyeva, and Douglas S. Goodin, "Pilot Trial of Low-Dose Naltrexone and Quality of Life in Multiple Sclerosis," *Annals of Neurology* 68, no. 2 (August 2010), https://doi.org/10.1002/ana.22006; Jill P. Smith et al., "Therapy with the Opioid Antagonist Naltrexone Promotes Mucosal Healing in Active Crohn's Disease: A Randomized Placebo-Controlled Trial," *Digestive Diseases and Sciences* 56, no. 7 (August 2011): 2088–97, https://doi.org/10.1007 /s10620-011-1653-7; Daniel J. Clauw, Lesley M. Arnold, and Bill H. McCarberg, "The Science of Fibromyalgia," *Mayo Clinic Proceedings* 86, no. 9 (2011): 907–11, https://doi.org/10.4065/mcp.2011.0206; Jarred Younger and Sean Mackey, "Fibromyalgia Symptoms Are Reduced by Low-Dose Naltrexone: A Pilot Study," *Pain Medicine* 10, no. 4 (2009): 663–72, https://doi.org/10.1111/j.1526-4637 .2009.00613.x; Brandon R. Selfridge et al., "Structure–Activity Relationships of (+)-Naltrexone-Inspired Toll-Like Receptor 4 (TLR4) Antagonists," *Journal of Medicinal Chemistry* 58, no. 12 (May 2015): 5038–52, https://doi.org/10.1021/acs .jmedchem.5b00426; Xiaohui Wang, "Pharmacological Characterization of the Opioid Inactive Isomers (+)-Naltrexone and (+)-Naloxone as Toll-Like Receptor 4 Antagonists," *Drug and Alcohol Dependence* 171 (February 2017): e212, https://doi.org/10.1016/j.drugalcdep.2016.08.580; Mark R. Hutchinson et al., "Non-Stereoselective Reversal of Neuropathic Pain by Naloxone and Naltrexone: Involvement of Toll-Like Receptor 4 (TLR4)," *European Journal of Neuroscience*

28, no. 1 (2008): 20–29, https://doi.org/10.1111/j.1460-9568.2008.06321.x; Luke Parkitny and Jarred Younger, "Reduced Pro-Inflammatory Cytokines after Eight Weeks of Low-Dose Naltrexone for Fibromyalgia," *Biomedicines* 5, no. 4 (2017): 16, https://doi.org/10.3390/biomedicines5020016.

70. Guus Wolswijk, "Oligodendrocyte Survival, Loss and Birth in Lesions of Chronic-Stage Multiple Sclerosis," *Brain* 123, no. 1 (2000): 105–15, https://doi.org/10.1093/brain/123.1.105; Antoine Lampron et al., "Inefficient Clearance of Myelin Debris by Microglia Impairs Remyelinating Processes," *Journal of Experimental Medicine* 212, no. 4 (2015): 481–95, https://doi.org/10.1084/jem.20141656; Elizabeth Gray et al., "Elevated Myeloperoxidase Activity in White Matter in Multiple Sclerosis," *Neuroscience Letters* 444, no. 2 (2008): 195–98, https://doi.org/10.1016/j.neulet.2008.08.035; Judy S. H. Liu et al., "Expression of Inducible Nitric Oxide Synthase and Nitrotyrosine in Multiple Sclerosis Lesions," *American Journal of Pathology* 158, no. 6 (2001): 2057–66, https://doi.org/10.1016/s0002-9440(10)64677-9; Marie T. Fischer et al., "NADPH Oxidase Expression in Active Multiple Sclerosis Lesions in Relation to Oxidative Tissue Damage and Mitochondrial Injury," *Brain* 135, no. 3 (2012): 886–99, https://doi.org/10.1093/brain/aws012; Marie T. Fischer et al., "Disease-Specific Molecular Events in Cortical Multiple Sclerosis Lesions," *Brain* 136, no. 6 (2013): 1799–815, https://doi.org/10.1093/brain/awt110; Thomas Zeis et al., "Molecular Changes in White Matter Adjacent to an Active Demyelinating Lesion in Early Multiple Sclerosis," *Brain Pathology* 19, no. 3 (2009): 459–66, https://doi.org/10.1111/j.1750-3639.2008.00231.x.

71. M. Gironi et al., "A Pilot Trial of Low-Dose Naltrexone in Primary Progressive Multiple Sclerosis," *Multiple Sclerosis Journal* 14, no. 8 (2008): 1076–83, https://doi.org/10.1177/1352458508095828; Anthony P. Turel et al., "Low Dose Naltrexone for Treatment of Multiple Sclerosis," *Journal of Clinical Psychopharmacology* 35, no. 5 (2015): 609–11, https://doi.org/10.1097/jcp.0000000000000373; Cree, Kornyeyeva, and Goodin, "Pilot Trial of Low-Dose Naltrexone"; Michael D. Ludwig et al., "Long-Term Treatment with Low Dose Naltrexone Maintains Stable Health in Patients with Multiple Sclerosis," *Multiple Sclerosis Journal—Experimental, Translational and Clinical* 2 (2016): 1–11, https://doi.org/10.1177/2055217316672242; Guttorm Raknes and Lars Småbrekke, "Low Dose Naltrexone in Multiple Sclerosis: Effects on Medication Use. A Quasi-Experimental Study," *PloS One* 12, no. 11 (March 2017), https://doi.org/10.1371/journal.pone.0187423; Michael D. Ludwig, Ian S. Zagon, and Patricia J. McLaughlin, "Featured Article: Serum [Met5]-Enkephalin Levels Are Reduced in Multiple Sclerosis and Restored by Low-Dose Naltrexone," *Experimental Biology and Medicine* 242, no. 15 (February 2017): 1524–33, https://doi.org/10.1177/1535370217724791.

72. Liu, Du, and Hong, "Naloxone Protects Rat Dopaminergic Neurons against Inflammatory Damage."

73. Yuxin Liu et al., "Inhibition by Naloxone Stereoisomers of β-Amyloid Peptide (1–42)-Induced Superoxide Production in Microglia and Degeneration of

Cortical and Mesencephalic Neurons," *Journal of Pharmacology and Experimental Therapeutics* 302, no. 3 (January 2002): 1212–19, https://doi.org/10.1124/jpet .102.035956; Qingshan Wang et al., "Naloxone Inhibits Immune Cell Function by Suppressing Superoxide Production through a Direct Interaction with gp91 Phox Subunit of NADPH Oxidase," *Journal of Neuroinflammation* 9, no. 1 (2012): 32, https://doi.org/10.1186/1742-2094-9-32.

74. Thomas Guttuso Jr., Naomi Salins, and David Lichter, "Abstract #13: Low-Dose Naltrexone's Tolerability and Effects in Fatigued Patients with Parkinson's Disease: An Open-Label Study," *Neurotherapeutics* 7, no. 3 (2010): 332, https://doi.org /10.1016/j.nurt.2010.06.015.

75. Bernard Bihari, "Low-Dose Naltrexone for Normalizing Immune System Function," *Alternative Therapies in Health and Medicine* 19, no. 2 (March–April 2013): 56–65.

76. Xuan Liang et al., "Opioid System Modulates the Immune Function: A Review," *Translational Perioperative and Pain Medicine* 1, no. 1 (March 2016): 5–13; Jana Ninković and Sabita Roy, "Role of the Mu-Opioid Receptor in Opioid Modulation of Immune Function," *Amino Acids* 45, no. 1 (2011): 9–24, https:// doi.org/10.1007/s00726-011-1163-0; Patricia J. McLaughlin and Ian S. Zagon, "The Opioid Growth Factor–Opioid Growth Factor Receptor Axis: Homeostatic Regulator of Cell Proliferation and Its Implications for Health and Disease," *Biochemical Pharmacology* 84, no. 6 (2012): 746–55, https://doi.org/10.1016/j .bcp.2012.05.018.

77. Astrid Nehlig, "The Neuroprotective Effects of Cocoa Flavanol and Its Influence on Cognitive Performance," *British Journal of Clinical Pharmacology* 75, no. 3 (May 2013): 716–27, https://doi.org/10.1111/j.1365-2125.2012.04378.x; Paul W. Bosland, "Hot Stuff—Do People Living in Hot Climates Like Their Food Spicy Hot or Not?" *Temperature* 3, no. 1 (February 2016): 41–42, https://doi.org/10 .1080/23328940.2015.1130521; P. C. Dinas, Y. Koutedakis, and A. D. Flouris, "Effects of Exercise and Physical Activity on Depression," *Irish Journal of Medical Science* 180, no. 2 (2010): 319–25, https://doi.org/10.1007/s11845-010-0633-9; Jan G. Veening and Henk P. Barendregt, "The Effects of Beta-Endorphin: State Change Modification," *Fluids and Barriers of the CNS* 12, no. 1 (2015): 3, https:// doi.org/10.1186/2045-8118-12-3; University of Turku, "Social Laughter Releases Endorphins in the Brain," *Neuroscience News*, June 2, 2017, http://neuroscience news.com/endorphins-social-laughter-6825; Ji-Sheng Han, "Acupuncture and Endorphins," *Neuroscience Letters* 361, no. 1–3 (2004): 258–61, https://doi .org/10.1016/j.neulet.2003.12.019; Tongjian You et al., "Effects of Tai Chi on Beta Endorphin and Inflammatory Markers in Older Adults with Chronic Pain: An Exploratory Study," *Aging Clinical and Experimental Research* (2019), https://doi .org/10.1007/s40520-019-01316-1.

78. Helle Mørch and Bente Klarlund Pedersen, "β-Endorphin and the Immune System—Possible Role in Autoimmune Diseases," *Autoimmunity* 21, no. 3 (1995): 161–71, https://doi.org/10.3109/08916939509008013; T. G. Shrihari, "Beta-Endorphins: Anti-Inflammatory Activity in Holistic Treatment of Diseases," *EC*

Microbiology 14, no. 11 (October 2018): 732–35, https://www.ecronicon.com
/ecmi/pdf/ECMI-14-00557.pdf; Junichi Hosoi, Hiroaki Ozawa, and Richard D.
Granstein, "β-Endorphin Binding and Regulation of Cytokine Expression in
Langerhans Cells," *Annals of the New York Academy of Sciences* 885, no. 1 (June
2006): 405–13, https://doi.org/10.1111/j.1749-6632.1999.tb08700.x.

79. Massimo Franceschi et al., "Plasma β-Endorphin and β-Lipotropin in Patients with
Parkinson's Disease," *Clinical Neuropharmacology* 9, no. 6 (1986): 549–55, https://
doi.org/10.1097/00002826-198612000-00006; G. Nappi et al., "Beta-Endorphin
Cerebrospinal Fluid Decrease in Untreated Parkinsonian Patients," *Neurology*
35, no. 9 (January 1985): 1371, https://doi.org/10.1212/wnl.35.9.1371; H. Khalil
et al., "The Circulatory Levels of Serotonin, Beta Endorphin and Dopamine and
Their Relations to Pain Perception in People with Parkinson's Disease [abstract],"
Movement Disorders 34, supplement 2 (2019), https://www.mdsabstracts.org
/abstract/the-circulatory-levels-of-serotonin-beta-endorphin-and-dopamine
-and-their-relations-to-pain-perception-in-people-with-parkinsons-disease.

80. Jarred Younger and Sean Mackey, "Fibromyalgia Symptoms Are Reduced by Low-Dose
Naltrexone: A Pilot Study," *Pain Medicine* 10, no. 4 (2009): 663–72, https://doi
.org/10.1111/j.1526-4637.2009.00613.x; Guttorm Raknes and Lars Småbrekke,
"Correction: Low Dose Naltrexone: Effects on Medication in Rheumatoid and
Seropositive Arthritis. A Nationwide Register-Based Controlled Quasi-Experimental
Before-After Study," *PloS One* 14, no. 10 (January 2019), https://doi.org/10.1371
/journal.pone; Kirbie M. Bostick, Andrew G. McCarter, and Diane Nykamp, "The
Use of Low-Dose Naltrexone for Chronic Pain," *Senior Care Pharmacist* 34, no. 1
(January 2019): 43–46, https://doi.org/10.4140/tcp.n.2019.43.

81. Ketaki S. Bhalsing, Masoom M. Abbas, and Louis C. S. Tan, "Role of Physical
Activity in Parkinson's Disease," *Annals of Indian Academy of Neurology* 21, no. 4
(October–December 2018): 242–49, https://doi.org/10.4103/aian.AIAN_169_18;
Barbara Pickut et al., "Mindfulness Training among Individuals with Parkinson's
Disease: Neurobehavioral Effects," *Parkinson's Disease* 2015 (2015): 1–6, https://
doi.org/10.1155/2015/816404; Corjena Cheung et al., "Effects of Yoga on Oxidative
Stress, Motor Function, and Non-Motor Symptoms in Parkinson's Disease: A Pilot
Randomized Controlled Trial," *Pilot and Feasibility Studies* 4, no. 1 (2018): 162, https://
doi.org/10.1186/s40814-018-0355-8; Sook-Hyun Lee and Sabina Lim, "Clinical
Effectiveness of Acupuncture on Parkinson's Disease," *Medicine* 96, no. 3 (2017):
e5836, https://doi.org/10.1097/md.0000000000005836; Sujung Yeo et al., "A Study of
the Effects of 8-Week Acupuncture Treatment on Patients with Parkinson's Disease,"
Medicine 97, no. 50 (2018): e13434, https://doi.org/10.1097/md.0000000000013434;
Jaung-Geng Lin et al., "Electroacupuncture Promotes Recovery of Motor Function
and Reduces Dopaminergic Neuron Degeneration in Rodent Models of Parkinson's
Disease," *International Journal of Molecular Sciences* 18, no. 9 (2017): 1846, https://
doi.org/10.3390/ijms18091846; Karishma Smart et al., "A Potential Case of Remission
of Parkinson's Disease," *Journal of Complementary and Integrative Medicine* 13, no.
3 (January 2016): 311–15, https://doi.org/10.1515/jcim-2016-0019; Marieke Van
Puymbroeck et al., "Functional Improvements in Parkinson's Disease Following a

Randomized Trial of Yoga," *Evidence-Based Complementary and Alternative Medicine* 2018 (March 2018): 1–8, https://doi.org/10.1155/2018/8516351; Barbara A. Pickut et al., "Mindfulness Based Intervention in Parkinson's Disease Leads to Structural Brain Changes on MRI," *Clinical Neurology and Neurosurgery* 115, no. 12 (2013): 2419–25, https://doi.org/10.1016/j.clineuro.2013.10.002; Long Zhang et al., "A Review Focused on the Psychological Effectiveness of Tai Chi on Different Populations," *Evidence-Based Complementary and Alternative Medicine* 2012 (2012): 1–9, https://doi.org/10.1155/2012/678107; Madeleine E. Hackney and Gammon M. Earhart, "Effects of Dance on Balance and Gait in Severe Parkinson's Disease: A Case Study," *Disability and Rehabilitation* 32, no. 8 (August 2009): 679–84, https://doi.org/10.3109/09638 280903247905; M. E. Mcneely, R. P. Duncan, and G. M. Earhart, "Impacts of Dance on Non-Motor Symptoms, Participation, and Quality of Life in Parkinson's Disease and Healthy Older Adults," *Maturitas* 82, no. 4 (2015): 336–41, https://doi.org/10.1016/j.maturitas.2015.08.002; Gammon M. Earhart, "Dance as Therapy for Individuals with Parkinson's Disease," *European Journal of Physical and Rehabilitation Medicine* 45, no. 2 (June 2009): 231–38, https://www.ncbi.nlm.nih.gov/pubmed/19532110.

82. Stefania Kalampokini et al., "Nonpharmacological Modulation of Chronic Inflammation in Parkinson's Disease: Role of Diet Interventions," *Parkinson's Disease* 2019 (2019): 1–12, https://doi.org/10.1155/2019/7535472; Valentina Caputi and Maria Giron, "Microbiome-Gut-Brain Axis and Toll-Like Receptors in Parkinson's Disease," *International Journal of Molecular Sciences* 19, no. 6 (June 2018): 1689, https://doi.org/10.3390/ijms19061689; Agata Mulak, "Brain-Gut-Microbiota Axis in Parkinson's Disease," *World Journal of Gastroenterology* 21, no. 37 (2015): 10609, https://doi.org/10.3748/wjg.v21.i37.10609; Lisa Klingelhoefer and Heinz Reichmann, "The Gut and Nonmotor Symptoms in Parkinson's Disease," *International Review of Neurobiology* 134 (2017): 787–809, https://doi.org/10.1016/bs.irn.2017.05.027; Meng-Fei Sun and Yan-Qin Shen, "Dysbiosis of Gut Microbiota and Microbial Metabolites in Parkinson's Disease," *Ageing Research Reviews* 45 (2018): 53–61, https://doi.org/10.1016/j.arr.2018.04.004; Meng-Fei Sun et al., "Neuroprotective Effects of Fecal Microbiota Transplantation on MPTP-Induced Parkinson's Disease Mice: Gut Microbiota, Glial Reaction and TLR4/TNF-α Signaling Pathway," *Brain, Behavior, and Immunity* 70 (May 2018): 48–60, https://doi.org/10.1016/j.bbi.2018.02.005; Feng Lai et al., "Intestinal Pathology and Gut Microbiota Alterations in a Methyl-4-Phenyl-1,2,3,6-Tetrahydropyridine (MPTP) Mouse Model of Parkinson's Disease," *Neurochemical Research* 43, no. 10 (2018): 1986–99, https://doi.org/10.1007/s11064-018-2620-x; Javier Campos-Acuña, Daniela Elgueta, and Rodrigo Pacheco, "T-Cell-Driven Inflammation as a Mediator of the Gut-Brain Axis Involved in Parkinson's Disease," *Frontiers in Immunology* 10 (2019), https://doi.org/10.3389/fimmu.2019 .00239; Rodrigo Pacheco, "Cross-Talk between T-Cells and Gut-Microbiota in Neurodegenerative Disorders," *Neural Regeneration Research* 14, no. 12 (2019): 2091, https://doi.org/10.4103/1673-5374.262582; Xiao-Lu Niu et al., "Prevalence of Small Intestinal Bacterial Overgrowth in Chinese Patients with

Parkinson's Disease," *Journal of Neural Transmission* 123, no. 12 (February 2016): 1381–86, https://doi.org/10.1007/s00702-016-1612-8; Zhi-Lan Zhou et al., "Neuroprotection of Fasting Mimicking Diet on MPTP-Induced Parkinson's Disease Mice via Gut Microbiota and Metabolites," *Neurotherapeutics* 16, no. 3 (2019): 741–60, https://doi.org/10.1007/s13311-019-00719-2.

83. Ai Huey Tan et al., "Small Intestinal Bacterial Overgrowth in Parkinson's Disease," *Parkinsonism & Related Disorders* 20, no. 5 (2014): 535–40, https://doi.org/10.1016/j.parkreldis.2014.02.019.

84. Xiao-Lu Niu et al., "Prevalence of Small Intestinal Bacterial Overgrowth."

85. Luca Magistrelli et al., "Probiotics May Have Beneficial Effects in Parkinson's Disease: In Vitro Evidence," *Frontiers in Immunology* 10 (July 2019), https://doi.org/10.3389/fimmu.2019.00969; Parisa Gazerani, "Probiotics for Parkinson's Disease," *International Journal of Molecular Sciences* 20, no. 17 (2019): 4121, https://doi.org/10.3390/ijms20174121; E. Cassani et al., "Use of Probiotics for the Treatment of Constipation in Parkinson's Disease Patients," *Minerva Gastroenterologica e Dietologica* 57, no. 2 (2011): 117–21, https://www.ncbi.nlm.nih.gov/pubmed/21587143; Stefania Kalampokini et al., "Nonpharmacological Modulation of Chronic Inflammation in Parkinson's Disease: Role of Diet Interventions," *Parkinson's Disease* 2019 (2019): 1–12, https://doi.org/10.1155/2019/7535472; Małgorzata Kujawska and Jadwiga Jodynis-Liebert, "What Is the Evidence That Parkinson's Disease Is a Prion Disorder, Which Originates in the Gut?" *International Journal of Molecular Sciences* 19, no. 11 (December 2018): 3573, https://doi.org/10.3390/ijms19113573; Ying Chen et al., "Prion-Like Propagation of α-Synuclein in the Gut-Brain Axis," *Brain Research Bulletin* 140 (2018): 341–46, https://doi.org/10.1016/j.brainresbull.2018.06.002; Paula Perez-Pardo et al., "The Gut-Brain Axis in Parkinson's Disease: Possibilities for Food-Based Therapies," *European Journal of Pharmacology* 817 (2017): 86–95, https://doi.org/10.1016/j.ejphar.2017.05.042; Dongming Yang et al., "The Role of the Gut Microbiota in the Pathogenesis of Parkinson's Disease," *Frontiers in Neurology* 10 (June 2019), https://doi.org/10.3389/fneur.2019.01155; Michal Lubomski et al., "Parkinson's Disease and the Gastrointestinal Microbiome," *Journal of Neurology* 2019, https://doi.org/10.1007/s00415-019-09320-1; Sarah M. O'Donovan et al., "Nigral Overexpression of αSynuclein in a Rat Parkinson's Disease Model Indicates Alterations in the Enteric Nervous System and the Gut Microbiome," *Neurogastroenterology & Motility* 32, no. 1 (February 2019), https://doi.org/10.1111/nmo.13726; Visonneau Leclair et al., "The Gut in Parkinson's Disease: Bottomup, Topdown, or Neither?" *Neurogastroenterology & Motility* 32, no. 1 (2019), https://doi.org/10.1111/nmo.13777; Arthur Lionnet et al., "Does Parkinson's Disease Start in the Gut?" *Acta Neuropathologica* 135, no. 1 (2017): 1–12, https://doi.org/10.1007/s00401-017-1777-8; David K. Simon, Caroline M. Tanner, and Patrik Brundin, "Parkinson's Disease Epidemiology, Pathology, Genetics, and Pathophysiology," *Clinics in Geriatric Medicine* 36, no. 1 (2020): 1–12, https://doi.org/10.1016/j.cger.2019.08.002.

86. Mitchell R.K.L. Lie et al., "Low Dose Naltrexone for Induction of Remission in Inflammatory Bowel Disease Patients," *Journal of Translational Medicine* 16, no. 1 (September 2018): 55, https://doi.org/10.1186/s12967-018-1427-5; J. Ploesser, L. B.

Weinstock, and E. Thomas, "Low Dose Naltrexone: Side Effects and Efficacy in Gastrointestinal Disorders," *International Journal of Pharmaceutical Compounding* 14, no. 2 (2010): 171–73, https://www.ncbi.nlm.nih.gov/pubmed/23965429.

87. Robert A. Hauser et al., "Randomized, Double-Blind, Pilot Evaluation of Intravenous Glutathione in Parkinson's Disease," *Movement Disorders* 24, no. 7 (2009): 979–83, https://doi.org/10.1002/mds.22401.

Chapter 6: Pediatrics

1. Centers for Disease Control and Prevention, "Data and Statistics on Children's Mental Health," April 2019, https://www.cdc.gov/childrensmentalhealth/data.html.

2. Jon Baio et al., "Prevalence of Autism Spectrum Disorder among Children Aged 8 Years—Autism and Developmental Disabilities Monitoring Network, 11 Sites, United States, 2014," *Morbidity and Mortality Weekly Report. Surveillance Summaries* 67, no. 6 (April 27, 2018): 1–23.

3. Interactive Autism Network, "Diagnostic Criteria for Autism Spectrum Disorder," in American Psychiatric Association, *Diagnostic and Statistical Manual of Mental Disorders*, 5th ed. (Arlington, VA: American Psychiatric Association, 2013), pp. 50–51.

4. Baio et al., "Prevalence of Autism Spectrum Disorder."

5. Interactive Autism Network, "Diagnostic Criteria for Autism Spectrum Disorder," 52.

6. Audrey Thurm et al., "State of the Field: Differentiating Intellectual Disability from Autism Spectrum Disorder," *Frontiers in Psychiatry* 10 (July 2019): 526, https://doi.org/10.3389/fpsyt.2019.00526.

7. M. Harada et al., "Non-Invasive Evaluation of the Gabaergic/Glutamatergic System in Autistic Patients Observed by MEGA-Editing Proton MR Spectroscopy Using a Clinical 3 Tesla Instrument," *Journal of Autism and Developmental Disorders* 41, no. 4 (April 2011): 447–54.

8. S. Braat and R. F. Kooy, "The GABAA Receptor as a Therapeutic Target for Neurodevelopmental Disorders," *Neuron* 86, no. 5 (June 2015): 119–30.

9. Marvin Boris et al., "Association of MTHFR Gene Variants with Autism," *Journal of American Physicians and Surgeons* 9, no. 4 (2004): 106–08.

10. David Rosenberg, "Obsessive-Compulsive Disorder in Children and Adolescents: Epidemiology, Pathogenesis, Clinical Manifestations, Course, Assessment and Diagnosis," *UpToDate*, https://www.uptodate.com/contents/obsessive-compulsive -disorder-in-children-and-adolescents-epidemiology-pathogenesis-clinical -manifestations-course-assessment-and-diagnosis, last edited June 7, 2019.

11. Sandra Meier et al., "Obsessive-Compulsive Disorder and Autism Spectrum Disorders: Longitudinal and Offspring Risk," *PLoS One*, https://doi.org/10.1371/journal.pone.0141703.

12. Helen E. Vuong et al., "Emerging Roles for the Gut Microbiome in Autism Spectrum Disorder," *Biological Psychiatry* 81, no. 5 (March 2017): 411–23; Jennifer G. Mulle et al., "The Gut Microbiome: A New Frontier in Autism Research," *Current Psychiatry Reports* 15, no. 2 (February 2013): 337; S. M. O'Mahony et al., "Serotonin, Tryptophan Metabolism and the Brain-Gut-Microbiome Axis," *Behavioural Brain Research* 277 (2015): 32–48.

13. Centers for Disease Control and Prevention, "Anxiety and Depression in Children: Get the Facts," April 2019, CDC.gov.

14. Centers for Disease Control and Prevention, "Data and Statistics on Children's Mental Health," April 2019, https://www.cdc.gov/childrensmentalhealth/data.html.

15. Jean-Philippe Boulenger et al., "Increased Sensitivity to Caffeine in Patients with Panic Disorders. Preliminary Evidence," *Archives of General Psychiatry* 41, no. 11 (1984): 1067–71.

16. US Food and Drug Administration, "Questions and Answers on Monosodium Glutamate (MSG)," https://www.fda.gov/food/food-additives-petitions /questions-and-answers-monosodium-glutamate-msg, November 19, 2012.

17. S. E. Jacob and S. Stechschulte, "Formaldehyde, Aspartame, and Migraines: A Possible Connection," *Dermatitis* 19, no. 3 (May 2008): E10–E11.

18. Karol Rycerz and J. E. Jaworska-Adamu, "Effects of Aspartame Metabolites on Astrocytes and Neurons," *Folia Neuropathologica* 51, no. 1 (2013): 10–17.

19. Dana L. McMakin and Candice A. Alfano, "Sleep and Anxiety in Late Childhood and Early Adolescence," *Current Opinion in Psychiatry* 28, no. 6 (November 2015): 483–89.

20. T. A. Mellman and T. W. Uhde, "Sleep Panic Attacks: New Clinical Findings and Theoretical Implications," *American Journal of Psychiatry* 146, no. 9 (September 1989): 1204–07.

21. Cara A. Palmer et al., "Co-Sleeping Among School-Aged Anxious and Non-Anxious Children: Associations with Sleep Variability and Timing," *Journal of Abnormal Child Psychology* 46, no. 6 (August 2018): 1321–32.

22. Dr. Siri Carpenter, "That Gut Feeling," *American Psychological Association* 43, no. 8 (September 2012): 50.

23. Pandasnetwork.org, "PANDAS/PANS Prevalence," http://pandasnetwork.org/statistics.

24. Maryann P. Platt et al., "Hello from the Other Side: How Autoantibodies Circumvent the Blood-Brain Barrier in Autoimmune Encephalitis," *Frontiers in Immunology* 8, no. 442 (2017).

25. Carol Cox et al., "Brain Human Monoclonal Autoantibody from Sydenham Chorea Targets Dopaminergic Neurons in Transgenic Mice and Signals Dopamine D2 Receptor: Implications in Human Disease," *Journal of Immunology* 191, no. 11 (December 2013): 5524–41; Linor Brimberg et al., "Behavioral, Pharmacological, and Immunological Abnormalities after Streptococcal Exposure: A Novel Rat Model of Sydenham Chorea and Related Neuropsychiatric Disorders," *Neuropsychopharmacology* 37, no. 9 (August 2012): 2076–87; Christine A. Kirvan et al., "Streptococcal Mimicry and Antibody-Mediated Cell Signaling in the Pathogenesis of Sydenham's Chorea," *Autoimmunity* 39, no. 1 (February 2006): 21–29; Christine A. Kirvan et al., "Tubulin Is a Neuronal Target of Autoantibodies in Sydenham's Chorea," *Journal of Immunology* 178, no. 11 (June 2007): 7412–21.

26. H. S. Singer et al., "Neuronal Antibody Biomarkers for Sydenham's Chorea Identify a New Group of Children with Chronic Recurrent Episodic Acute Exacerbations of Tic and Obsessive Compulsive Symptoms Following a Streptococcal Infection," *PLoS One* 10, no. 3 (March 2015): e0120499.

27. PANDAS Physicians Network, "Symptom Severity Based Treatment," https://www
.pandasppn.org/symptom-severity.

28. Gina Chun Kost et al., "Clavulanic Acid Increases Dopamine Release in Neuronal
Cells through a Mechanism Involving Enhanced Vesicle Trafficking," *Neuroscience
Letters* 504, no. 2 (October 2011): 170–75.

29. Jennifer Frankovich et al., "Overview of Treatment of Pediatric Acute-Onset
Neuropsychiatric Syndrome," *Journal of Child and Adolescent Psychopharmacology*
27, no. 7 (September 2017).

30. B. Muhammad et al., "Juvenile Primary Fibromyalgia Syndrome. A Clinical Study of
Thirty-Three Patients and Matched Normal Controls," *Arthritis and Rheumatology*
28, no. 2 (February 1985): 137–45.

31. B. Muhammad et al., "Juvenile Primary Fibromyalgia Syndrome."

32. B. Muhammad et al., "Primary Fibromyalgia (Fibrositis): Clinical Study of 50
Patients with Matched Normal Controls," *Seminars in Arthritis and Rheumatism*
11, no. 1 (August 1981): 151–71.

33. J. Younger and S. Mackey, "Fibromyalgia Symptoms Are Reduced by Low-Dose
Naltrexone: A Pilot Study," *Pain Medicine* 10, no. 4 (May 2009): 663–72.

Chapter 7: Women's Health

1. "What Is Endometriosis?" Endometriosis, American College of Obstetricians and
Gynecologists, updated January 2019, https://www.acog.org/patient-resources
/faqs/gynecologic-problems/endometriosis.

2. N. Gleicher et al., "Is Endometriosis an Autoimmune Disease?" *Obstetrics and Gynecology*
70, no. 1 (July 1987): 115–22, https://www.ncbi.nlm.nih.gov/pubmed/3110710.

3. "Polycystic Ovary Syndrome: ACOG Practice Bulletin Summary, Number 194,"
Obstetrics and Gynecology 131, no. 6 (June 2018): 1174–76, https://doi.org
/10.1097/AOG.0000000000002657.

4. Brigitte J. Roozenburg et al., "Successful Induction of Ovulation in
Normogonadotrophic Clomiphene Resistant Anovulatory Women by Combined
Naltrexone and Clomiphene Citrate Treatment," *Human Reproduction* 12, no. 8
(August 1997): 1720–22, https://doi.org/10.1093/humrep/12.8.1720.

5. L. Wildt et al., "Treatment with Naltrexone in Hypothalamic Ovarian Failure:
Induction of Ovulation and Pregnancy," *Human Reproduction* 8, no. 3 (March
1993): 350–58, https://doi.org/10.1093/oxfordjournals.humrep.a138050.

Chapter 8: Traumatic Brain Injury

1. Suzanne Polinder et al., "A Multidimensional Approach to Post-Concussion
Symptoms in Mild Traumatic Brain Injury," *Frontiers in Neurology* 9 (December
2018): Article 1113, http://doi.org/10.3389/fneur.2018.01113.

2. Daniel Laskowitz and Gerald Grant, eds., *Translational Research in Traumatic Brain
Injury* (Boca Raton, FL: CRC Press/Taylor and Francis Group, 2016), 2–12.

3. Kathryn E. Saatman et al., "Classification of Traumatic Brain Injury for Targeted
Therapies," *Journal of Neurotrauma* 25, no. 7 (July 2008): 719–38, https://doi.org
/10.1089/neu.2008.0586.

4. Laskowitz and Grant, *Translational Research in Traumatic Brain Injury*.

5. Laskowitz and Grant, *Translational Research in Traumatic Brain Injury*.

6. Zoe M. Tapp, Jonathan P. Godbout, and Olga N. Kokiko-Cochran, "A Tilted Axis: Maladaptive Inflammation and HPA Axis Dysfunction Contribute to Consequences of TBI," *Frontiers in Neurology* 10 (April 2019): Article 345, https://doi.org/10.3389/fneur.2019.00345.

7. David J. Sharp and Peter O. Jenkins, "Concussion Is Confusing Us All," *Practical Neurology* 15, no. 3 (June 2015): 172–86, https://doi.org/10.1136/practneurol-2015-001087.

8. Polinder et al., "A Multidimensional Approach."

9. Polinder et al., "A Multidimensional Approach."

10. Polinder et al., "A Multidimensional Approach."

11. Laskowitz and Grant, *Translational Research in Traumatic Brain Injury*.

12. Polinder et al., "A Multidimensional Approach."

13. Jerrold R. Turner, "Intestinal Mucosal Barrier Function in Health and Disease," *Nature Reviews Immunology* 9, no. 11 (November 2009): 799–809, https://doi.org/10.1038/nri2653.

14. Mark E. M. Obrenovich, "Leaky Gut, Leaky Brain?" *Microorganisms* 6, no. 4 (October 2018): 107, https://doi.org/10.3390/microorganisms6040107.

15. Datis Kharrazian, *Why Isn't My Brain Working?: A Revolutionary Understanding of Brain Decline and Effective Strategies to Recover Your Brain's Health* (Carlsbad, CA: Elephant Press, July 2013).

16. Kharrazian, *Why Isn't My Brain Working?*

17. Gerwyn Morris et al., "Leaky Brain in Neurological and Psychiatric Disorders: Drivers and Consequences," *Australian and New Zealand Journal of Psychiatry* 52, no. 10 (October 2018): 924–48, https://doi.org/10.1177/0004867418796955.

18. Kharrazian, *Why Isn't My Brain Working?*

19. Obrenovich, "Leaky Gut, Leaky Brain?"

20. Anthony Samsel and Stephanie Seneff, "Glyphosate, Pathways to Modern Diseases II: Celiac Sprue and Gluten Intolerance," *Interdisciplinary Toxicology* 6, no. 4 (2013): 159–84, https://doi.org/10.2478/intox-2013-0026.

21. Obrenovich, "Leaky Gut, Leaky Brain?"

22. Kharrazian, *Why Isn't My Brain Working?*

23. Obrenovich, "Leaky Gut, Leaky Brain?"

24. Khalafalla O. Bushara, "Neurologic Presentation of Celiac Disease," *Gastroenterology* 128, no. 4 (April 2005): S92–S97, https://doi.org/10.1053/j.gastro.2005.02.018.

25. David J. Wallace et al., "Spinal Cord Injury and the Human Microbiome: Beyond the Brain-Gut Axis," *Neurosurgical Focus* 46, no. 3 (March 2019): E11, https://doi.org/10.3171/2018.12.FOCUS18206.

26. Kiran V. Sandhu et al., "The Microbiota-Gut-Brain Axis: Diet, Microbiome, and Neuropsychiatry," *Translational Research* 179 (January 2017): 223–44, https://doi.org/10.1016/j.trsl.2016.10.002.

27. Ana Agustí et al., "Interplay between the Gut-Brain Axis, Obesity and Cognitive Function," *Frontiers in Neuroscience* 12 (March 2018): Article 155, https://doi.org/10.3389/fnins.2018.00155.

28. Julia König et al., "Human Intestinal Barrier Function in Health and Disease," *Clinical and Translational Gastroenterology* 7, no. 10 (2016): e196, https://doi.org/10.1038/ctg.2016.54.

29. Tapp, Godbout, and Kokiko-Cochran, "A Tilted Axis."

30. Tapp, Godbout, and Kokiko-Cochran, "A Tilted Axis."

31. Elisa Bisicchia et al., "Plasticity of Microglia in Remote Regions after Focal Brain Injury," *Seminars in Cell & Developmental Biology* 94 (October 2019): 104–11, https://doi.org/10.1016/j.semcdb.2019.01.011.

32. M. E. Tremblay et al., "The Role of Microglia in the Healthy Brain," *Journal of Neuroscience* 9, no. 31 (November 2011): 16064–69, https://doi.org/10.1523/JNEUROSCI.4158-11.2011.

33. Sudhakar R. Subramaniam and Howard J. Federoff, "Targeting Microglial Activation States as a Therapeutic Avenue in Parkinson's Disease," *Frontiers in Aging Neuroscience* 9, no. 176 (June 2017), https://doi.org/10.3389/fnagi.2017.00176.

34. A. Dalgleish, "The Role of LDN in the Management of Cancer," Research presented at the LDN AIIC 2018 Conference, Glasgow, Scotland, July 7, 2018.

35. Jarred Younger, Luke Parkitny, and David McLain, "The Use of Low-Dose Naltrexone (LDN) as a Novel Anti-Inflammatory Treatment for Chronic Pain," *Clinical Rheumatology* 33, no. 4 (April 2014): 451–59, https://doi.org/10.1007/s10067-014-2517-2.

36. Jacqueline R. Kulbe and James W. Geddes, "Current Status of Fluid Biomarkers in Mild Traumatic Brain Injury," *Experimental Neurology* 275, no. 3 (January 2016): 334–52, https://doi.org/10.1016/j.expneurol.2015.05.004.

37. Si Yun Ng and Alan Yiu Wah Lee, "Traumatic Brain Injuries: Pathophysiology and Potential Therapeutic Targets," *Frontiers in Cellular Neuroscience* 13 (November 2019): Article 528, https://doi.org/fncel.2019.00528.

38. Maria Teresa Viscomi, "The Plasticity of Plasticity: Lesson from Remote Microglia Induced by Focal Central Nervous System Injury," *Neural Regeneration Research* 15, no. 1 (2020): 57–58, https://doi.org/10.4103/1673-5374.264448.

39. Xiangrong Chen et al., "Omega-3 Polyunsaturated Fatty Acid Supplementation Attenuates Microglial-Induced Inflammation by Inhibiting the HMGB1/TLR4/NF-κB Pathway Following Experimental Traumatic Brain Injury," *Journal of Neuroinflammation* 14, no. 1 (July 2017): Article 143, https://doi.org/10.1186/s12974-017-0917-3.

40. Bisicchia et al., "Plasticity of Microglia in Remote Regions."

41. "Ketogenic Diet," in *Nutrition and Traumatic Brain Injury: Improving Acute and Subacute Health Outcomes in Military Personnel*, ed. John Erdman, Maria Oria, and Laura Pillsbury (Washington, DC: National Academies Press, 2011), p. 11, https://doi.org/10.17226/13121.

42. Jama Lambert, Soledad Mejia, and Aristo Vojdani, "Plant and Human Aquaporins: Pathogenesis from Gut to Brain," *Immunology Research* 67 (February 2019): 12–20, https://doi.org/10.1007/s12026-018-9046-z.

43. Kharrazian, *Why Isn't My Brain Working?*

44. Heather M. Wilkins and Jill K. Morris, "New Therapeutics to Modulate Mitochondrial Function in Neurodegenerative Disorders," *Current Pharmaceutical Design* 23, no. 5 (2017): 731–52, https://doi.org/10.2174/1381612822666161230144517.

45. "Brain Basics: Understanding Sleep," National Institutes of Health: National Institute of Neurological Disorders and Strokes, last updated August 13, 2019, https://www.ninds.nih.gov/Disorders/patient-caregiver-education/Understanding-sleep.

46. M. S. Cooper, "LDN, Endosomes, and the Nanophysiology of Autoimmune Movement Disorders." Research presented at the LDN AIIC 2019 Conference, Portland, OR, June 7–9, 2019, https://www.ldnresearchtrust.org/conference-2019/ldn-endosomes-and-nanophysiology-autoimmune-movement-disorders; Aamir Hadanny et al., "Effect of Hyperbaric Oxygen Therapy on Chronic Neurocognitive Deficits of Post-Traumatic Brain Injury Patients: Retrospective Analysis," *BMJ Open* 8, no. 9 (2018): e023387, https://doi.org/10.1136/bmjopen-2018-023387.

47. David J. Eve et al., "Hyperbaric Oxygen Therapy as a Potential Treatment for Post-Traumatic Stress Disorder Associated with Traumatic Brain Injury," *Neuropsychiatric Disease and Treatment* 12 (October 2016): 2689–705, https://doi.org/10.2147/NDT.S110126.

48. Rahav Boussi-Gross et al., "Hyperbaric Oxygen Therapy Can Improve Post Concussion Syndrome Years after Mild Traumatic Brain Injury—Randomized Prospective Trial," *PLoS One* 8, no. 11 (November 2013): e79995, https://doi.org/10.1371/journal.pone.0079995.

49. Paul G. Harch et al., "Case Control Study: Hyperbaric Oxygen Treatment of Mild Traumatic Brain Injury Persistent Post-Concussion Syndrome and Post-Traumatic Stress Disorder," *Medical Gas Research* 7, no. 3 (October 2017): 156–74, https://doi.org/10.4103/2045-9912.215745.

Chapter 9: Dissociative Disorders

1. David Spiegel et al., "Dissociative Disorders in DSM-5," *Depression and Anxiety* 28, no. 9 (September 2011): 824–52, http://doi.org/10.1002/da.20874.

2. Marlene Steinberg, *Interviewer's Guide to the Structured Clinical Interview for DSM-IV Dissociative Disorders: Revised* (Washington, DC: American Psychiatric Press, 1994), 11.

3. American Psychiatric Association, *Diagnostic and Statistical Manual of Mental Disorders*, 5th ed. (Arlington, VA: American Psychiatric Association, 2013); also see American Psychiatric Association, "What Are Dissociative Disorders?," https://www.psychiatry.org/patients-families/dissociative-disorders/what-are-dissociative-disorders.

4. Emily A. Holmes et al., "Are There Two Qualitatively Distinct Forms of Dissociation? A Review and Some Clinical Implications," *Clinical Psychology Review* 25, no. 1 (January 2005): 1–23, http://doi.org/10.1016/j.cpr.2004.08.006.

5. Spiegel et al., "Dissociative Disorders in DSM-5."

6. Marlene Steinberg, "In-Depth: Understanding Dissociative Disorders," *Psych Central*, last updated January 14, 2020, http://psychcentral.com/disorders/dissociative-identity-disorder/in-depth.

7. Chris R. Brewin, "Complex Post-Traumatic Stress Disorder: A New Diagnosis in ICD-11," *BJPsych Advances* (2019), 1–8, https://doi.org/10.1192/bja.2019.48.

8. Ulrich Lanius, "Opioid Antagonists and Dissociation: Pharmacological Interventions," in *Neurobiology and Treatment of Traumatic Dissociation: Toward*

an Embodied Self, ed. Ulrich F. Lanius, Sandra L. Paulsen, and Frank M. Corrigan (New York: Springer, 2014), pp. 471–98.

9. Ulrich F. Lanius, "Dissociation and Endogenous Opioids: A Foundational Role," in *Neurobiology and Treatment of Traumatic Dissociation*, ed. Lanius, Paulsen, and Corrigan, pp. 81–104.

10. Henry Krystal, *Massive Psychic Trauma* (New York: International Universities Press, 1968), 117.

11. Martin J. Bohus et al., "Naltrexone in the Treatment of Dissociative Symptoms in Patients with Borderline Personality Disorder: An Open-Label Trial," *Journal of Clinical Psychiatry* 60, no. 9 (1999): 598–603, https://doi.org/10.4088/jcp.v60 n0906; Christian Schmahl et al., "Evaluation of Naltrexone for Dissociative Symptoms in Borderline Personality Disorder," *International Clinical Psychopharmacology* 27, no. 1 (2012): 61–68.

12. Gad Lubin et al., "Short-Term Treatment of Post-Traumatic Stress Disorder with Naltrexone: An Open-Label Preliminary Study," *Human Psychopharmacology* 17, no. 4 (2002): 181–85, http://doi.org/10.1002/hup.395; Ulrich F. Lanius, "EMDR Processing with Dissociative Clients: Adjunctive Use of Opioid Antagonists," in *EMDR Solutions: Pathways to Healing*, ed. Robin Shapiro (New York: W. W. Norton, 2005), pp. 121–46.

13. W. Pape and W. Wöller, "Niedrig Dosiertes Naltrexon in Der Behandlung Dissoziativer Symptome," *Der Nervenarzt* 86 (2015): 346–51.

Chapter 10: Post-Traumatic Stress Disorder

1. Dean G. Kilpatrick et al., "National Estimates of Exposure to Traumatic Events and PTSD Prevalence Using DSM-IV and DSM-5 Criteria," *Journal of Traumatic Stress* 26, no. 5 (2013): 537–47, https://doi.org/10.1002/jts.21848.

2. T. Karatzias et al., "Risk Factors and Comorbidity of ICD-11 PTSD and Complex PTSD: Findings from a Trauma-Exposed Population Based Sample of Adults in the United Kingdom," *Depression and Anxiety* 36, no. 7 (July 2019): https://doi .org/10.1002/da.22934.

3. Jytte van Huijstee and Eric Vermetten, "The Dissociative Subtype of Post-Traumatic Stress Disorder: Research Update on Clinical and Neurobiological Features," in *Behavioral Neurobiology of PTSD*, ed. Eric Vermetten, Dewleen G. Baker, and Victoria B. Risbrough (Cham, Switzerland: Springer International, 2017), pp. 229–48.

4. Vincent J. Felitti et al., "Relationship of Childhood Abuse and Household Dysfunction to Many of the Leading Causes of Death in Adults. The Adverse Childhood Experiences (ACE) Study," *American Journal of Preventive Medicine* 14, no. 4 (1998): 245–58, https://doi.org/10.1016/S0749-3797(98)00017-8.

5. Bessel A. van der Kolk, "The Compulsion to Repeat the Trauma," *Psychiatric Clinics of North America* 12, no. 2 (1989): 389–411, https://doi.org/10.1016/s0193 -953x(18)30439-8.

6. Marc Schmid et al., "Developmental Trauma Disorder: Pros and Cons of Including Formal Criteria in the Psychiatric Diagnostic Systems," *BMC Psychiatry* 13, no. 3 (January 2013): https://bmcpsychiatry.biomedcentral.com/articles/10.1186/1471 -244X-13-3.

7. Philip Hyland et al., "The Relationship between ICD-11 PTSD, Complex PTSD and Dissociative Experiences," *Journal of Trauma & Dissociation* 21, no. 1 (October 2019): 1–11, https://doi.org/10.1080/15299732.2019.1675113.

8. Hiroaki Hori and Yoshiharu Kim, "Inflammation and Post-Traumatic Stress Disorder," *Psychiatry and Clinical Neurosciences* 73, no. 4 (2019): 143–53, https://doi.org/10.1111/pcn.12820.

9. Joseph A. Boscarino, "Posttraumatic Stress Disorder and Physical Illness: Results from Clinical and Epidemiologic Studies," *Annals of the New York Academy of Sciences* 1032, no. 1 (January 2005): 141–53, https://doi.org/10.1196/annals.1314.011.

10. Aoife O'Donovan et al., "Elevated Risk for Autoimmune Disorders in Iraq and Afghanistan Veterans with Posttraumatic Stress Disorder," *Biological Psychiatry* 77, no. 4 (2015): 365–74, https://doi.org/10.1016/j.biopsych.2014.06.015.

11. Mark W. Miller et al., "Oxidative Stress, Inflammation, and Neuroprogression in Chronic PTSD," *Harvard Review of Psychiatry* 26, no. 2 (April 2018): 57–69, htpps://doi.org/10.1097/HRP.0000000000000167.

12. Martin R. Cohen et al., "Studies of the Endogenous Opioid System in the Human Stress Response," in *Enkephalins and Endorphins*, ed. N. P. Plotnikoff et al. (Boston, MA: Springer, 1986); Paula P. Schnurr and Bonnie L. Green, "Understanding Relationships among Trauma, Posttraumatic Stress Disorder and Health Outcomes," in *Trauma and Health: Physical Health Consequences of Exposure to Extreme Stress*, ed. Paula P. Schnurr and Bonnie L. Green (American Psychological Association, 2004), pp. 247–75, https://doi.org/10.1037/10723-010; Ruth A. Lanius, Eric Vermetten, and Clare Pain, eds., *The Impact of Early Life Trauma on Health and Disease: The Hidden Epidemic* (Cambridge, U.K.: Cambridge University Press, 2010), https://doi.org/10.1017/CBO9780511777042.

13. Ulrich F. Lanius, "Dissociation and Endogenous Opioids: A Foundational Role," in *Neurobiology and Treatment of Traumatic Dissociation: Toward an Embodied Self*, ed. Ulrich F. Lanius, Sandra L. Paulsen, and Frank M. Corrigan (New York: Springer, 2014), pp. 471–98; J. Douglas Bremner and Elizabeth Brett, "Trauma-Related Dissociative States and Long-Term Psychopathology in Posttraumatic Stress Disorder," *Journal of Traumatic Stress* 10 (January 1997): 37–49, https://doi.org/10.1023/A:1024804312978.

14. Henry K. Beecher, "Pain in Men Wounded in Battle," *Annals of Surgery* 123, no. 1 (1946): 96–105, https://doi.org/10.1097/00000658-194601000-00008.

15. R. F. Mucha, "Effect of Naloxone and Morphine on Guinea Pig Tonic Immobility," *Behavioral and Neural Biology* 28, no. 1 (1980): 111–15, https://doi.org/10.1016/s0163-1047(80)93230-6.

16. Jaak Panksepp, *Affective Neuroscience: The Foundations of Human and Animal Emotions* (Oxford, U.K.: Oxford University Press, 1998).

17. Jaak Panksepp and Lucy Biven, *The Archaeology of Mind: Neuroevolutionary Origins of Human Emotions* (New York: W. W. Norton, 2012).

18. Claudia Regina Monassi, Andrade Leite-Panissi, and Leda Menescal-de-Oliveira, "Ventrolateral Periaqueductal Gray Matter and the Control of Tonic Immobility,"

Brain Research Bulletin 50, no. 3 (1999): 201–08, https://doi.org/10.1016/S0361 -9230(99)00192-6.

19. Osamu Sakurada, Louis Sokoloff, and Yasuko F. Jacquet, "Local Cerebral Glucose Utilization Following Injection of β-Endorphin into Periaqueductal Gray Matter in the Rat," *Brain Research* 153, no. 2 (1978): 403–07, https://doi.org/10.1016 /0006-8993(78)90423-7.

20. Monassi, Leite-Panissi, and Menescal-de-Oliveira, "Ventrolateral Periaqueductal Gray Matter."

21. Rebecca Valle, Negin Mohammadmirzaei, and Dayan Knox, "Single Prolonged Stress Alters Neural Activation in the Periacqueductal Gray and Midline Thalamic Nuclei during Emotional Learning and Memory," *Learning and Memory* 26 (2019): 403–11, https://doi.org/10.1101/lm.050310.119.

22. Francesca Farabollini et al., "Immune and Neuroendocrine Response to Restraint in Male and Female Rats," *Psychoneuroendocrinology* 18, no. 3 (1993): 175–82, https://doi.org/10.1016/0306-4530(93)90002-3.

23. A. Kling and Horst D. Steklis, "A Neural Substrate for Affiliative Behavior in Nonhuman Primates," *Brain, Behavior and Evolution* 13, no. 2–3 (1976): 216–38, https://doi.org/10.1159/000123811.

24. John D. Newman, M. R. Murphy, and C. R. Harbough, "Naloxone-Reversible Suppression of Isolation Call Production after Morphine Injections in Squirrel Monkeys [abstract]," *Society of Neuroscience* 8 (1982): 940.

25. Bessel A. van der Kolk, "Developmental Trauma Disorder: Toward a Rational Diagnosis for Children with Complex Trauma Histories," *Psychiatric Annals* 35, no. 5 (January 2005): 401–08, https://doi.org/10.3928/00485713-20050501-06.

26. Allan N. Schore, "The Effects of Early Relational Trauma on Right Brain Development, Affect Regulation, and Infant Mental Health," *Infant Mental Health Journal* 22, no. 1–2 (2003): 201–69, https://doi.org/10.1002/1097-0355(200101/04)22:1<201::AID-IMHJ8>3.0.CO;2-9.

27. K. A. Bonnet et al., "The Effects of Chronic Opiate Treatment and Social Isolation Receptors in the Rodent Brain," in *Opiate and Endogenous Opioid Peptides*, ed. H. W. Kosterlitz (Amsterdam: North Holland Publishing, 1976).

28. Schore, "The Effects of Early Relational Trauma."

29. Kathleen T. Brady et al., "Comorbidity of Psychiatric Disorders and Posttraumatic Stress Disorder," *Journal of Clinical Psychiatry* 61, supplement 7 (2000): 22–32; Deborah S. Lipschitz et al., "Posttraumatic Stress Disorder in Hospitalized Adolescents: Psychiatric Comorbidity and Clinical Correlates," *Journal of the American Academy of Child and Adolescent Psychiatry* 38, no. 4 (1999): 385–92, https://doi.org/10.1097/00004583-199904000-00010.

30. Israel Liberzon et al., "Altered Central μ-Opioid Receptor Binding after Psychological Trauma," *Biological Psychiatry* 61, no. 9 (2007): 1030–38, https:// doi.org/10.1016/j.biopsych.2006.06.021.

31. Ulrich F. Lanius and Frank. M. Corrigan, "Opioid Antagonists and Dissociation: Adjunctive Pharmacological Interventions," in *Neurobiology and Treatment of Traumatic Dissociation*, ed. Lanius, Paulsen, and Corrigan, pp. 471–98.

32. Monica Bolton et al., "Serious Adverse Events Reported in Placebo Randomised Controlled Trials of Oral Naltrexone: A Systematic Review and Meta-Analysis," *BMC Medicine* 17, no. 1 (2019), https://doi.org/10.1186/s12916-018-1242-0.

33. Martin J. Bohus et al., "Naltrexone in the Treatment of Dissociative Symptoms in Patients with Borderline Personality Disorder," *Journal of Clinical Psychiatry* 60, no. 9 (1999): 598–603, https://doi.org/10.4088/jcp.v60n0906; David Mischoulon et al., "Randomized, Proof-of-Concept Trial of Low Dose Naltrexone for Patients with Breakthrough Symptoms of Major Depressive Disorder on Antidepressants," *Journal of Affective Disorders* 208 (2017): 6–14, https://doi.org/10.1016/j.jad .2016.08.029; Wiebke Pape and Wolfgang Wöller, "Niedrig Dosiertes Naltrexon in Der Behandlung Dissoziativer Symptome," *Der Nervenarzt* 86, no. 3 (2014): 346–51, https://doi.org/10.1007/s00115-014-4015-9.

34. Claudio Castellano and Stefano Puglisi-Allegra, "Effects of Naloxone and Naltrexone on Locomotor Activity in C57BL/6 and DBA/2 Mice," *Pharmacology Biochemistry and Behavior* 16, no. 4 (1982): 561–63, https://doi.org/10.1016 /0091-3057(82)90415-4.

35. James Belluzzi and Larry Stein, "Brain Endorphins: Possible Role in Long-Term Memory," *Annals of the New York Academy of Sciences* 398, no. 1 (1982): 221–29, https://doi.org/10.1111/j.1749-6632.1982.tb39496.x.

36. E. S. Collin et al., "κ-opioid Receptor Stimulation Abolishes μ- but Not δ-Mediated Inhibitory Control of Spinal Met-Enkephalin Release," *Neuroscience Letters* 134, no. 2 (1992): 238–42, https://doi.org/10.1016/0304-3940(92)90525-c.

37. Liberzon et al., "Altered Central μ-Opioid Receptor Binding."

38. Leigh McCullough et al., eds., *Treating Affect Phobia: A Manual for Short-Term Dynamic Psychotherapy* (New York: Guilford Press, 2003).

39. Lanius and Corrigan, "Opioid Antagonists and Dissociation."

40. Lanius and Corrigan, "Opioid Antagonists and Dissociation."

41. Mark Hyman Rapaport et al., "Beneficial Effects of Nalmefene Augmentation in Neuroleptic-Stabilized Schizophrenic Patients," *Neuropsychopharmacology* 9 (September 1993): 111–15, https://doi.org/10.1038/npp.1993.49.

42. Mischoulon et al., "Randomized, Proof-of-Concept Trial of Low Dose Naltrexone."

43. Revital Amiaz et al., "Resolution of Treatment-Refractory Depression with Naltrexone Augmentation of Paroxetine—A Case Report," *Psychopharmacology* 143, no. 4 (1999): 433–34, https://doi.org/10.1007/s002130050969.

44. Daniel J. Siegel, *The Developing Mind: How Relationships and the Brain Interact to Shape Who We Are* (New York: Guilford Press, 1999).

45. Luby Elliot and Mary Ann Marrazzi, "A Panic Attack Precipitated by Opiate Blockade—A Case Study," *Journal of Clinical Psychology* 7, no. 5 (October 1987): 361, https://doi.org/10.1097/00004714-198710000-00025.

46. Lanius and Corrigan, "Opioid Antagonists and Dissociation."

47. R. B. Hemingway and T. G. Reigle, "The Involvement of Endogenous Opiate Systems in Learned Helplessness and Stress-Induced Analgesia," *Psychopharmacology* 93, no. 3 (1987), https://doi.org/10.1007/bf00187256.

Chapter 11: Lyme Disease and Other Tick-Borne Illnesses

1. Christina A. Nelson et al., "Incidence of Clinician-Diagnosed Lyme Disease, United States, 2005–2010," *Emerging Infectious Diseases* 21, no. 9 (September 2015): 1625–31, https://doi.org/10.3201/eid2109.150417.

2. Elisabeth Baum, Fong Hue, and Alan G. Barbour, "Experimental Infections of the Reservoir Species *Peromyscus Leucopus* with Diverse Strains of *Borrelia Burgdorferi*, a Lyme Disease Agent," *mBio* 3, no. 6 (November–December 2012): e00434-12, https://doi.org/10.1128/mBio.00434-12; Kit Tilly, Patricia A. Rosa, and Philip E. Stewart, "Biology of Infection with *Borrelia Burgdorferi*," *Infectious Disease Clinics of North America* 22, no. 2 (June 2008): 217–34, http://doi.org/10.1016/j.idc.2007.12.013.

3. C. M. Shih and A. Spielman, "Accelerated Transmission of Lyme Disease Spirochetes by Partially Fed Vector Ticks," *Journal of Clinical Microbiology* 31, no. 11 (November 1993): 2878–81.

4. "Lyme In 80+ Countries Worldwide," Lyme Disease Association, August 27, 2013, https://lymediseaseassociation.org/about-lyme/cases-stats-maps-a-graphs/lyme-in-more-than-80-countries-worldwide.

5. Lisa A. Waddell et al., "A Systematic Review on the Impact of Gestational Lyme Disease in Humans on the Fetus and Newborn," *PLoS One* 13, no. 11 (November 2018): e0207067, https://doi.org/10.1371/journal.pone.0207067.

6. Raphael B. Stricker and Marianne J. Middelveen, "Sexual Transmission of Lyme Disease: Challenging the Tickborne Disease Paradigm," *Expert Review of Anti-Infective Therapy* 13, no. 11 (August 2015): 1303–06, https://doi.org/10.1586/14787210.2015.1081056.

7. Lachlan McIver et al., "Health Impacts of Climate Change in Pacific Island Countries: A Regional Assessment of Vulnerabilities and Adaptation Priorities," *Environmental Health Perspective* 124, no. 11 (November 2016): 1707–14, https://doi.org/10.1289/ehp.1509756.

8. S. M. Engstrom, E. Shoop, and R. C. Johnson, "Immunoblot Interpretation Criteria for Serodiagnosis of Early Lyme Disease," *Journal of Clinical Microbiology* 33, no. 2 (February 1995): 419–27.

9. Centers for Disease Control and Prevention, "Lyme Disease," last updated November 20, 2019, https://www.cdc.gov/lyme/diagnosistesting/index.html.

10. Sam T. Donta, "Late and Chronic Lyme Disease," *Medical Clinics of North America* 86, no. 2 (March 2002): 341–49, https://doi.org/10.1016/S0025-7125(03)00090-7.

11. Robert B. Nadelman et al., "Prophylaxis with Single-Dose Doxycycline for the Prevention of Lyme Disease after an *Ixodes Scapularis* Tick Bite," *New England Journal of Medicine* 345 (July 2001): 79–84, https://doi.org/10.1056/NEJM200107123450201.

12. Leena Meriläinen et al., "Morphological and Biochemical Features of *Borrelia Burgdorferi* Pleomorphic Forms," *Microbiology* 161, no. 3 (March 2015): 516–27, https://doi.org/10.1099/mic.0.000027.

13. R. B. Stricker and L. Johnson, "Lyme Disease: The Promise of Big Data, Companion Diagnostics and Precision Medicine," *Infection and Drug Resistance* 2016, no. 9 (September 2016): 215–19, http://doi.org/10.2147/IDR.S114770.

14. Nadelman et al., "Prophylaxis with Single-Dose Doxycycline," 79–84.

15. Darin Ingels, *The Lyme Solution: A 5-Part Plan to Fight the Inflammatory Autoimmune Response and Beat Lyme Disease* (New York: Penguin Random House, 2018).

16. A. M. Ercolini and S. D. Miller, "The Role of Infections in Autoimmune Disease," *Clinical and Experimental Immunology* 155, no. 1 (December 2008): 1–15, https://doi.org/10.1111/j.1365-2249.2008.03834.x.

17. A. C. Steere et al., "Autoimmune Mechanisms in Antibiotic Treatment-Resistant Lyme Arthritis," *Journal of Autoimmunity* 16, no. 3 (May 2001): 263–68.

18. A. Pianta et al., "Annexin A2 Is a Target of Autoimmune T and B Cell Responses Associated with Synovial Fibroblast Proliferation in Patients with Antibiotic-Refractory Lyme Arthritis," *Clinical Immunology* 160, no. 2 (October 2015): 336–41, https://doi.org/10.1016 /j.clim.2015.07.005.

19. L. H. Sigal and S. Williams, "A Monoclonal Antibody to *Borrelia Burgdorferi* Flagellin Modifies Neuroblastoma Cell Neuritogenesis in Vitro: A Possible Role for Autoimmunity in the Neuropathy of Lyme Disease," *Infection and Immunity* 65, no. 5 (May 1997): 1722–28.

20. R. Kaiser, "Intrathecal Immune Response in Patients with Neuroborreliosis: Specificity of Antibodies for Neuronal Proteins," *Journal of Neurology* 242, no. 5 (May 1995): 319–25, https://doi.org/10.1007/bf00878875.

21. Kristen A. Rahn, Patricia J. McLaughlin, and Ian S. Zagon, "Prevention and Diminished Expression of Experimental Autoimmune Encephalomyelitis by Low Dose Naltrexone (LDN) or Opioid Growth Factor (OGF) for an Extended Period: Therapeutic Implications for Multiple Sclerosis," *Brain Research* 1381 (March 2011): 243–53, https://doi.org/10.1016/j.brainres.2011.01.036.

22. Jarred Younger and Sean Mackey, "Fibromyalgia Symptoms Are Reduced by Low-Dose Naltrexone: A Pilot Study," *Pain Medicine* 10, no. 4 (May 2009): 663–72, http://doi.org/10.1111/j.1526-4637.2009.00613.x.

Appendix: Dosing Protocols

1. Pierre Dayer, Jules Desmeules, and Laurence Collart, "Pharmacologie du Tramadol [Pharmacology of Tramadol]," *Drugs* 53, supplement 2 (October 2012): 18–24, https://doi.org/10.2165/00003495-199700532-00006.

2. Karlo Toljan and Bruce Vrooman, "Low-Dose Naltrexone (LDN)—Review of Therapeutic Utilization," *Medical Sciences* 6, no. 4 (September 2018): 82, https://doi.org/10.3390/medsci6040082.

3. Toljan and Vrooman, "Low-Dose Naltrexone."

4. Ginevra Liptan, "Combine Opioid and Opioid Blocker for Less Fibromyalgia Pain?," March 7, 2016, http://www.drliptan.com/blog/2016/3/7/combine-opiate-and -opiate-blocker-for-less-fibromyalgia-pain.

5. Stewart B. Leavitt, "Opioid Antagonists in Pain Management," *Practical Pain Management* 9, no. 3 (December 2011).

CONTRIBUTORS

Apple Bodemer, MD

Apple Bodemer is an associate professor in the Dermatology Department at the University of Wisconsin–Madison. After finishing her residency, she completed a fellowship in integrative medicine through the University of Arizona. She was the first dermatologist to be board-certified in integrative medicine and now sits on the American Board of Integrative Medicine. She is passionate about teaching and works with both dermatology residents at the University of Wisconsin and integrative medicine fellows both in Wisconsin and Arizona. She has authored chapters in the primary integrative medicine textbook and written curriculum for the University of Arizona Integrative Medicine Fellowship program as well as for the National Veterans Association Whole Health Initiative.

Along with her academic teaching, she is committed to prevention and believes that the best way to impact health is to empower people to take their health into their own hands. She has significant experience interacting with people through a variety of media outlets, including radio, television, and print, and has worked with a number of schools to educate children about skin cancer prevention.

Her passion in this area is exploring how lifestyle impacts both chronic and acute skin conditions with a particular focus on diet and nutrition.

Darin Ingels, ND, FAAEM, FMAPS

Dr. Ingels is a respected leader in natural medicine with numerous publications, international lectures, and almost 30 years of experience in the health care field. He received his BS degree in medical technology from Purdue University and his doctorate in naturopathic medicine from Bastyr University in Seattle, Washington, completing a residency program at the Bastyr Center for Natural Health. He is a fellow with both the American

Academy of Environmental Medicine and the Medical Academy of Pediatric Special Needs.

Dr. Ingels authored *The Lyme Solution: A 5-Part Plan to Fight the Inflammatory Auto-Immune Response and Beat Lyme Disease* (Avery, 2018), which covers an integrative, natural approach to the treatment and management of Lyme disease. He overcame his own three-year battle with Lyme disease and applied the same principles to more than 6,000 Lyme and co-infection patients over the past 20 years. Dr. Ingels has been featured on numerous podcasts, articles, and docuseries as one of the leading experts in Lyme disease.

Dr. Ingels's practice focuses on environmental medicine with special emphasis on Lyme disease and co-infections and chronic immune dysfunction. He treats both children and adults using diet, nutrients, herbs, homeopathy, and immunotherapy to help his patients achieve better health.

Galyn Forster, MS

Galyn Forster is a licensed professional counselor practicing in Eugene, Oregon, since 1988.

He earned an MS in counseling psychology from the University of Oregon. He works with adults, youth, and couples, focusing on a wide range of issues, including complex trauma, dissociation, anxiety, attachment issues, physical pain, and traumatic brain injury.

His clinical, theoretical orientation is eclectic, with an eye to integrating recent neurobiological finding into his treatment. Central to his practice are eye movement desensitization and reprocessing therapy (EMDR), coherence therapy, acceptance and commitment therapy (ACT), sensorimotor therapy, and LENS neurofeedback. He began working with patients prescribed low dose naltrexone as an adjunctive treatment to psychotherapy in 2010. Since then he has helped over 60 of his clients in their exploration of LDN as an adjunctive treatment for mental health issues and presented locally and internationally on the topic.

Jill Cottel, MD

Dr. Cottel is native to Southern California and grew up in San Diego. She received her bachelor's degree with honors at the University of California–San Diego (UCSD) in biochemistry and cell biology. She received her medical degree from UCSD School of Medicine in 1995. She completed her internship and residency in internal medicine in Portland, Oregon, and returned home to San Diego, where sunshine and family beckoned.

Dr. Cottel has over 20 years of internal medicine experience, which has led to her current focus on integrative care and holistic health. She became a diplomate of the American Board of Holistic Medicine Integrative in 2007. Recently transplanted to Virginia, she sees patients in clinical practice and is the medical director at the Lackey Clinic in Yorktown.

Kirsten Singler, NMD

Kirsten Singler is native to the verdant hills of Kentucky. Making her way westward, she received her bachelor's degree with honors at the University of Texas in Austin. She obtained her naturopathic medical degree at Southwest College of Naturopathic Medicine and Health Sciences in Arizona. She received additional training and certification in botanical medicine and holistic nutrition under the mentorship of JoAnn Sanchez at Southwest Institute for Healing Arts. She is currently the clinical director and naturopathic doctor at Lee Regenerative Medical Institute in California.

She is passionate about her role as clinician and collaborator, empowering patients to have increased vitality, capability, and energy to realize their dreams.

Kristen Blasingame, MA

Kristen Blasingame, MA, has served in the medical field in a variety of capacities, particularly in medical research and patient care. Kristen is a graduate of Washington University, St. Louis, for master of arts, and Lake Forest College, Lake Forest, Illinois, for a BA. She continues to further her education, currently being in pursuit of a medical degree at Avalon University. In August 2019 she married her husband, Benton, and the two are expecting their first child to be born in June 2020. In her spare time Kristen enjoys visiting family, hiking, and choral singing.

Leonard B. Weinstock, MD

Dr. Leonard B. Weinstock is board-certified in gastroenterology and internal medicine. He is president of Specialists in Gastroenterology and the Advanced Endoscopy Center. He is an associate professor of clinical medicine and surgery at Washington University School of Medicine.

Dr. Weinstock received a BA magna cum laude from the University of Vermont and a medical degree from University of Rochester School of Medicine. He completed his postgraduate training and was chief resident in internal medicine at Rochester General Hospital. His gastroenterology fellowship was performed at Washington University School of Medicine.

Dr. Weinstock is an active lecturer and has published more than 80 articles, abstracts, editorials, and book chapters. He is an investigator at Sundance Clinical Research and has participated in over 30 research studies. He is currently researching the role and treatment of small intestinal bacterial overgrowth in restless legs syndrome, irritable bowel syndrome, and rosacea. Low dose naltrexone as treatment for a variety of inflammatory conditions is a topic of clinical research. He is interested in new syndromes that involve the gastrointestinal tract, including mast cell activation syndrome. A complete CV is available at www.gidoctor.net.

Mark Mandel, PharmD

Mark Mandel is a registered pharmacist who specializes in bio-identical hormone replacement therapy (BHRT), pain management, and the treatment of chronic health conditions with natural pharmaceutical alternatives and complementary medicine (CAM). He has been a proponent of LDN since 2007, counsels patients and clinicians from around the world on its uses and potential benefits, and compounds LDN in a variety of forms and strengths. He is a graduate of the University of Illinois College of Pharmacy (1983) and completed his doctorate of pharmacy at Midwestern University in Downers Grove, Illinois, in 2007. He is the host of the weekly radio health show the *Doctor and the Pharmacist*, which airs at 10 AM central time, Saturdays on WYLL AM 1160, and may be heard online at www.1160hope.com.

Mark has educated hundreds of student pharmacists on the topics of CAM, compounding, and durable medical equipment. He speaks regularly to health care professionals, providing insights on how natural pharmaceutical alternatives and prescription compounding can enhance patient care and quality of life.

Mark believes that many chronic health conditions can be ameliorated and potentially eliminated by complementing allopathic medicine with combinations of natural pharmaceutical alternatives and lifestyle changes that are easy to use, safe, and effective.

Neel D. Mehta, MD

Dr. Mehta is the director of the Weill Cornell Pain Management Center and an associate professor of clinical anesthesiology at Weill Cornell Medical College. He also serves as a co-director of the Center for Comprehensive Spine Care, medical director of Greenberg 14 South's amenities unit, and advisory board member to the Patient Experience Task Force and Integrative Medicine Center. He is a director-at-large of the New York Society of Interventional Pain Physicians and president-elect of the Eastern Pain Association.

Embodying Weill Cornell's tripartite mission, Dr. Mehta delivers superior patient care, conducts groundbreaking research, and educates doctors-in-training in the field of pain medicine. His work has been featured on television as well as National Public Radio. Dr. Mehta was an invited expert on Facebook Patient Chats for the Neuropathy Association of America and has led courses in Barcelona, Spain, and Mumbai, India, training the next generation of international pain medicine physicians.

Dr. Mehta is leading efforts to help improve the patient experience for those undergoing surgery while advancing the field of knowledge in chronic pain and spinal cord stimulation. He has authored over 30 peer-reviewed papers, chapters, and abstracts.

Olga L. Cortez, MD, OB-GYN, FACOG

Dr. Olga L. Cortez is a board-certified ob-gyn who provides personalized care for women and men at Cross Roads Hormonal Health & Wellness. In addition to the obstetric and gynecologic care she provides, Dr. Cortez offers medically supervised weight loss plans and hormonal therapies for both women and men.

Dr. Cortez began her education in medicine at the University of North Texas. She earned her medical degree in 2002 from the University of Texas Southwestern Medical School. Dr. Cortez completed her internship and residency at Parkland Memorial Hospital in Dallas, where she provided comprehensive care for women of all ages.

After her medical training Dr. Cortez returned to Denton, Texas, to start her practice and to raise her family. Over the years she learned from personal experience the difficulties of weight loss and hormonal imbalance. That led her to devote herself to helping others with these same issues. Dr. Cortez has since done post graduate training on hormone and thyroid management.

As a passionate advocate for the overall health of each person, Dr. Cortez aims to support the path of each patient to optimal well-being.

Phil Boyle, MD

Dr. Boyle is a general practitioner with a special interest in infertility, miscarriage, and women's health. He is the founder and director of Neo Fertility, Dublin, Ireland.

Dr. Boyle graduated in Medicine from the National University of Ireland, Galway, in 1992. He is a member of both the Irish (MICGP) and Royal (MRCGP) College of General Practitioners, as well as the Irish Fertility Society. He is currently president of the International Institute for Restorative Reproductive Medicine (www.iirrm.org), a doctors' group that aims to publish and scientifically validate restorative reproduction.

Dr. Boyle had helped over 3,500 couples achieve successful pregnancies since commencing practice in 1998. He has published papers in peer-reviewed medical journals on restorative reproduction to treat couples with infertility, previous failed IVF, and recurrent miscarriage. Dr. Boyle has prescribed LDN for infertility patients since 2004 and has safely treated over 500 women with LDN during pregnancy.

Sarah J. Zielsdorf, MD

Above all, health is not simply the absence of disease, but is living a life of passionate vitality. Dr. Sarah Zielsdorf attended Miami University (in Ohio—not Florida), where she received a BA in microbiology, minors in molecular biology and religious studies, and a concentration in oboe performance. She earned an MS in public health, microbiology, and emerging infectious diseases from The George Washington University in Washington, DC, and her MD at Loyola University Chicago Stritch School of Medicine. Dr. Z completed her residency at Loyola and the Hines VA Hospital. She is an Institute for Functional Medicine–certified practitioner and board-certified in internal medicine. She is proud to serve patients worldwide, having quickly attained her reputation as both a skilled diagnostician and a passionate teacher. She values the transformative power of the patient-physician relationship, and understands that every individual is biochemically and genetically unique. Dr. Zielsdorf refines her craft on a daily basis, learns from her patients, and is never satisfied with her knowledge base. She truly believes in the art of medicine, which keeps her relentlessly searching for answers.

Dr. Zielsdorf is the owner and medical director of Motivated Medicine (www.motivatedmedicine.com), an innovative consultative medical practice in the western suburbs of Chicago.

J. Stephen Dickson BSC (hons) MRPharmS

J. Stephen Dickson has been working with LDN for over a decade in the U.K., working together with pharma partners in the industry to stabilize the supply chain and standardize methods of obtaining prescriptions in a safe and compliant manner. As well as running the well-established private medical department of Dickson Chemist, he runs seven NHS pharmacies in Glasgow.

Stephen also works in several other businesses, owning a technology company responsible for dispensing the majority of the methadone in the U.K. in community pharmacy (MethaMeasure), and one of the largest online controlled drugs systems in the U.K. (CDRx). He is an adviser to Canidol Pharmaceutics, a company dedicated to furthering the cause for medical cannabis in the U.K., and helped design the U.K. Cannabis Clinic Model for use in community pharmacy and primary care.

In his spare time, Stephen plays guitar in several bands (including a ceilidh band), is on the board of directors of a semi-professional theater group (where he generally functions as the costume guru), oversees their MethaMeasure North American operation, and is a frequent speaker at the LDN conferences internationally.

Ulrich Lanius, PhD

Dr. Ulrich F. Lanius is a registered psychologist in West Vancouver, British Columbia, with a practice in clinical and neuropsychology. He has a particular interest in brain-behavior relationships and the effects of acquired brain injury, as well as trauma and dissociation. He has worked with clients with psychiatric symptoms who have been prescribed opioid antagonists, including naltrexone in a variety of doses, including low dose naltrexone (LDN), since 1999 and has written multiple book chapters on the subject. Dr. Lanius specializes in therapeutic interventions for traumatic brain injury / mild traumatic brain injury, as well as the treatment of trauma stress syndromes, dissociation, and attachment-related issues. Dr. Lanius has presented both in North America and internationally, and he has authored a recent book on trauma and dissociation.

Vivian F. DeNise, DO, ABAARM, FAARFM

Dr. Vivian DeNise has been practicing pediatric medicine for 35 years and integrative medicine since 2009. Although her passion has always been to care for children, she became acutely aware of the need to explore other treatment modalities when the traditional therapies were simply ineffective. At that time she began on her journey of studying integrative medicine with the American Academy of Anti-Aging Medicine. She completed her training in 2009. Dr. DeNise currently has a pediatric medical practice as well as an integrative medical practice for all ages in Long Island, New York.

Dr. DeNise graduated cum laude from Hofstra University in 1980 with a bachelor of arts in biology. She then went to New York College of Osteopathic Medicine and graduated in 1984. She completed a rotating internship at Baptist Medical Center in Brooklyn, New York, and a pediatric residency at NYU–Winthrop Hospital in 1988. She is a diplomate of the American Academy of Anti-Aging and Regenerative Medicine and is board-certified by the American Academy of Anti-Aging and Regenerative Medicine.

Wiebke Pape, MD

Wiebke Pape, MD, is the senior consultant in the department of trauma-related disorders at the Rhein-Klinik in Bad Honnef, Germany (a clinic for psychosomatic diseases offering inpatient treatment).

She studied medicine at the Georg-August-Universität Göttingen, Germany. She specialized in psychiatry, psychosomatic medicine, and psychotherapy after spending her medical education in the fields of neurology, internal medicine, and psychiatry. She completed her psychotherapeutic education in psychodynamic and systemic therapy and is a certified EMDR therapist. She is especially interested in the treatment of patients with complex PTSD and severe dissociative symptoms.

Publication: W. Pape and W. Wöller, "Low Dose Naltrexone in the Treatment of Dissociative Symptoms," *Der Nervenarzt* 86 (2015): 346–52 (in German).

INDEX

Note: Page numbers followed by "*n*" refer to footnotes. Page numbers followed by "t" refer to tables.

ABOUT THE EDITOR

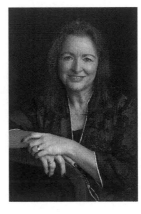

Photo by Julia Holland

L inda Elsegood is the founder of the LDN
Research Trust, which was set up in the U.K.
as a registered charity in 2004, and is the editor
of *The LDN Book, Volume 1* and *2*. Diagnosed
with multiple sclerosis in August of 2000, she
started LDN therapy in December of 2003, and
now has a better quality of life and hope for the
future. Through the Trust, she has connected
thousands of patients, doctors, and pharmacists
around the world with information, articles, and
patient stories about LDN , and helped organize
conferences, seminars, and the Trust's *LDN
Radio Show*.